Lippincott's
CONCISE ILLUSTRATED ANATOMY:

Back, Upper Limb &
Lower Limb

OTHER TITLES IN THIS SERIES:

Lippincott's Concise Illustrated Anatomy: Thorax, Abdomen & Pelvis

Lippincott's Concise Illustrated Anatomy: Head & Neck

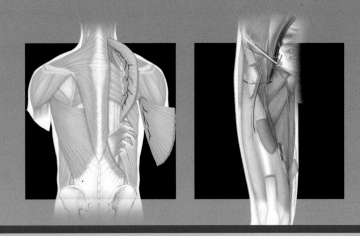

Lippincott's
CONCISE ILLUSTRATED ANATOMY:
Back, Upper Limb & Lower Limb

VOLUME 1

Ben Pansky, PhD, MD

Professor Emeritus
Department of Surgery
University of Toledo College of Medicine
and Life Sciences
Toledo, Ohio

Thomas R. Gest, PhD

Associate Professor of Anatomy
University of Michigan Medical School
Ann Arbor, Michigan

Trine University
Health Education Center - FWRC
1819 Carew Street
Fort Wayne, IN 46805

Wolters Kluwer | Lippincott Williams & Wilkins
Health

Philadelphia • Baltimore • New York • London
Buenos Aires • Hong Kong • Sydney • Tokyo

Acquisitions Editor: Crystal Taylor
Product Manager: Julie Montalbano
Marketing Manager: Joy Fisher Williams
Designer: Steve Druding
Compositor: SPi Global

351 West Camden Street
Baltimore, MD 21201

Two Commerce Square
2001 Market Street
Philadelphia, PA 19103

Printed in China

Library of Congress Cataloging-in-Publication Data
Pansky, Ben.
    Lippincott's concise illustrated anatomy. Back, upper limb & lower limb / authors, Ben Pansky and Thomas Gest. — 1st ed.
      p. ; cm.
    Concise illustrated anatomy
    Back, upper limb & lower limb
    Includes index.
    ISBN 978-1-60831-383-9
  1. Extremities (Anatomy) 2. Back—Anatomy. I. Gest, Thomas R. II. Title. III. Title: Concise illustrated anatomy. IV. Title: Back, upper limb & lower limb.
    [DNLM: 1. Back—anatomy & histology—Atlases. 2. Lower Extremity—anatomy & histology—Atlases. 3. Upper Extremity—anatomy & histology—Atlases. WE 17]
    QM548.P36   2011
    611.9—dc22

        2011005093

DISCLAIMER
Care has been taken to confirm the accuracy of the information present and to describe generally accepted practices. However, the authors, editors, and publisher are not responsible for errors or omissions or for any consequences from application of the information in this book and make no warranty, expressed or implied, with respect to the currency, completeness, or accuracy of the contents of the publication. Application of this information in a particular situation remains the professional responsibility of the practitioner; the clinical treatments described and recommended may not be considered absolute and universal recommendations.

The authors, editors, and publisher have exerted every effort to ensure that drug selection and dosage set forth in this text are in accordance with the current recommendations and practice at the time of publication. However, in view of ongoing research, changes in government regulations, and the constant flow of information relating to drug therapy and drug reactions, the reader is urged to check the package insert for each drug for any change in indications and dosage and for added warnings and precautions. This is particularly important when the recommended agent is a new or infrequently employed drug.

Some drugs and medical devices presented in this publication have Food and Drug Administration (FDA) clearance for limited use in restricted research settings. It is the responsibility of the health care provider to ascertain the FDA status of each drug or device planned for use in their clinical practice.

To purchase additional copies of this book, call our customer service department at (800) 638-3030 or fax orders to (301) 223-2320. International customers should call (301) 223-2300.

Visit Lippincott Williams & Wilkins on the Internet: http://www.lww.com. Lippincott Williams & Wilkins customer service representatives are available from 8:30 am to 6:00 pm, EST.

9 8 7 6 5 4 3 2 1

I dedicate this new endeavor to my dearly beloved wife **JULIE**, who will live in my loving memory forever, after our more than 50 years together, whose love, patience, understanding, encouragement and constant inspiration, supported me through the seasons of my maturation and productive life.

And to my loving son, **JONATHAN**, who grew up and matured along with me, my writings, illustrations, and stories. He is ever present by my side with love and encouragement helping me maintain the "Spark of Life and Creativity" which has forever glowed brightly within me.

—BEN PANSKY

For my children, **MADISON** and **TAYLOR**, the most important people in my life.

—THOMAS GEST

Medical education continues to be in a constant state of change. Dedicated teachers experiment with teaching methods and curricula, always striving to refine, to define, to update, and to narrow the gap between the what, the how, and the why of what is being taught and the state of our present knowledge. Academic traditions are often quite rigid, cemented into place by a "yardstick of established time (hours)," so any effort to change becomes formidable and medical, clinical, and scientific relevance may receive secondary consideration. What the art of medicine always requires, no matter how much manipulating is done, is a strong foundation in the basic sciences. To fully appreciate and understand the complexities and nuances of variation in us all, Anatomy is the keystone in that foundation.

Lippincott's Concise Illustrated Anatomy series presents human gross anatomy in more than a synopsis form and far less than one encounters in a massive traditional text. Each title in the series is a highly illustrated, complete, functionally oriented, clinically informative text, concerned with "living" anatomy and stressing the importance of the relationship between structure and function. Repetition only occurs as needed to emphasize particular points or to demonstrate continuity between regions.

Terminology adheres to the *Terminologia Anatomica* (1998) approved by the Federative Committee on Anatomical Nomenclature (FCAT) of the International Federation of Associations of Anatomists (IFAA). Official English-equivalent terms are used throughout this edition.

Anatomy requires one to think three-dimensionally, which is often a new concept for students and a difficult one for practitioners desiring to review. Studying and palpating a body at a dissection table may be the best way to comprehend the three-dimensional fundamentals of anatomy and the relationships of many of its parts. However, lacking the physical body, this text maintains a tradition utilized in six editions of *Review of Gross Anatomy* by Ben Pansky of being planned and written around its illustrations, which come predominantly from the highly acclaimed *Lippincott Williams & Wilkins Atlas of Anatomy* by Drs. Tank and Gest, together with a reworking of a number of illustrations from Dr. Pansky's 6th edition of *Review of Gross Anatomy*, into beautiful, full-color illustrations closely coordinated with those of the *Atlas*.

The illustrations present anatomical images concisely in a logical sequence, making them easier and faster to use, a critical and essential need in this era of compressed anatomical curricula.

The hundreds of illustrations in full color combined with an abbreviated, outlined, but comprehensive and detailed text convey a simplified, multi-faceted, three-dimensional aspect of the beauty and function of the human body not found in other texts.

Because the overall volume of material (in text and illustration) needed to present the true, complete reality of the human body is so massive, many texts have become larger and larger over the years. It was felt that a huge "tome" of 1,000 or more pages would be too overwhelming and formidable as well as difficult for students to tackle without great trepidation. Thus, we have decided to present three volumes for the seven chapters or units of associated areas of the body—namely, Volume I: Back, Upper Limb & Lower Limb; Volume II: Thorax, Abdomen & Pelvis; and Volume III: Head & Neck. Each volume is approximately 300 pages. Thus, as one studies a respective body region, one needs to essentially carry, transport and study from a single volume at a time. Furthermore, if a student or practitioner is predominantly involved only in one or two major body areas, they may be able to concentrate on the essentials of her/his study or review (i.e., orthopedics, dentistry, ophthalmology, physical therapy, surgery, etc.) without carrying around a large tome. He or she would still have the other volume(s) for reference since the body functions as a unit and one part depends on or is related to the other.

Progression from region to region, from the Back to the Upper and Lower Limbs, to the Thorax, Abdomen, and Pelvis, and to the Head and Neck, allows one to fully appreciate the continuity between the regions. The regional approach duplicates that used in many human anatomy courses and laboratories of dissection as well as in surgical areas of concentration. However, the illustrations show some overlapping of structures to allow the student to move easily from one region to the next.

The body is discussed from its superficial layers to its deep structures, except for the osteology. Because the bones form the framework of the body and lend themselves to the attachment of soft parts, they tend to appear early in the text and are also to be studied early in most courses. This makes understanding of the relationships of the soft body parts more easily and clearly understood.

By extracting information from within the living organism, the student and practitioner are better able to describe and define both normal and abnormal states. Increasingly, sophisticated tools help them understand that continuum. At first, students of the medical arts used only observations and palpation, then they undertook dissection, and now "tools" have gained momentum, moving quickly from the stethoscopes and ophthalmoscopes to powerful x-rays and imaging technologies. To put this in perspective, x-rays were discovered at the close of the 19th century; nuclear medicine and ultrasonography were introduced in the 1950s; and computed tomography (CT), positron emission tomography (PET), single-photon emission computed tomography (SPECT), digital radiography, and nuclear magnetic resonance (NMR) became available in the 1970s.

Thus, an anatomy text would be incomplete without some discussion and illustration of radiography, CT, PET, SPECT and NMR, which provide a good clinical introduction to the current state of the patient's health. This has been included in our books since the sooner one learns to identify normal anatomy on x-ray film and computer imaging, the easier it becomes to locate and understand the changes brought on by genetics, disease, or trauma and thus, anatomy becomes a "keystone" to all of medicine and its many related fields.

Although much basic and essential clinical consideration has been presented in many areas of our texts, all clinically relevant material cannot be fully discussed for each anatomical region. However, its importance in one's understanding of basic anatomy and how that can be altered is essential for truly appreciating what is generally "normal" before it becomes altered and creates clinical signs and symptoms.

Since walking plays such a strong role in our present concept of physical fitness and health, several units on walking have been included in our discussion of the lower extremity, which correlate structure with kinesiology.

In the same vein, the ability to "get about" from place to place and take care of oneself, handle objects, shower, drive a car, make meals and eat in comfort without stress or pain makes our discussion of range of motion (ROM) of essential body parts and joints very important and essential not only as we age and flexibility diminishes, but in all stages of life. Thus, much effort has been made to outline the ROM of the essential anatomy of the body and delineate, to some degree, what the "normal" ranges are that may be necessary for adequate function.

We, as educators in the anatomical sciences, are aware of the fact that gross anatomy is a subject quickly memorized and just as easily forgotten, unless the student or practitioner constantly reviews the material. Time can be an adversary and multiple duties are often overwhelming. It is our hope that in this series we have been concise, direct, and meaningful, without "running on and on" with excessive nonessentials, and that we have been able to create books that will guide the reader easily and thoughtfully through the very complex detail that makes up the human body and its many parts.

ACKNOWLEDGMENTS

Many thanks to those at Lippincott Williams & Wilkins who participated in the development of this textbook, including Acquisitions Editor Crystal Taylor, Product Manager Julie Montalbano, Art Director Jennifer Clements, and Designer Steve Druding. Additional thanks goes to Kelly Horvath for her editorial guidance.

Marcelo Oliver and Body Scientific International did a superb job of converting many of Dr. Pansky's original black-and-white illustrations into full color, managing to duplicate the tone, color, and beauty of the illustrations from the *Lippincott Williams & Wilkins Atlas of Anatomy* by Drs. Tank and Gest.

Much gratitude is extended to Danelle Mooi, Secretary, Department of Surgery, Division of Neurosurgery, University of Toledo Medical Center for her persistent encouragement, understanding, and great help to Dr. Pansky with her knowledge of the computer and digital world, which made his transgression into the realm of computers and wireless connections possible and a great learning experience; and to Jason W. Levine, M.D., Assistant Professor of Orthopedics, Department of Surgery, Division of Sports Medicine, University of Toledo Medical Center for his discussions with Dr. Pansky on joint movements and range of motion (ROM), and his suggestions for references, which helped Dr. Pansky fully understand the complexities of "living with our bones, muscles, and joints."

And special thanks goes to Patrick Tank, PhD, Professor of Neurobiology and Developmental Sciences, University of Arkansas for Medical Sciences. His inspiration and hard work on the initial chapter of this book helped to get this project underway.

Ben Pansky
Thomas Gest

CONTENTS

Preface   vii
Acknowledgments   ix

Chapter 1: The Back

1.1	Superficial Anatomy of the Back	2
1.2	The Vertebral Column	7
1.3	Vertebrae: Cervical and Thoracic	10
1.4	Vertebrae: Lumbar, Sacrum, and Coccyx	16
1.5	Atlanto-Occipital and Atlantoaxial Joints	20
1.6	Intervertebral Joints	22
1.7	Costovertebral Joints	25
1.8	Clinical Considerations: Vertebral Column	28
1.9	Fascia of the Back	30
1.10	Superficial Muscles of the Back	32
1.11	Deep Muscles of the Back, Part 1	36
1.12	Deep Muscles of the Back, Part 2	40
1.13	Movements of the Vertebral Column and Head	42
1.14	Spinal Meninges	46
1.15	Spinal Cord	50
1.16	Spinal Nerves and Their Branches	53
1.17	Blood Supply of the Spinal Cord	58
1.18	Veins of Spinal Cord and Vertebral Column	60

Chapter 2: Upper Limb

2.1	Introduction to the Upper Limb	64
2.2	Cutaneous Innervation of the Upper Limb	66
2.3	Superficial Veins and Deep Fascial Specializations of the Upper Limb	68
2.4	Lymphatics of the Upper Limb	70
2.5	Bones of the Pectoral (Shoulder) Girdle	72
2.6	Bone of the Arm: Humerus	74
2.7	Bones of the Forearm	76
2.8	Bones of the Wrist and Hand	79

2.9	Muscles of the Anterior Shoulder	82
2.10	Muscles of the Posterior Shoulder and the Rotator Cuff	84
2.11	Axilla and Brachial Plexus	87
2.12	Axillary Artery and Blood Supply to the Shoulder	92
2.13	Muscles of the Arm	95
2.14	Neurovasculature of the Arm	98
2.15	Muscles of the Anterior Forearm	100
2.16	Neurovasculature of the Anterior Forearm	103
2.17	Muscles of the Posterior Forearm	106
2.18	Neurovasculature of the Posterior Forearm	108
2.19	Dorsum of the Hand	110
2.20	Palm of the Hand, Superficial	114
2.21	Muscles of the Palmar Hand	119
2.22	Vessels of the Hand	123
2.23	Nerves of the Hand	126
2.24	Articulations of the Shoulder and Pectoral Girdle	129
2.25	Elbow Joint	133
2.26	Joints of the Wrist and Hand	136
2.27	Specific Nerve Injury: Median Nerve (C5-T1)	141
2.28	Specific Nerve Injury: Ulnar Nerve (C8, T1)	144
2.29	Specific Nerve Injury: Radial Nerve (C5-T1)	146

Chapter 3: Lower Limbs

3.1	Introduction to the Lower Limb	150
3.2	Cutaneous Innervation of the Lower Limb	152
3.3	Superficial Veins and Deep Fascia of the Lower Extremity	155
3.4	Lymphatic Drainage of the Lower Extremity	158
3.5	The Pelvic Girdle	160
3.6	Articulations of the Pelvic Girdle	164
3.7	Bones of the Thigh	166
3.8	Bones of the Leg	169
3.9	Bones of the Ankle and Foot	172
3.10	Compartments of the Thigh	176
3.11	Muscles of the Anterior Thigh	178
3.12	Femoral Triangle and Femoral Sheath	180
3.13	Muscles of the Medial Thigh	182
3.14	Femoral and Obturator Vessels and Nerves	184
3.15	Muscles of the Gluteal Region	188

3.16	Vessels and Nerves of the Gluteal Region	190
3.17	Muscles of the Posterior Thigh	194
3.18	Popliteal Region and Anastomosis Around the Knee	196
3.19	Compartments of the Leg	198
3.20	Muscles of the Posterior Leg	200
3.21	Muscles of the Lateral and Anterior Leg	204
3.22	Vessels and Nerves of the Leg	207
3.23	Dorsum of the Foot	211
3.24	Plantar Aponeurosis and Cutaneous Nerves of the Sole of the Foot	214
3.25	Muscles of the Sole of the Foot	216
3.26	Vessels and Nerves of the Sole of the Foot	220
3.27	The Hip Joint	222
3.28	The Knee Joint	226
3.29	Bursae of the Knee Joint and the Tibiofibular Joints	233
3.30	Joints of the Ankle and Foot	236
3.31	Arches of the Foot	242
3.32	Disorders of the Feet	244
3.33	Walking (Bipedal Locomotion), Part 1	246
3.34	Walking (Bipedal Locomotion), Part 2	248
3.35	Walking (Bipedal Locomotion), Part 3	250
3.36	Nerve Injuries in the Lower Limb	254

Appendix A: Essential Terms of Direction and Movement   261
Appendix B: Fundamentals of Joints   263

Index   267

The Back

1.1	Superficial Anatomy of the Back	2
1.2	The Vertebral Column	7
1.3	Vertebrae: Cervical and Thoracic	10
1.4	Vertebrae: Lumbar, Sacrum, and Coccyx	16
1.5	Atlanto-Occipital and Atlantoaxial Joints	20
1.6	Intervertebral Joints	22
1.7	Costovertebral Joints	25
1.8	Clinical Considerations: Vertebral Column	28
1.9	Fascia of the Back	30
1.10	Superficial Muscles of the Back	32
1.11	Deep Muscles of the Back, Part 1	36
1.12	Deep Muscles of the Back, Part 2	40
1.13	Movements of the Vertebral Column and Head	42
1.14	Spinal Meninges	46
1.15	Spinal Cord	50
1.16	Spinal Nerves and Their Branches	53
1.17	Blood Supply of the Spinal Cord	58
1.18	Veins of Spinal Cord and Vertebral Column	60

Superficial Anatomy of the Back

I. Surface Anatomy (Fig. 1.1A, B)

- **A.** **Erector spinae muscle:** bulge on either side of the midline parallel to the vertebral column, best seen in the lumbar region
- **B.** **Median furrow:** groove in the midline between the erector spinae muscles
- **C.** **Spinous processes:** vertebrae from the C7 to L5 can be palpated in the median furrow
- **D.** **Median sacral crest:** equivalent to the spines of the sacral vertebrae
- **E.** **Trapezius muscle:** superior border is palpable on the lateral side of the neck and shoulder
- **F.** **Latissimus dorsi muscle:** lateral border is palpable on the side of the back
- **G.** **Ribs**
- **H.** **Iliac crest**
- **I.** **Posterior superior iliac spine:** has a "dimple" overlying it
- **J.** Important vertebral levels
  1. **T3:** base of the spine of the scapula
  2. **T7:** inferior angle of the scapula
  3. **L4:** iliac crest
  4. **S2:** posterior superior iliac spine

II. Dermatomes of the Back (Fig. 1.1C)

- **A.** A dermatome is the area of the skin supplied by the afferent nerve fibers of the posterior and anterior rami of a spinal nerve
- **B.** In the back, the dermatomes form regular strips of the skin supplied by posterior rami
- **C.** A dermatome in the limbs is innervated by contributions from several named cutaneous nerves

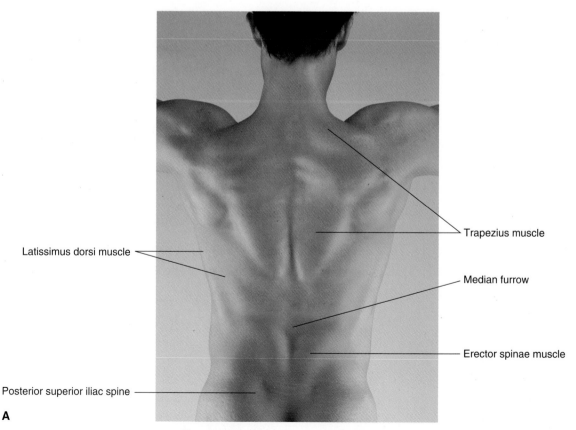

Latissimus dorsi muscle

Posterior superior iliac spine

Trapezius muscle

Median furrow

Erector spinae muscle

A

Figure 1.1A. Surface Anatomy of the Back

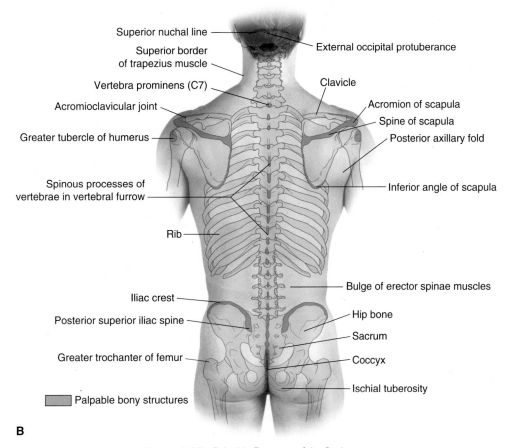

Superior nuchal line —
Superior border of trapezius muscle —
Vertebra prominens (C7) —
Acromioclavicular joint —
Greater tubercle of humerus —
Spinous processes of vertebrae in vertebral furrow —
Rib —
Iliac crest —
Posterior superior iliac spine —
Greater trochanter of femur —

— External occipital protuberance
— Clavicle
— Acromion of scapula
— Spine of scapula
— Posterior axillary fold
— Inferior angle of scapula
— Bulge of erector spinae muscles
— Hip bone
— Sacrum
— Coccyx
— Ischial tuberosity

Palpable bony structures

B

Figure 1.1B. Palpable Features of the Back

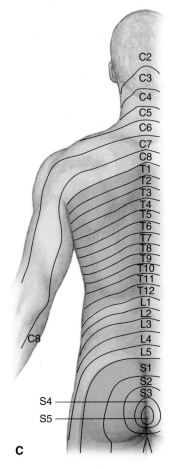

C2
C3
C4
C5
C6
C7
C8
T1
T2
T3
T4
T5
T6
T7
T8
T9
T10
T11
T12
L1
L2
L3
L4
L5
S1
S2
S3
S4
S5

C8

C

Figure 1.1C. Dermatomes of the Back

III. Cutaneous Nerves of the Back (Fig. 1.1D,E)

A. Pierce the back muscles and deep fascia over the muscles to enter the superficial fascia

B. All are branches of posterior rami containing sensory and autonomic (postsynaptic sympathetic) nerve fibers

　　1. **Sensory fibers** carry general sensory (afferent) information from the skin

　　2. **Sympathetic fibers** supply the smooth muscle of blood vessels, erector pili muscles, and sweat glands

C. Thoracic cutaneous nerves display the typical pattern of cutaneous nerves of the back

　　1. Branches of posterior rami of thoracic spinal nerves

　　2. Each posterior ramus divides into a medial branch and a lateral branch

　　3. In the upper half of the back, the lateral branch remains in the muscles, whereas the medial branch supplies muscles and continues superficially to become a cutaneous nerve (cutaneous nerves are found close to the midline in the upper back)

　　4. In the lower half of the back, the medial branch remains in the muscles, whereas the lateral branch continues to become a cutaneous nerve (cutaneous nerves appear approximately 3 to 4 in away from the midline in the lower back)

D. Cervical cutaneous nerves to the back of the neck may vary from the typical pattern; all are branches of posterior rami

　　1. 1st cervical (C1) spinal nerve: usually has no cutaneous branches; its posterior ramus supplies motor fibers to suboccipital muscles

　　2. 2nd cervical (C2) nerve: posterior ramus has a very large medial branch called the greater occipital nerve that supplies the posterior scalp (also supplies deep neck muscles before scalp)

　　3. 3rd cervical (C3) nerve: posterior ramus has a medial branch called occipitalis tertius, which supplies the skin of the neck and a small area of the scalp

　　4. 4th cervical (C4) nerve: medial branch of the posterior ramus provides a cutaneous nerve with a pattern typical of cutaneous nerves in the upper back

　　5. 5th to 8th cervical (C5-8) spinal nerves: posterior rami may lack cutaneous nerves because they are small and may end in the muscles of the back

E. Lumbar cutaneous nerves

　　1. 1st to 3rd lumbar (L1-3) spinal nerves: lateral branches of the posterior rami become cutaneous nerves called superior cluneal nerves; they enter the superficial fascia just lateral to the erector spinae muscles and are distributed over the gluteal region

　　2. 4th and 5th lumbar (L4-5) spinal nerves: posterior rami have no cutaneous branches because they supply only muscular branches

F. Sacral cutaneous nerves

　　1. 1st to 3rd sacral (S1-3) spinal nerves: lateral branches of posterior rami become cutaneous nerves called middle cluneal nerves; they are distributed over the gluteal region as well as on the posterior surface of the sacral region

　　2. 4th and 5th sacral (S4-5) spinal nerves and the single coccygeal (Co) nerve: do not divide into medial and lateral branches; instead, a cutaneous nerve is formed from this complex, which is distributed to the coccygeal region (**inferior cluneal nerves** are branches of posterior femoral cutaneous nerve [from anterior rami] and is discussed with the inferior extremity)

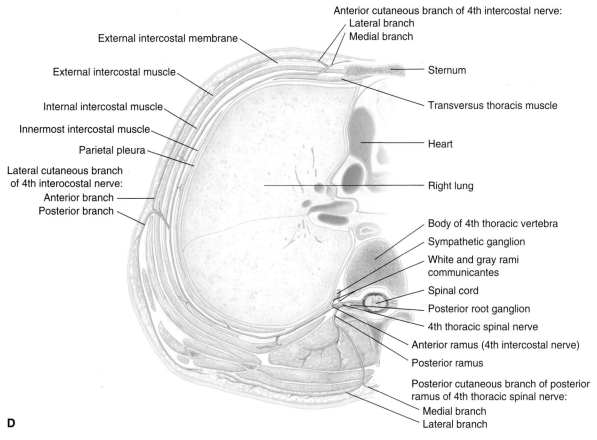

Figure 1.1D. Pattern of a Typical Spinal Nerve

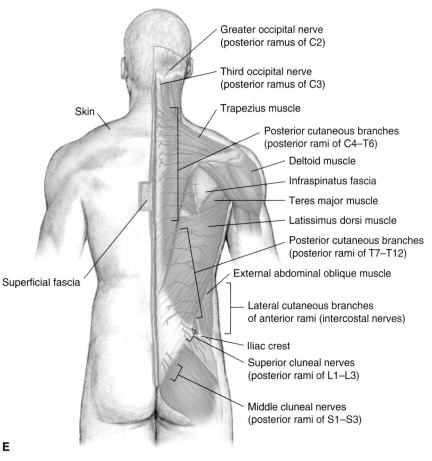

Figure 1.1E. Cutaneous Innervation of the Back

IV. Fasciae of the Back (Fig. 1.1F)

A. Superficial fascia

1. A layer of fat-filled loose connective tissue located under the skin
2. Varies in thickness from person to person
3. Thicker in females than in males
4. Thicker in the lumbar region of the back than in other back regions

B. Deep fascia

1. Located deep to the superficial fascia
2. A thin layer of loose connective tissue without fat
3. Surrounds each muscle and separates groups of muscles

V. Cutaneous Arteries and Veins of the Back

A. Cutaneous vessels accompany the cutaneous nerves and have similar branches

B. Origins of vessels to the skin of the back

1. Occipital artery (from external carotid): back of the head and back of the neck
2. Transverse cervical artery (from thyrocervical trunk of the subclavian): back of the neck
3. Posterior intercostal arteries (from thoracic aorta): thoracic region
4. Lumbar segmental arteries (from abdominal aorta): lower back
5. Lateral sacral arteries (from internal iliac): sacrococcygeal region

VI. Lymphatics of the Back

A. Scalp drains to occipital and mastoid nodes

B. Skin of the neck drains into cervical nodes

C. Superficial structures of the back above the iliac crests drain into axillary nodes

D. Superficial structures of the back below the iliac crests drain into superficial inguinal nodes

E. Deeper structures of the back tend to follow the veins, such as posterior intercostal and lumbar, to drain into deep cervical, posterior mediastinal, lateral aortic, and sacral nodes

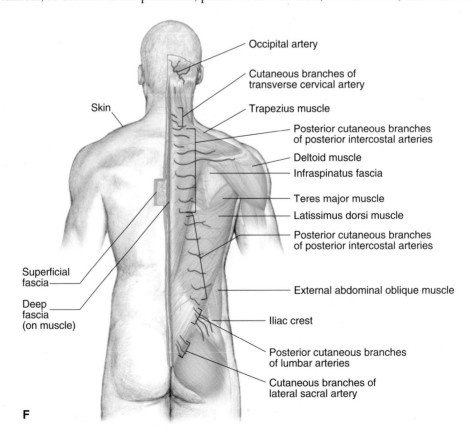

Figure 1.1F. Fascia and Cutaneous Vessels of the Back

The Vertebral Column

I. Composition and Length (Fig. 1.2A)

A. 32 to 34 vertebrae
   1. 7 cervical
   2. 12 thoracic
   3. 5 lumbar
   4. 5 sacral (fused)
   5. 3 to 5 coccygeal (fused)
B. In male, 71 cm; in female, 61 cm

II. Normal Curvatures

A. **Cervical:** concave posteriorly
B. **Thoracic:** convex posteriorly
C. **Lumbar:** concave posteriorly
D. **Sacral:** convex posteriorly
E. Developmental changes
   1. **Primary curvatures** (thoracic and sacral) are present at birth
   2. **Secondary curvatures** (cervical and lumbar) develop after birth
   3. **Cervical:** from elevation and extension of the head in infancy
   4. **Lumbar:** from assumption of erect position when a child begins to walk

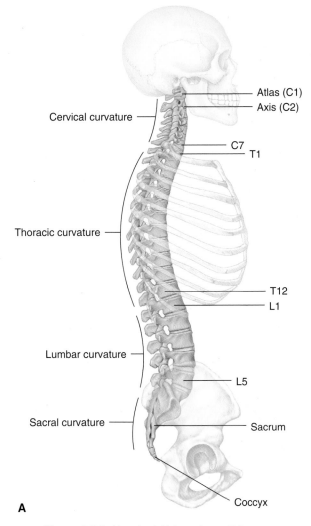

Atlas (C1)
Axis (C2)
Cervical curvature
C7
T1
Thoracic curvature
T12
L1
Lumbar curvature
L5
Sacral curvature
Sacrum
Coccyx

A

Figure 1.2A. Vertebral Column. Lateral View

III. Features of the Articulated Vertebral Column (Fig. 1.2B–D)

A. Lateral view
  1. Sides of bodies of vertebrae show articular facets for ribs in the thorax
  2. Intervertebral foramina formed by the opposition of notches in adjoining vertebrae (increase in size from above downward)
  3. Tips of spines are below the level of the bodies of the corresponding vertebrae in the midthoracic region
B. Anterior view
  1. Vertebral bodies are seen in the anterior view
  2. In general, the width of vertebral bodies gradually broadens with the widest point at the base of the sacrum, then tapers sharply to the apex at the tip of the coccyx
C. Posterior view
  1. Spinous processes are seen in the midline
    a. Cervical (except for C2 and C7): short and horizontal, have bifid tip
    b. Thoracic: long, upper spines directed obliquely caudally with some separation; middle spines, almost vertical in direction with overlapping; lower spines, shorter and directed almost posteriorly with separation between them
    c. Lumbar: short, thick, and separated by interval
  2. Vertebral groove
    a. On either side of spinous processes, formed by laminae and transverse processes
    b. Shallow in cervical and lumbar areas
    c. Deep in thoracic area
D. **Vertebral canal** consists of the vertebral foramina of adjoining vertebrae

IV. Clinical Considerations

A. Abnormal curvatures
  1. **Kyphosis:** increased backward curvature of spine (most frequent in the thorax)
  2. **Lordosis:** exaggerated forward curvature of the lumbar segment
  3. **Scoliosis:** lateral bending of the spine (most frequent in the thorax) of more than 10°
B. Dislocations without fracture occur only in the cervical region due to the inclination of articular processes, commonly between C4 and C5 or C5 and C6

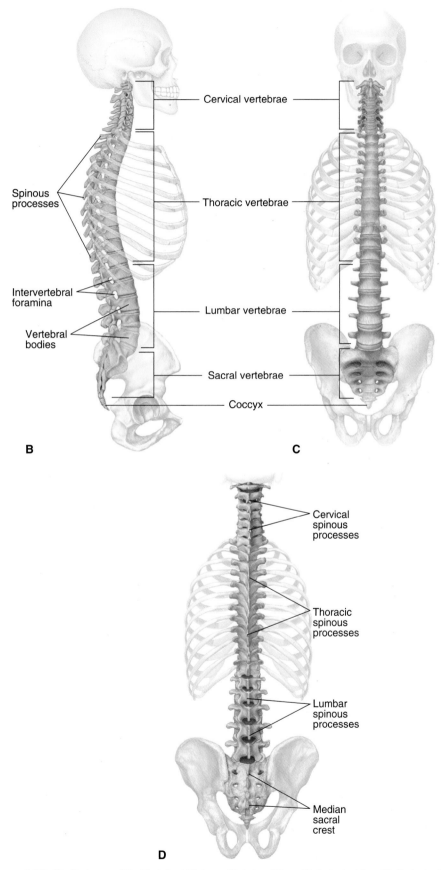

Figure 1.2B–D. Features of the Vertebral Column. **B.** Lateral View. **C.** Anterior View. **D.** Posterior View

Vertebrae: Cervical and Thoracic

I. General Features of Vertebrae (Fig. 1.3A,B)

A. Vertebral body
1. Anterior, drum-shaped part of the vertebra
2. Size increases from superior to inferior

B. Vertebral arch: located posteriorly; consists of
1. **Pedicles (2)**
   a. Pedicle: joins the arch to the body
   b. **Vertebral notches:** concavities in upper and lower surfaces of the pedicle
2. **Laminae (2):** plates extending medially from the pedicle to meet in the midline

C. Vertebral foramen: opening surrounded by the body and the vertebral arch

D. Processes (7 total)
1. **Spinous process:** directed posteriorly and caudally from the union of laminae
2. **Articular processes (2 pair)** extend upward and downward from the point where pedicles and laminae join
   a. **Superior (2):** articular surfaces face posteriorly
   b. **Inferior (2):** articular surfaces face anteriorly
3. **Transverse processes (2):** project laterally between the superior and the inferior articular processes

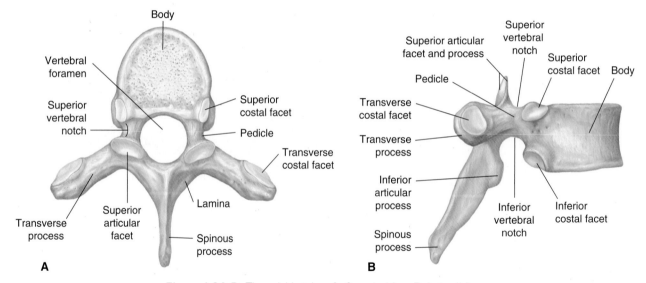

Figure 1.3A,B. Thoracic Vertebra. **A.** Superior View. **B.** Lateral View

II. Cervical Vertebrae (Fig. 1.3C–H)

A. Small in size

B. Short spinous processes
1. C1 has no spinous process
2. C3 through C6 are usually bifid
3. Spines of C6 and C7 are much longer

C. General characteristics
1. Small body
2. Large, triangular vertebral foramen
3. Bifid spinous process
4. **Transverse foramen** in transverse process

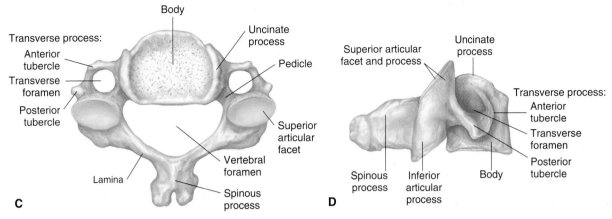

Figure 1.3C,D. Cervical Vertebra. **C.** Superior View. **D.** Lateral View

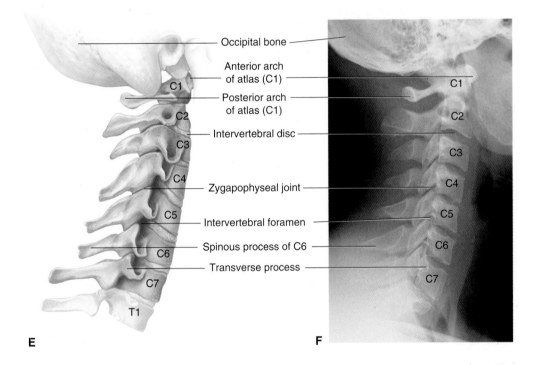

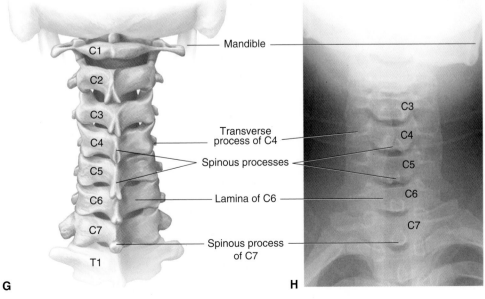

Figure 1.3E–H. Articulated Cervical Vertebrae. **E,F.** Lateral View. **G,H.** Posterior View

D. Unique cervical vertebrae (Fig. 1.31–K)

   1. **C1: atlas**
      a. Has no body; is more or less circular
      b. **Anterior arch** has an anterior tubercle, posterior to which is an oval articular facet
      c. **Posterior arch** has a posterior tubercle
      d. Superior articular facets are large concave ovals
         i. Face upward
         ii. Articulate with occipital condyles
      e. Inferior articular facets are circular and articulate with axis

   2. **C2: axis**
      a. **Dens:** long projection directed cranially
      b. **Anterior articular facet:** on anterior surface of dens for articulation with anterior arch of the atlas
      c. Transverse processes: small, end in single tubercle
      d. Transverse foramina: set obliquely

   3. **C7: vertebra prominens**
      a. Spinous process: thick, directed posteriorly; is not bifid, but ends in tubercle to which is attached the lower end of the ligamentum nuchae
      b. Transverse processes: large
      c. Transverse foramina: do not contain vertebral arteries

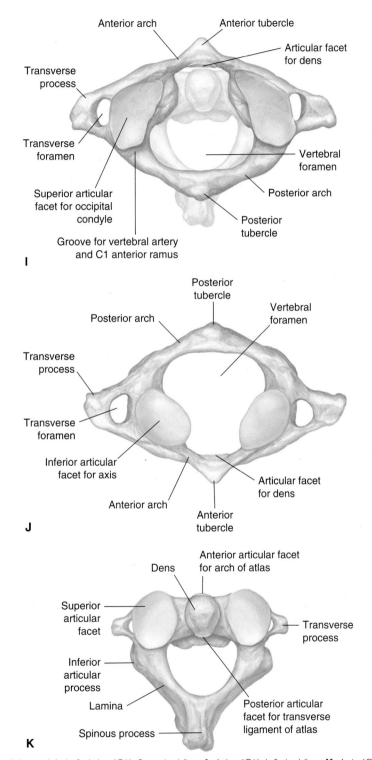

Figure 1.3I–K. Atlas and Axis. **I.** Atlas (C1), Superior View. **J.** Atlas (C1), Inferior View. **K.** Axis (C2), Superior View

III. Thoracic Vertebrae (Fig. 1.3L–O)

A. General characteristics
   1. Bodies: increase in size from above downward
   2. **Costal facets** or demifacets for rib articulation
   3. Laminae: broad and thick
   4. Spinous processes: long and directed obliquely inferiorly
   5. Superior articular processes: thin with facets facing posteriorly
   6. Inferior articular processes: short with facets facing anteriorly
   7. Transverse processes: thick, strong, and have transverse costal facets for rib tubercles
B. Unique features
   1. T1: single costal facet on each side of the body for the 1st rib
   2. T10: single pair of costal facets on each side for the 10th rib
   3. T11: similar to a lumbar vertebra: large body, large articular facet; spinous process is short and almost horizontal, whereas transverse process has no transverse costal facet; however, it has a single pair of costal facets for articulation with the 11th rib
   4. T12: resembles both T11 and L1; inferior articular facet faces laterally; transverse process has superior, inferior, and lateral tubercles; transverse process has no transverse costal facet; 1 costal facet on each side of body articulates with the 12th rib

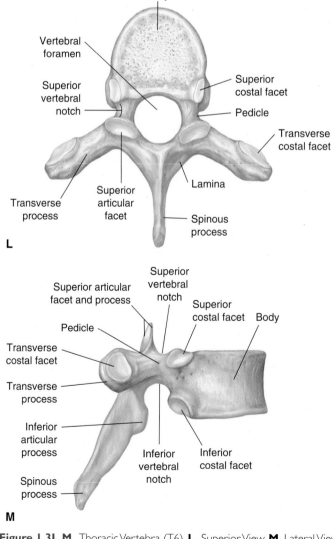

Figure 1.3L,M. Thoracic Vertebra (T6). **L.** Superior View. **M.** Lateral View

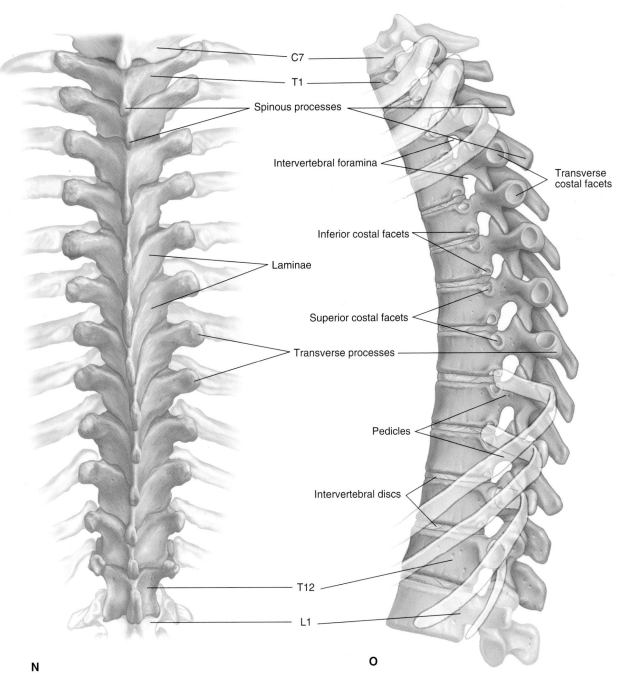

C7

T1

Spinous processes

Intervertebral foramina

Transverse costal facets

Inferior costal facets

Laminae

Superior costal facets

Transverse processes

Pedicles

Intervertebral discs

T12

L1

N

O

Figure 1.3N,O. Articulated Thoracic Vertebrae. **N.** Lateral View. **O.** Posterior View

Vertebrae: Lumbar, Sacrum, and Coccyx

I. Lumbar Vertebrae (Fig. 1.4A–F)

A. General characteristics
   1. Largest vertebrae
   2. Bodies: large, wide, and thick
   3. Pedicles: strong
   4. Laminae: thick and strong
   5. Spinous processes: thick, broad, and directed posteriorly
   6. Superior articular processes: directed medially
   7. Inferior articular processes: directed anteriorly
   8. Transverse processes: long, slender
   9. **Mammillary process:** posterior projection from the superior articular process

B. Unique features
   1. Laminae of adjacent lumbar vertebrae do not overlap
   2. Spines do not overlap

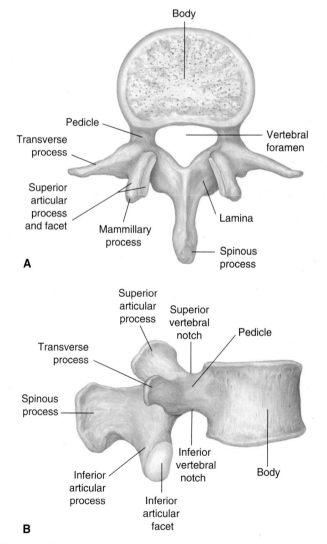

Figure 1.4A,B. Lumbar Vertebra (L3). **A.** Superior View. **B.** Lateral View

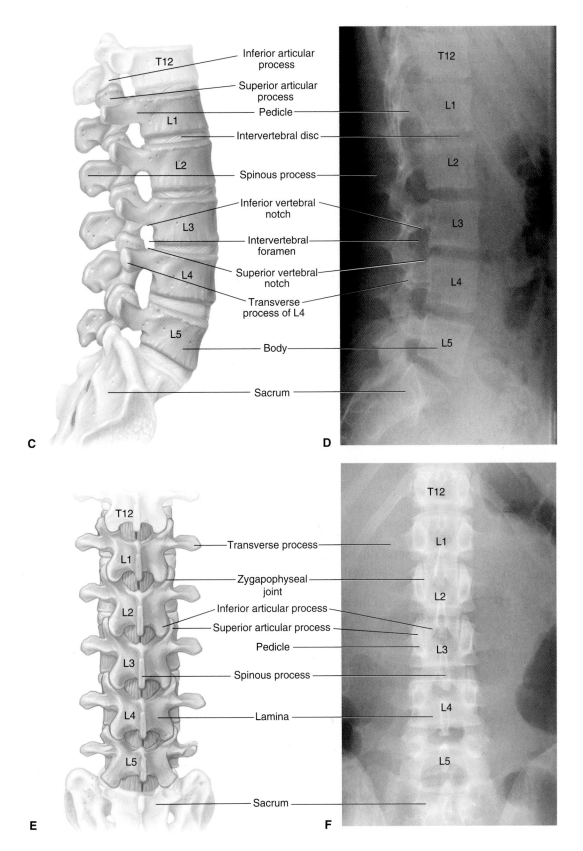

Figure 1.4C–F. Articulated Lumbar Vertebrae. **C,D.** Lateral View. **E,F.** Posterior View

II. Sacrum (Fig. 1.4G,H)

A. 5 vertebrae fused together during development
B. Anterior surface
   1. Concave
   2. Crossed by 4 transverse ridges
   3. **Anterior (pelvic) sacral foramina:** seen at ends of the ridges
C. Posterior surface
   1. Convex
   2. **Median sacral crest:** in midline
   3. **Intermediate sacral crests (2):** terminating as the sacral cornua
   4. **Posterior sacral foramina (4):** lateral to the intermediate sacral crest
   5. **Lateral sacral crests (2):** lateral to the posterior sacral foramina
D. Lateral surface
   1. **Auricular surface:** upper half of the lateral surface
   2. **Sacral tuberosity:** posterior to the auricular surface
   3. **Inferolateral angle:** lower half of the lateral surface
E. Base
   1. Composed of the body of S1 vertebra and the 2 alae
   2. **Lumbosacral articular surface**
   3. **Sacral canal** is located posterior to the body
   4. **Sacral promontory:** sharp anterior projection from the superior surface of the 1st sacral vertebral body
   5. Superior articular processes are supported by short, heavy pedicles and laminae that enclose the sacral canal
F. Apex
   1. Narrow inferior end of the sacrum
   2. Has oval articular facet at its end for articulation with the coccyx

III. Coccyx

A. 3 to 5 rudimentary vertebrae fused together during development
B. Anterior surface
   1. Slightly concave
   2. Has transverse ridges
C. Posterior surface
   1. Convex
   2. Has transverse ridges
   3. Has an articular crest in the midline
D. Base
   1. Superior end of the coccyx
   2. Articular facet: oval, to articulate with the sacrum
   3. **Coccygeal cornua:** projections on the lateral surface of the base
E. Apex
   1. Inferior tip of the coccyx
   2. Rounded, but may be bifid

IV. Clinical Considerations: Coccygeal Injury

A. **Coccydynia:** Pain in the coccygeal region
B. Injuries include a fall onto the buttocks that may result in painful bruising or fracture of the coccyx, or a fracture dislocation of the sacrococcygeal joint; displacement is common; a difficult childbirth may also result in injuries to the mother's coccyx

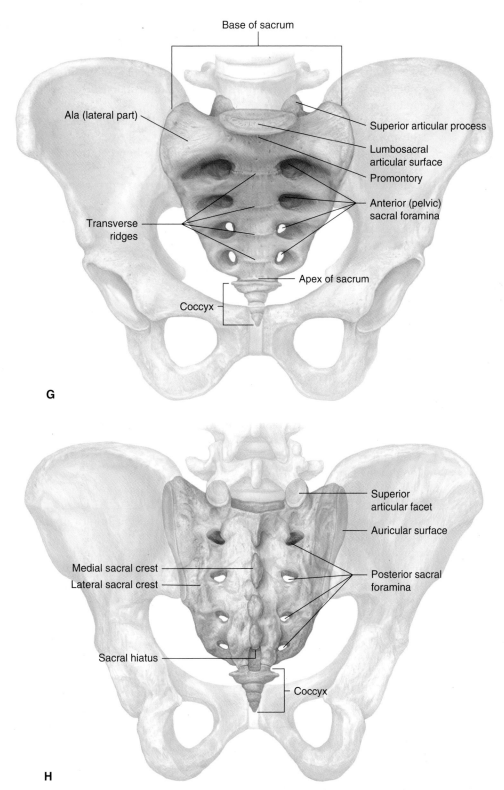

Figure 1.4G,H. Articulated Pelvis. **G.** Anterior View. **H.** Posterior View

Atlanto-Occipital and Atlantoaxial Joints (Fig. 1.5A–F)

I. Atlanto-Occipital Joint

A. Type: condyloid synovial joint
B. Movements: flexion, extension, and lateral bending (abduction)
C. Bones: condyles of occipital bone and superior facets of atlas
D. Articular capsules: surround condyles and superior articular processes of the atlas
E. Ligaments and membranes
   1. **Anterior atlanto-occipital membrane:** membrane between the foramen magnum and the anterior arch of the atlas
   2. **Posterior atlanto-occipital membrane:** membrane between the margin of the foramen magnum and posterior arch of the atlas
   3. **Lateral atlanto-occipital ligament:** connects transverse processes of the atlas to jugular processes of the occipital bone

II. Atlantoaxial Joint

A. Type: pivot (trochoid) synovial joint
B. Movement: rotation
C. Bones: dens of axis articulates with the anterior arch of the atlas
D. Ligaments
   1. **Anterior atlantoaxial ligament:** from the body of the axis to the border of the anterior arch of the atlas
   2. **Posterior atlantoaxial ligament:** from the lamina of the axis to the posterior arch of the atlas
   3. **Transverse ligament:** spans across the arch of the atlas to hold dens against the anterior arch of the atlas
      a. **Superior longitudinal band:** upward prolongation to the occipital bone
      b. **Inferior longitudinal band:** inferior extension to the posterior surface of the body of the axis
   4. **Cruciate ligament of the atlas:** combination of the transverse ligament and the superior longitudinal and inferior longitudinal band

III. Ligaments Connecting Axis with Occipital Bone

A. **Tectorial membrane:** cephalic extension of the posterior longitudinal ligament from the body of axis to occipital bone
B. **Alar ligaments (2):** from sides of dens to condyles of occipital bone
C. **Apical ligament of dens:** from apex of dens to anterior margin of foramen magnum

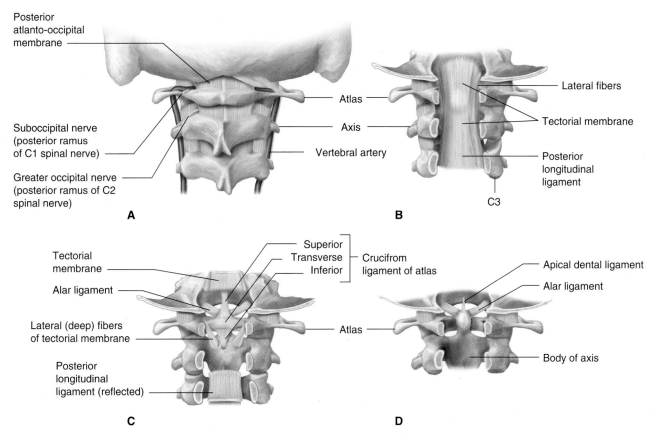

Posterior atlanto-occipital membrane

Suboccipital nerve (posterior ramus of C1 spinal nerve)

Greater occipital nerve (posterior ramus of C2 spinal nerve)

Atlas

Axis

Vertebral artery

A

Lateral fibers

Tectorial membrane

Posterior longitudinal ligament

C3

B

Tectorial membrane

Alar ligament

Lateral (deep) fibers of tectorial membrane

Posterior longitudinal ligament (reflected)

Superior
Transverse
Inferior
Crucifrom ligament of atlas

Atlas

C

Apical dental ligament

Alar ligament

Body of axis

D

Figure 1.5A–D. Atlanto-Occipital and Atlantoaxial Joints. **A.** Posterior View. **B–D.** Posterior View, Posterior Arch and Laminae Removed

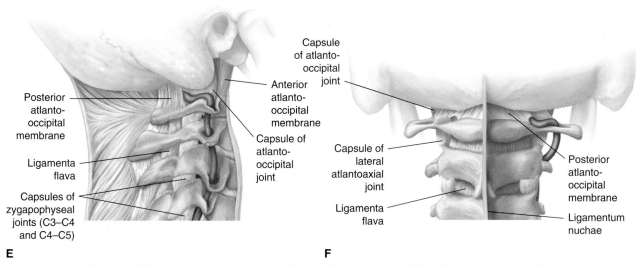

Posterior atlanto-occipital membrane

Ligamenta flava

Capsules of zygapophyseal joints (C3–C4 and C4–C5)

Capsule of atlanto-occipital joint

Anterior atlanto-occipital membrane

Capsule of atlanto-occipital joint

E

Capsule of lateral atlantoaxial joint

Ligamenta flava

Posterior atlanto-occipital membrane

Ligamentum nuchae

F

Figure 1.5E,F. Ligaments of the Vertebral Column. **E.** Cervical, Lateral View. **F.** Cervical, Posterior View

Intervertebral Joints

I. Intervertebral Joints (Fig. 1.6A–C)

A. Joints between vertebral bodies

1. Type: symphysis
2. Ligaments
   a. **Anterior longitudinal ligament**
      i. Covers anterior surfaces of vertebral bodies from the basilar part of occipital bone to the sacrum
      ii. Attached to intervertebral discs and margins of vertebral bodies
   b. **Posterior longitudinal ligament**
      i. In the vertebral canal over the posterior surface of vertebral bodies, extending from the axis to the sacrum
      ii. Closely adherent to discs and margins of vertebral bodies
3. **Intervertebral discs**
   a. Located between adjacent vertebral bodies from C2 to lumbosacral joint
   b. **Nucleus pulposus:** soft, pulpy, yellowish elastic material lying in the center of the disc; a remnant of the embryonic notochord
   c. **Anulus fibrosus (fibrous ring):** concentric ring of fibrous tissue and fibrocartilage
   d. Size varies according to the size of vertebral bodies
   e. In cervical and lumbar regions, it is thicker in front than behind, thus helping to form the convex curvatures in these regions
   f. Where disc contacts bones, cartilage is hyaline; in the center is the fibrocartilage
   g. Absorb shock
   h. Discs contribute about 25% of the length of the vertebral column above the sacrum
      i. Disc dehydration accounts for as much as 1.875 cm (0.75 in) in loss of height by a man, and 1.25 cm (0.5 in) by a woman, during the course of a day
      ii. Over a period of years, the discs gradually thin, accounting for part of the loss in height between young adulthood and old age

B. Joints between vertebral arches

1. **Zygapophyseal joints**
   a. Type: plane synovial joints
   b. Movements: gliding
   c. Bones: superior articular process with inferior articular process
   d. Articular capsule: attaches around articular facets of articular processes
2. Fibrous joints
   a. **Ligamenta flava:** interconnect laminae of vertebrae
   b. **Supraspinous ligament:** joins tips of vertebrae from C7 to sacrum
   c. **Ligamentum nuchae**
      i. Corresponds to the supraspinous ligament in the cervical region
      ii. Extends longitudinally from the external occipital protuberance and median nuchal line to the spine of C7
      iii. Attaches anteriorly to the posterior tubercle of atlas and spines of C2-6
   d. **Interspinous ligament**
      i. Interconnects spines of vertebrae
      ii. Extends from the root to the apex of the spinous process
   e. **Intertransverse ligament:** joins transverse processes of vertebrae

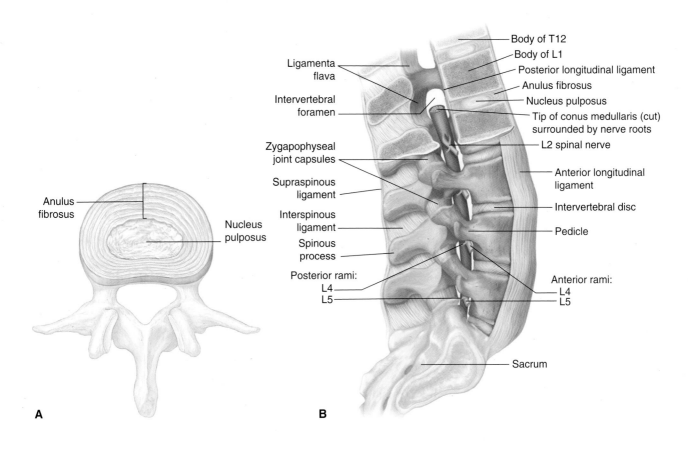

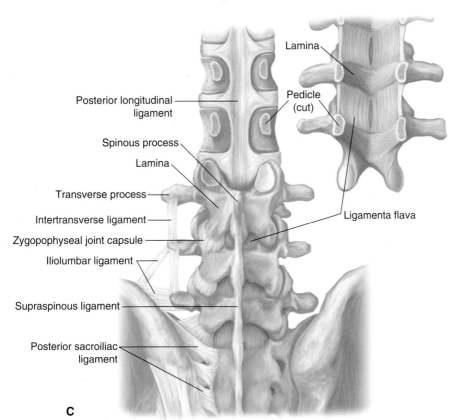

Figure 1.6A–C. Intervertebral Discs. **A.** Intervertebral Disc, Superior View. **B.** Ligaments of the Vertebral Column, Lumbar, Lateral View. **C.** Ligaments of the Vertebral Column, Lumbar, Posterior View

II. Clinical Considerations: Herniated (Slipped) Disc

A. Nucleus pulposus protrudes through a tear in the anulus fibrosus

B. Usually occurs in a posterolateral direction lateral to the posterior longitudinal ligament but may occur directly posteriorly

C. Herniation may occur at cervical, thoracic, or lumbar vertebral levels

   1. Most common location is low in the lumbar region (L4/5); most common in middle age with aging of discs as they become less vascular and lose water

   2. Cervical herniation is also common

D. May cause pressure on spinal nerve roots resulting in pain and paresthesia

   1. Cervical regions: spinal nerve affected is the one that exits the vertebral canal at the level of the herniated disc

   2. Lumbar regions: spinal nerve affected is usually the one that exits the vertebral canal below the herniated disc

E. Most herniated discs occur in the 3rd and 4th decades of life, which represent the most active period of adult life

F. Presents as back pain associated with pain in buttock or extremity, seen mostly with long sitting, flexion, or Valsalva maneuvers (with severity, if it involves the cauda equina, it can lead to back weakness, bowel, bladder, and sexual dysfunction)

Costovertebral Joints

I. Joints between Ribs and Vertebrae

A. Costovertebral joint (Fig. 1.7A, B)

1. Between the head of the rib and vertebral bodies
2. Type: plane synovial joint
3. Movements: gliding
4. Bones: head of the rib and superior and inferior costal facets on the side of 2 adjacent vertebral bodies
   a. Ribs 1, 10, 11, and 12 articulate with only 1 vertebra
5. Articular capsule reinforced by ligaments
   a. **Radiate ligament:** from anterior part of the head of the rib to bodies and intervertebral disc
   b. **Intra-articular ligament**
      i. From interarticular crest of the rib to the fibrocartilage
      ii. Located within the joint and divides synovial cavity into 2 cavities

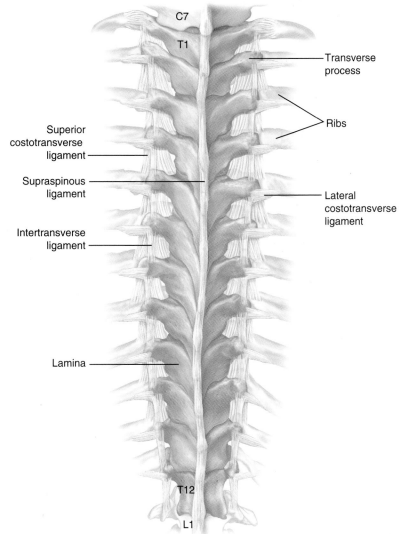

A

Figure 1.7A. Ligaments of the Vertebral Column. Thoracic, Posterior View

B. Costotransverse joint (Fig. 1.7C,D)
1. Between the rib and transverse process
2. Type: plane synovial joint
3. Movements: gliding
4. Bones: tubercle of the rib with the transverse process
5. Articular capsule is reinforced by ligaments
   a. **Costotransverse ligament:** from the posterior surface of the neck of the rib to the anterior surface of the adjacent transverse process
   b. **Superior costotransverse ligament:** from the superior border of the neck of the rib to the transverse process of the vertebra above
   c. **Lateral costotransverse ligament:** from the nonarticulated part of the tubercle of the rib to the tip of the transverse process of the same numbered vertebra

II. Movement of Ribs

A. Rotation of the head of the rib results from multiple small gliding motions so that the anterior part of the rib is raised or lowered
B. Muscles involved are those used in respiration

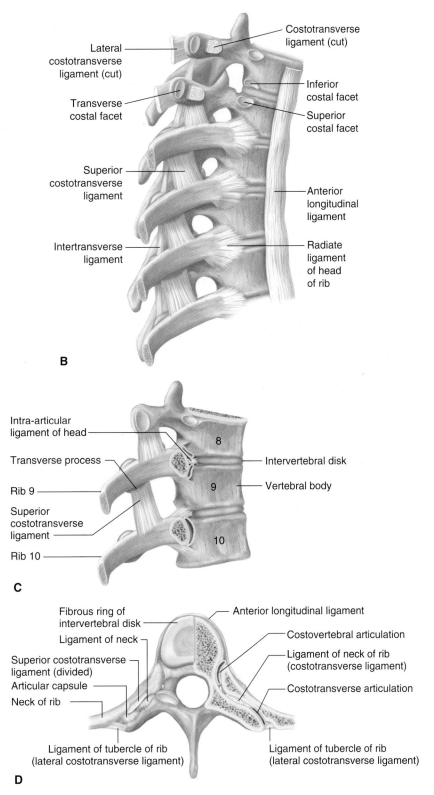

Lateral costotransverse ligament (cut)

Costotransverse ligament (cut)

Transverse costal facet

Inferior costal facet

Superior costal facet

Superior costotransverse ligament

Anterior longitudinal ligament

Intertransverse ligament

Radiate ligament of head of rib

B

Intra-articular ligament of head

Transverse process

Rib 9

Superior costotransverse ligament

Rib 10

8

9

10

Intervertebral disk

Vertebral body

C

Fibrous ring of intervertebral disk

Anterior longitudinal ligament

Ligament of neck

Costovertebral articulation

Superior costotransverse ligament (divided)

Ligament of neck of rib (costotransverse ligament)

Articular capsule

Costotransverse articulation

Neck of rib

Ligament of tubercle of rib (lateral costotransverse ligament)

Ligament of tubercle of rib (lateral costotransverse ligament)

D

Figure 1.7B–D. Ligaments of the Vertebral Column. **B.** Thoracic, Lateral View. **C.** Thoracic, Lateral View. **D.** Thoracic, Superior View

Clinical Considerations: Vertebral Column (Fig. 1.8A–E)

I. Fractures of the Vertebral Column

A. May lead to injury of the spinal cord or nerve roots
B. Cervical region
　1. Above C4 may lead to sudden death due to paralysis of the diaphragm
　2. Below C4 may result in quadriplegia
C. Thoracic region: may result in paraplegia
D. Lumbar region: may lead to variable sensory and motor loss in the lower extremities
E. Compression fractures of vertebral bodies
　1. Spondylomalacia: softening of vertebral bodies due to osteoporosis making them vulnerable to compression fractures
　2. Kyphosis (dowager hump): may result from compression fractures due to spondylomalacia
F. Spondylolysis: fracture of the intra-articular portion of the vertebral arch, which may result in spondylolisthesis (see below)

II. Dislocations of the Vertebral Column

A. Subluxation: partial displacement in which the normal relation of the articular surface is disturbed, although the surfaces may remain partly in contact
B. Spondylolisthesis
　1. Anterior displacement of a vertebral body onto the vertebral body below it
　2. May occur secondary to spondylolysis
　3. L5/S1 is the most common site of spondylolisthesis
C. Rotatory dislocation
　1. Most common in cervical region
　2. May result in fracture of the articular processes

III. Ankylosing Spondylitis

A. Inflammation of the joints of the vertebral column
　1. May lead to fusion of the intervertebral joints
　2. Begins in the lumbar region and, over time, spreads superiorly making the vertebral column rigid
　3. Also known as **Marie-Strümpell disease**

IV. Whiplash

A. Injury caused by a sudden forceful movement of the head in a posterior direction, commonly caused by a rear impact auto accident
B. Extent of cervical injuries depends on the degree of force of the posterior movement
C. Injuries may include muscle strain, cervical nerve root damage, subluxation of vertebrae, compression fractures, and herniation of an intervertebral disc

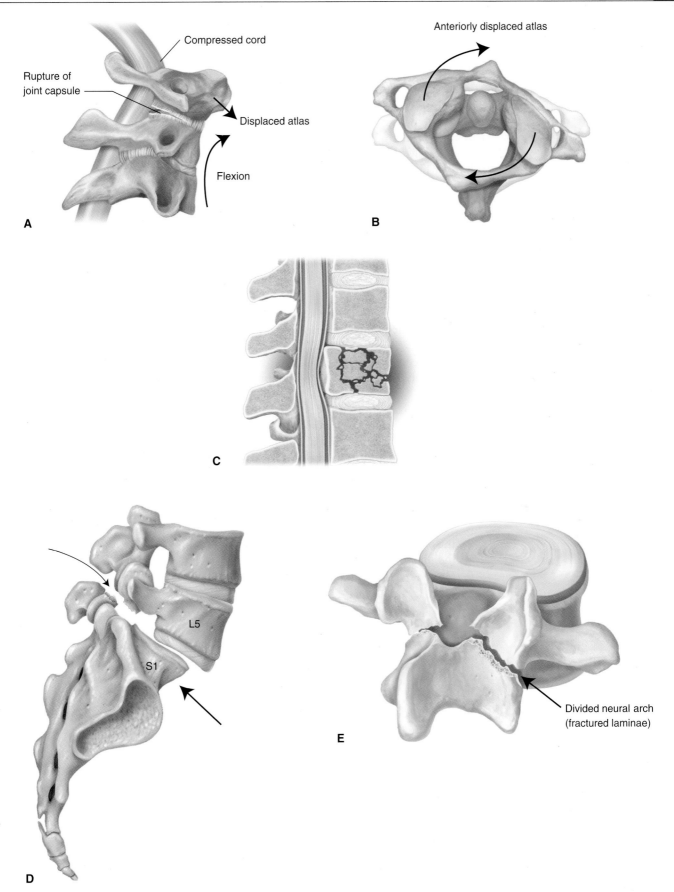

Figure 1.8. Clinical Considerations of the Vertebral Column. **A.** Anterior Subluxation of Atlas with Cord Compression. **B.** Rotary Dislocation of the Atlas on the Axis. **C.** Osteomalacia. **D.** Spondylolisthesis of L5 and S1. **E.** Spondylolysis

Fascia of the Back (Fig. 1.9)

I. Deep Fascia of the Back

A. Nuchal

1. Covers splenius muscles on the dorsum of the neck
2. Represents the posterior portion of the prevertebral fascia of the neck
3. Attaches in midline to ligamentum nuchae
4. Attaches laterally to transverse processes

B. Thoracolumbar fascia

1. Thoracic region
   a. Thin and transparent
   b. Covers the erector spinae muscles
   c. Attaches to tips of spinous processes and supraspinous ligament
   d. Attaches to angles of ribs lateral to the iliocostalis muscle
2. Lumbar region: 3 layers
   a. Superficial
      i. Dense and very strong
      ii. Attaches to spinous processes
      iii. Forms **thoracolumbar aponeurosis** for attachment of latissimus dorsi
   b. Intermediate
      i. Invests deep back muscles
      ii. Lies immediately deep to thoracolumbar aponeurosis
   c. Deep
      i. Attaches to transverse processes
      ii. Passes on deep surface of deep back muscles
      iii. Gives origin to transversus abdominis and internal abdominal oblique muscles
      iv. Also called quadratus lumborum fascia
3. Sacral region: attached to the median and lateral sacral crests

II. Clinical Considerations: Nodose Lumbago (Rheumatism)

A. Form of rheumatism characterized by nodule formation, often in areas where the posterior layer of the thoracolumbar fascia attaches to the bones (especially the iliac and sacral crests)

B. May lead to severe and incapacitating pain

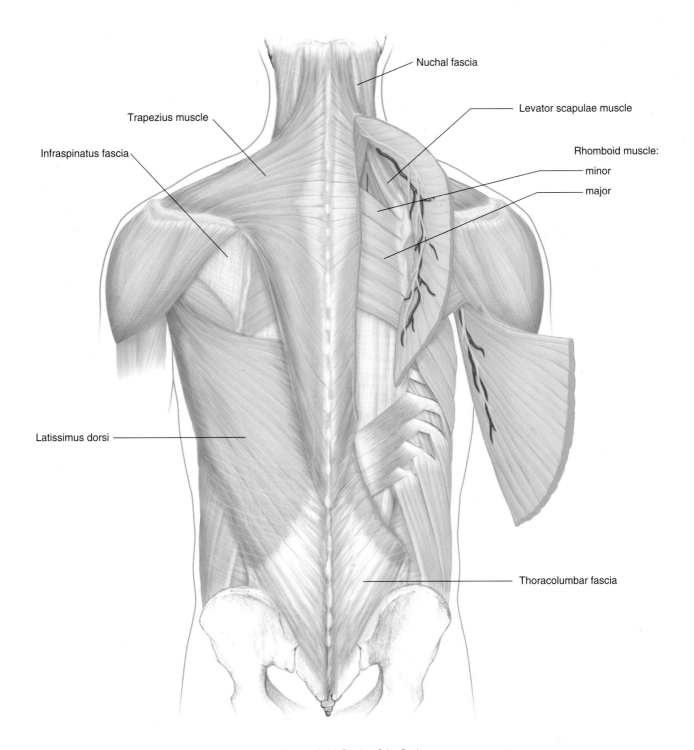

Nuchal fascia

Levator scapulae muscle

Rhomboid muscle:
minor
major

Trapezius muscle

Infraspinatus fascia

Latissimus dorsi

Thoracolumbar fascia

Figure 1.9. Fascia of the Back

Superficial Muscles of the Back (Fig. 1.10A)

I. General Characteristics

A. Arranged in 3 layers
   1. 1st layer: trapezius, latissimus dorsi
   2. 2nd layer: levator scapulae, rhomboideus major, rhomboideus minor
   3. 3rd layer: serratus posterior superior, serratus posterior inferior
B. Primarily concerned with movements of the upper limb
   1. May also move the head, vertebral column, or ribs, depending on attachments
C. Innervated by branches of anterior rami of spinal nerves, except trapezius (accessory nerve)

II. Superficial Back Muscles, 1st Layer

Muscle	Origin	Insertion	Action	Nerve
Trapezius	External occipital protuberance, medial 1/3 of the superior nuchal line, ligamentum nuchae, spinous process of C7 and T1-12 vertebrae, supraspinous ligament	Posterior border of the lateral 1/3 of the clavicle, medial border of the acromion, spine of scapula	Rotates glenoid cavity of scapula superiorly (raises point of shoulder), adducts scapula (draws medially), upper part acting alone elevates scapula, lower part acting alone depresses scapula	Accessory (CN XI), C3-4 (proprioceptive sensory)
Latissimus dorsi	Vertebral spines T6-L5 and median crest of sacrum via thoracolumbar aponeurosis, posterior 1/3 of iliac crest, lower 4 ribs, occasional attachment to inferior angle of scapula	Floor of the intertubercular groove of the humerus	Extends, adducts, and medially rotates arm	Thoracodorsal (middle subscapular), C6-8

III. Special Features (Fig. 1.10B)

A. Latissimus dorsi interdigitates with the costal origin of the external abdominal oblique muscle
B. Fibers of the latissimus dorsi twist as they converge to insert on humerus
C. When latissimus dorsi is paralyzed, patient is unable to raise the trunk as occurs during "chinning" oneself; also cannot use crutches because the shoulder is pushed superiorly by the crutch
D. Latissimus dorsi is active in crawl-stroke swimming and chopping wood
E. Trapezius rotates the scapula to assist the serratus anterior in abductions of more than 90°
F. **Triangle of auscultation**
   1. Borders
      a. Medial border: trapezius muscle
      b. Lateral border: scapula and rhomboid major muscle
      c. Inferior border: latissimus dorsi muscle
      d. Floor: chest wall
   2. Triangle can be enlarged by moving the scapula forward, exposing parts of the 6th and 7th ribs and the 6th intercostal space for auscultation of the lungs
G. **Lumbar triangle**
   1. Borders
      a. Medial border: latissimus dorsi muscle
      b. Lateral border: external abdominal oblique muscle
      c. Inferior border: iliac crest
      d. Floor: internal abdominal oblique muscle
   2. Site of infrequent lumbar herniation

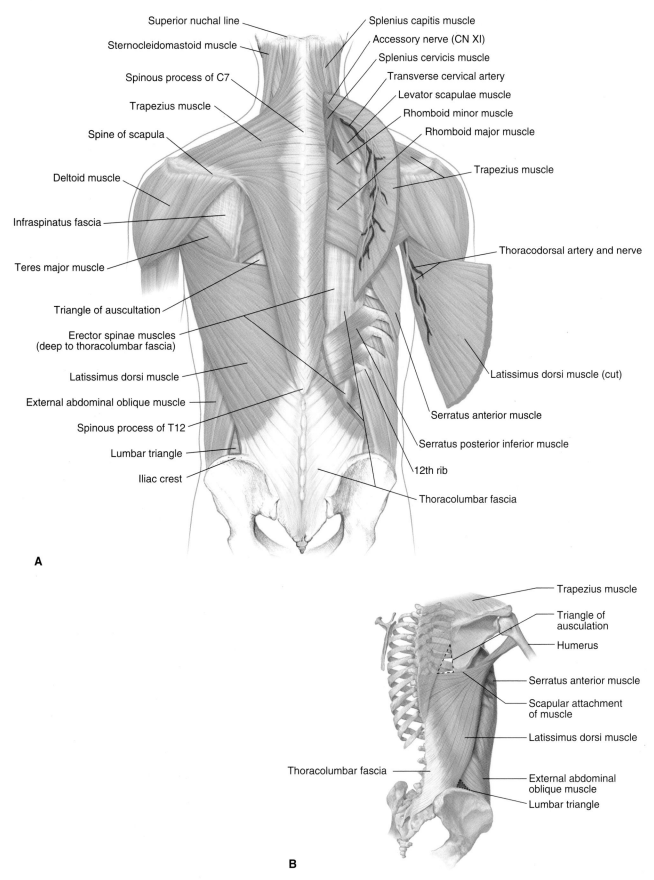

Superior nuchal line

Sternocleidomastoid muscle

Spinous process of C7

Trapezius muscle

Spine of scapula

Deltoid muscle

Infraspinatus fascia

Teres major muscle

Triangle of auscultation

Erector spinae muscles
(deep to thoracolumbar fascia)

Latissimus dorsi muscle

External abdominal oblique muscle

Spinous process of T12

Lumbar triangle

Iliac crest

Splenius capitis muscle

Accessory nerve (CN XI)

Splenius cervicis muscle

Transverse cervical artery

Levator scapulae muscle

Rhomboid minor muscle

Rhomboid major muscle

Trapezius muscle

Thoracodorsal artery and nerve

Latissimus dorsi muscle (cut)

Serratus anterior muscle

Serratus posterior inferior muscle

12th rib

Thoracolumbar fascia

A

Trapezius muscle

Triangle of
ausculation

Humerus

Serratus anterior muscle

Scapular attachment
of muscle

Latissimus dorsi muscle

External abdominal
oblique muscle

Lumbar triangle

Thoracolumbar fascia

B

Figure 1.10 A. Superficial Muscles of the Back: Superficial Dissection. **B.** Special Features of the Superficial Muscles of the Back

IV. Superficial Back Muscles, 2nd Layer (Fig. 1.10C)

Muscle	Origin	Insertion	Action	Nerve
Levator scapulae	Posterior tubercles of transverse processes of C1-4 vertebrae	Superior angle of scapula	Elevates the scapula, rotates the glenoid cavity of scapula inferiorly	C3, C4, dorsal scapular (C5)
Rhomboid minor	Ligamentum nuchae, spines of C7-T1 vertebrae	Medial border of scapula at the root of the spine	Adducts scapula, rotates glenoid cavity of scapula inferiorly	Dorsal scapular (C5)
Rhomboid major	Spines of T2-5 vertebrae	Medial border of scapula below the spine	Adducts scapula, rotates glenoid cavity of scapula inferiorly	Dorsal scapular (C5)

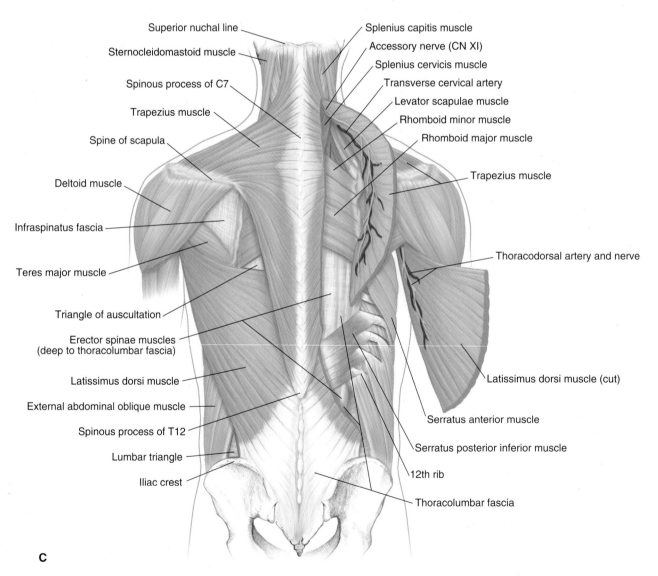

Figure 1.10C. Superficial Muscles of the Back: Intermediate Dissection

V. Superficial Back Muscles, 3rd Layer (Fig. 1.10D)

Muscle	Origin	Insertion	Action	Nerve
Serratus posterior superior	Ligamentum nuchae, spines of vertebrae C7 and T1-3	Ribs 1–4, lateral to the angles	Elevates the upper ribs	Branches of anterior rami of spinal nerves T1-4
Serratus posterior inferior	Thoracolumbar fascia, spines of vertebrae T11, T12 and L1, L2	Ribs 9–12, lateral to the angles	Pulls down lower ribs	Branches of anterior rami of spinal nerves T9-12

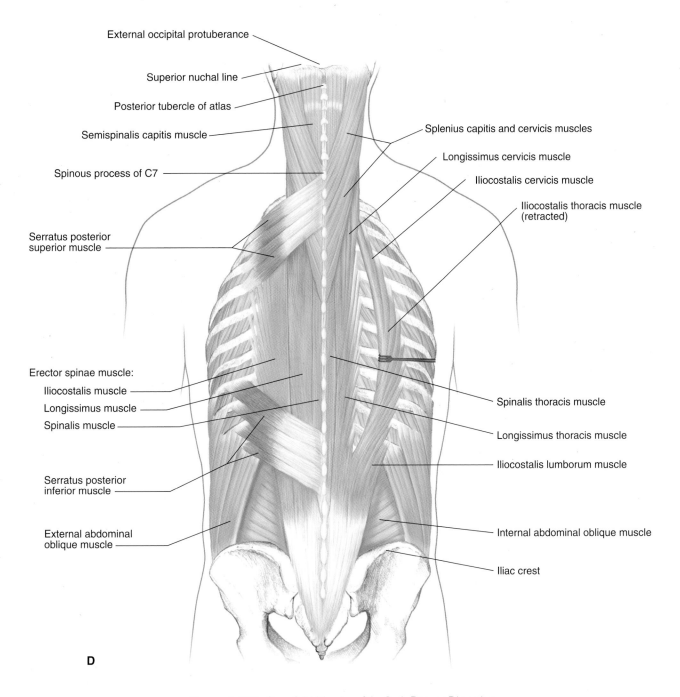

External occipital protuberance

Superior nuchal line

Posterior tubercle of atlas

Semispinalis capitis muscle

Spinous process of C7

Serratus posterior superior muscle

Erector spinae muscle:
Iliocostalis muscle
Longissimus muscle
Spinalis muscle

Serratus posterior inferior muscle

External abdominal oblique muscle

Splenius capitis and cervicis muscles

Longissimus cervicis muscle

Iliocostalis cervicis muscle

Iliocostalis thoracis muscle (retracted)

Spinalis thoracis muscle

Longissimus thoracis muscle

Iliocostalis lumborum muscle

Internal abdominal oblique muscle

Iliac crest

D

Figure 1.10D. Superficial Muscles of the Back: Deeper Dissection

Deep Muscles of the Back, Part 1 (Fig. 1.11A)

I. General Characteristics

A. All are innervated by branches of posterior rami of spinal nerves

B. Concerned with movements of the vertebral column (although some deep back muscles attach to ribs and may also be used in respiratory movements)

II. Splenius (Superficial Group)

Muscle	Origin	Insertion	Action
Splenius capitis	Ligamentum nuchae, spines of C7-T3 vertebrae	Lateral 1/3 of the superior nuchal line, mastoid process of the temporal bone	Extends and laterally bends the head, laterally rotates the head
Splenius cervicis	Spines T3-6 vertebrae	Posterior tubercles of transverse processes of C1-3 vertebrae	Extends and laterally bends the neck, laterally rotates the neck

III. Erector Spinae (Intermediate Group)

Muscle	Origin	Insertion	Action
Iliocostalis lumborum	Iliac crest and posterior surface of the sacrum	Angles of ribs 7–12	Extends and laterally bends the vertebral column
Iliocostalis thoracis	Upper borders of angles of ribs 7–12	Upper borders of angles of ribs 1–6, transverse process of the C7 vertebra	Extends and laterally bends the vertebral column
Iliocostalis cervicis	Angles of ribs 3–6	Posterior tubercles of transverse processes of C4-6 vertebrae	Extends and laterally bends the vertebral column
Longissimus thoracis	Transverse processes of lower thoracic and all lumbar vertebrae	Transverse processes of all thoracic vertebrae	Extends and laterally bends the vertebral column
Longissimus cervicis	Transverse processes T1-5 vertebrae	Posterior tubercles of transverse processes of C2-6 vertebrae	Extends and laterally bends the vertebral column
Longissimus capitis	Transverse processes T1-5 vertebrae	Mastoid process of temporal bone	Extends and laterally bends the head and vertebral column, rotates the head to the same side
Spinalis thoracis	Spines T11-L2 vertebrae	Spines of T1-8 vertebrae	Extends the vertebral column
Spinalis cervicis	Spine C7 (T1-2) vertebrae	Spine of C2 (occasionally C3-4) vertebrae	Extends the vertebral column

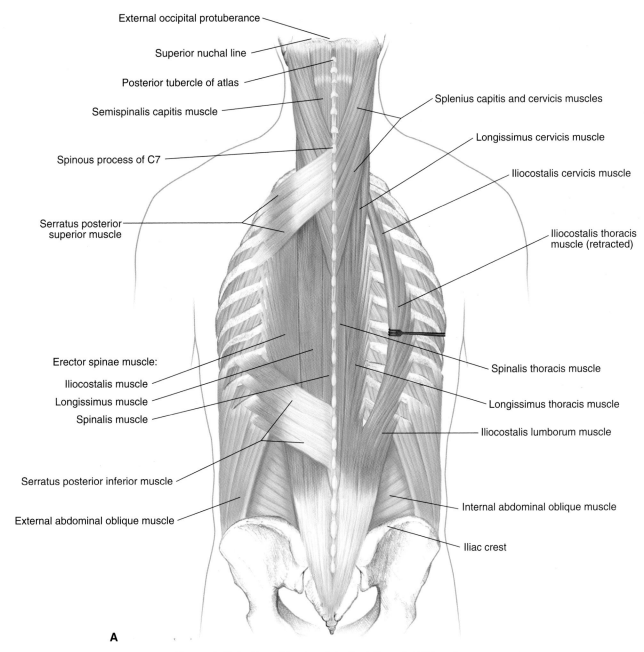

External occipital protuberance

Superior nuchal line

Posterior tubercle of atlas

Semispinalis capitis muscle

Spinous process of C7

Serratus posterior
superior muscle

Erector spinae muscle:

Iliocostalis muscle

Longissimus muscle

Spinalis muscle

Serratus posterior inferior muscle

External abdominal oblique muscle

Splenius capitis and cervicis muscles

Longissimus cervicis muscle

Iliocostalis cervicis muscle

Iliocostalis thoracis
muscle (retracted)

Spinalis thoracis muscle

Longissimus thoracis muscle

Iliocostalis lumborum muscle

Internal abdominal oblique muscle

Iliac crest

A

Figure 1.11A. Deep Muscles of the Back: Superficial Dissection

IV. Transversospinal Muscles (Deep Group) (Fig. 1.11B)

Muscle	Origin	Insertion	Action
Semispinalis group	Lateral part of transverse processes	In general, insertions are on spines 4–6 vertebral levels above origins	Rotates vertebral the column to the opposite side
Thoracis	Transverse process of T6-10 vertebrae	Spines C6-T4 vertebrae	Rotates the vertebral column to the opposite side
Cervicis	Transverse process of T1-6 vertebrae	Spines C2-5 vertebrae	Rotates the vertebral column to the opposite side
Capitis	Transverse process of C7-T7 vertebrae Articular process of C4-6 vertebrae	Occipital bone between superior and inferior nuchal lines	Extends the head, rotates the head to the opposite side
Multifidus	Medial part of transverse processes	In general, insertions are on spinous processes 2–4 vertebral levels above origins	Rotates the vertebral column to the opposite side
Sacral part	Posterior surface of the sacrum, thoracolumbar fascia, posterior superior iliac spine, posterior sacroiliac ligament	Muscle fascicles cross 2–4 vertebrae to insert on spines of vertebrae from C2-L5	
Lumbar part	From all mammillary processes		
Thoracic part	From all transverse processes		
Cervical part	Articular processes of C4-7 vertebrae		
Rotatores	Transverse process	Vertebral spine, 1–2 vertebral levels above the origin	Rotates the vertebral column to the opposite side
Longi	Transverse process	Spine, 2 vertebrae above	
Breves	Transverse process	Spine, next vertebra above	

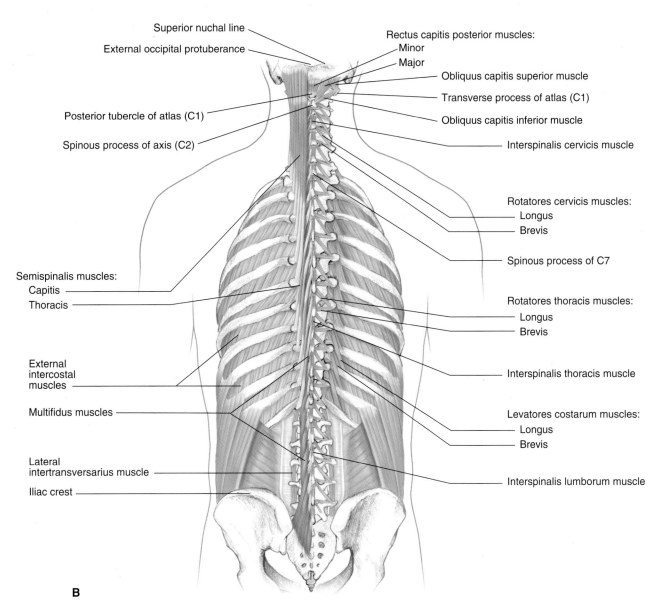

Figure 1.11B. Deep Muscles of the Back: Intermediate Dissection

Deep Muscles of the Back, Part 2

I. Minor Deep Back Muscles (Fig. 1.12A)

Muscle	Origin	Insertion	Action
Interspinalis	Spinous processes of 1 vertebra (C2-T2,T11-L5; muscles are paired)	Spinous process of the next vertebra above	Extends the vertebral column
Intertransversarii	Transverse processes of cervical and lumbar vertebrae	Transverse processes of the next vertebra above	Bends the vertebral column to the same side
Anterior	Interconnect the anterior tubercles of transverse processes from C1-T1,T10-L1		
Posterior	Interconnect posterior tubercles of transverse processes of lumbar vertebrae		
Lateral	Between adjoining transverse processes of lumbar vertebrae		
Medial	Between accessory process and mammillary processes of adjoining vertebrae of lumbar region		
Levatores costarum	Lateral ends of transverse processes from C7-T11	Upper borders of ribs below	Elevate ribs, bend the vertebral column to the same side

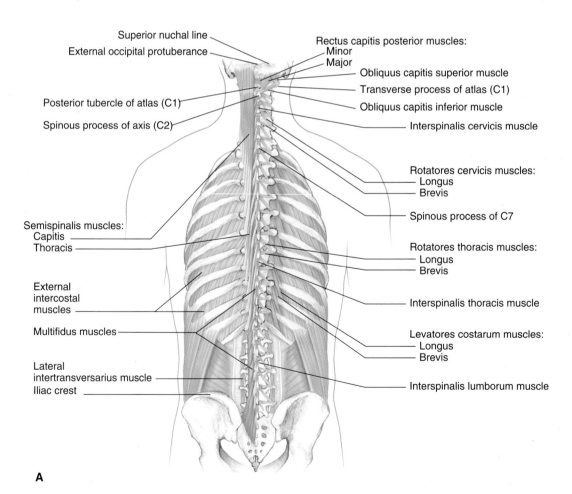

A

Figure 1.12A. Deep Muscles of the Back: Deeper Dissection

II. Suboccipital Muscles (Fig. 1.12B)

Muscle	Origin	Insertion	Action
Rectus capitis posterior major	Spinous process of the axis	Inferior nuchal line	Extends the head, rotates the head to the same side
Rectus capitis posterior minor	Posterior tubercle of the atlas	Inferior nuchal line	Extends the head
Obliquus capitis inferior	Tip of the spine of the axis	Transverse process of the atlas	Rotates the head to the same side
Obliquus capitis superior	Transverse process of the atlas	Occipital bone between superior and inferior nuchal lines	Extends the head, laterally bends the head

A. Suboccipital triangle: boundaries
   1. Superomedial: rectus capitis posterior major muscle
   2. Superolateral: obliquus capitis superior muscle
   3. Inferolateral: obliquus capitis inferior muscle
   4. Roof: semispinalis capitis muscle
   5. Floor: atlanto-occipital membrane and posterior arch of the atlas
B. Suboccipital triangle: contents
   1. Vertebral artery: lies on the upper surface of the arch of the atlas
   2. 1st cervical nerve
       a. Passes between the vertebral artery and the arch of the atlas
       b. Innervates all suboccipital muscles

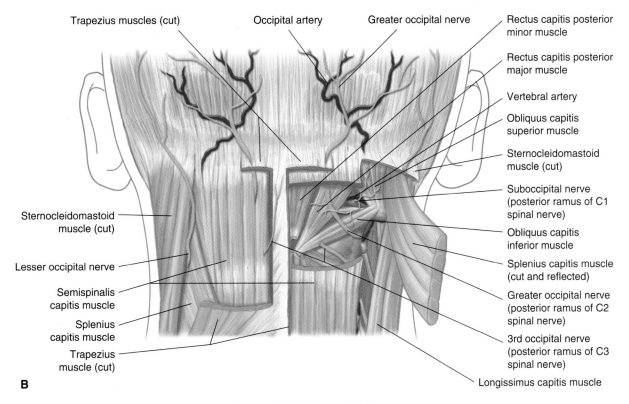

Figure 1.12B. Suboccipital Muscles

Movements of the Vertebral Column and Head

I. Nomenclature of Movements of the Vertebral Column

A. Flexion
1. Bending forward
2. Anterior parts of intervertebral discs compress; posterior parts expand
3. Motion limited by ligamenta flava, posterior longitudinal ligament, supraspinous ligament, interspinous ligaments, and deep back muscles (muscles are the primary limiting structure)

B. Extension
1. Bending backward
2. Anterior parts of discs expand; posterior parts compress
3. Motion limited by anterior longitudinal ligament, spinous processes

C. Lateral flexion
1. Bending to either side
2. Motion limited by ligamenta flava, intertransverse ligaments, part of anterior longitudinal ligament, and deep back muscles

D. Rotation
1. Rotation is limited between adjacent vertebrae
2. Summation of rotation at multiple intervertebral joints results in considerable rotational movement

II. Range of Motion (ROM) of Vertebral Segments

A. Joints are examined by performing active and passive motion
1. ROM is essential for fundamental task such as walking, climbing or descending stairs, sitting down or getting out of a chair
2. Noticing restricted ROM is essential in diagnosis
   a. Radiologic evidence may help
   b. Compare ROM between sides

B. Cervical spine
1. ROM is sum of movements at the atlanto-occipital and cervical intervertebral joints
2. Flexion: one should be able to place the chin on the chest (with mouth closed)
3. Extension: catches the examiner's finger between the occiput and C7 but does not "trap" it
4. Lateral bending: when the shoulders are steadied, ear toward shoulder movement should allow ROM that is just under 90° rotation
5. Rotation
   a. Normally brings the chin level with the shoulders (with shoulders steadied)
   b. Most of this ROM occurs at the atlanto-occipital joint
   c. Combined rotation with extension compresses the intervertebral foramina (can exaggerate nerve compression symptoms)

C. Thoracolumbar spine
1. General comments
   a. Rib cage and thinness of the intervertebral discs limit mobility of the thoracic spine in its upper and middle regions
   b. Flexion, extension, and lateral bending of the trunk occur mostly in the lumbar region; rotation occurs most freely in the thoracic region
2. Flexion: tested by bending forward as far as possible with the knees extended, measuring the movement of the distance between C7 and a fixed point on the sacrum (starting with the upright position)
3. Extension
   a. Normal lumbar curvature holds the lumbosacral angle in extension (even in the erect position)
   b. Range of extension is only approximately 15° to 30° and tends to exaggerate the normal "lordotic" lumbar curvature

4. Lateral bending
   a. Measured by sliding the hand down the side of the thigh as far as possible
   b. Normally, one can reach the head of the fibula without flexing the hip or knee
   c. Measure the distance between the fingertips and the fibular head (Note: If pain on the concave side is experienced during this test, nerve root compression may be suspected; pain on the convex side is usually related to muscle, tendon, or ligament abnormalities, such as arthritis)
5. Rotation
   a. Rotation of the trunk takes place primarily in the thoracic spine
   b. One must exclude hip rotation for an accurate measurement, because limitations in the lumbar region may be masked by movement of the hip joint; standing behind the patient, the examiner should hold the pelvis firmly at the iliac crests, while the patient twists the trunk in an attempt to look back at the examiner
   c. One may also attempt to rotate the trunk while the patient is seated; assess the change in position of the shoulders for evaluation

III. Range of Motion (ROM) of Vertebral Segments

| Level (Region) | Flexion/Extension (°) | | Lateral Bending (°) | | Rotation (°) | | Center of Movement |
	Per Segment[a]	Total	Per Segment[a]	Total	Per Segment[a]	Total	
Occiput–C1	0–13	Combined: 25	0–5	0	0–5	0	Skull: 2–3 cm below dens
C1-2	10	Combined: 20	0–5	0	40–45	40–45	"Waist" of dens (C2)
C2-T1 (C-spine)	10–15	Flex.: 40 Ext.: 0	8–10	40–45	0–10	45	Vertebral body below
T1-L1 (T-spine)	5–6	Flex.: 60–80 Ext.: 20–30	6	35	6–8	72	Vertebra below disc centrum
L1-5 (L-spine)	15–20	Flex.: 90 Ext.: 45	2–5	25	1–6	3–6	Anulus of disc
L5-S1 (S-spine)	10–20	10–20	2–5	2–5	0–2	0–2	Anulus of disc

[a]Motion segment involves 3 essential parts; namely, 2 vertebrae (facet joints) and their intervening soft tissues (intervertebral disc)

Total spine movement (from anatomical position): Flexion: 85° to 90°; Extension: 35° (Hyperextension + 30°); Lateral bending (flexion): 35° (right and left); Rotation: 30°

IV. Muscles Producing Movements of the Vertebral Column (Fig. 1.13)

Flexion[a]	Extension[a]	Lateral Bending[b]	Rotation[b]
Sternocleidomastoid	Erector spinae	Muscles listed under	All transversospinal muscles rotate
Longus coli	Semispinalis	flexion and extension	the spine toward the opposite side;
Scalenes	Splenius	when only 1 side acts,	external abdominal oblique and
Psoas major	Multifidus	quadratus lumborum	internal abdominal oblique rotate
External abdominal oblique	Rotatores		the spine toward the same side
Internal abdominal oblique	Interspinalis		
Rectus abdominis	Intertransversarii		

[a]Flexion and extension are accomplished when the bilateral muscles act together
[b]Lateral bending and rotation are accomplished when the muscles on 1 side contract unilaterally

V. Muscles Producing Movements of the Head

Flexion[a]	Extension[a]	Lateral Bending[b]	Rotation[b]
Longus capitis	Rectus capitis posterior major	Sternocleidomastoid	To opposite side:
Rectus capitis anterior	Rectus capitis posterior minor	Trapezius	Sternocleidomastoid
	Obliquus capitis superior	Splenius capitis	Trapezius
	Semispinalis capitis		To same side:
	Splenius capitis		Semispinalis capitis
	Sternocleidomastoid		Longus capitis
	Upper trapezius		Splenius capitis
			Longissimus capitis
			Rectus capitis posterior major
			Obliquus capitis superior and inferior

[a]Flexion and extension are accomplished when the bilateral muscles act together
[b]Lateral bending and rotation are accomplished when the muscles on 1 side contract unilaterally

VI. Testing Back Muscles

A. Evaluate muscles in groups

B. From the prone position, the patient is asked to raise his or her head and shoulders from the table; resistance may be applied by the examiner to the head and shoulders, testing the strength in the cervical and thoracolumbar regions, and the lumbar musculature may be tested by observation and palpation during the maneuver

C. Unless there is regional paralysis, generalized weakness of the spine extensors is rarely associated with back problems; more commonly, back symptoms are the result of weakness of trunk flexor muscles, especially the rectus abdominis and the muscles of the flank

D. Another test used to evaluate the back muscles should include attempted sit-ups, while the hips and knees are kept in the flexed position, because inability to do sit-ups in this position indicates a marked weakness of the abdominal musculature. Strengthening the abdominal musculature may relieve symptoms due to strains on the vertebral column

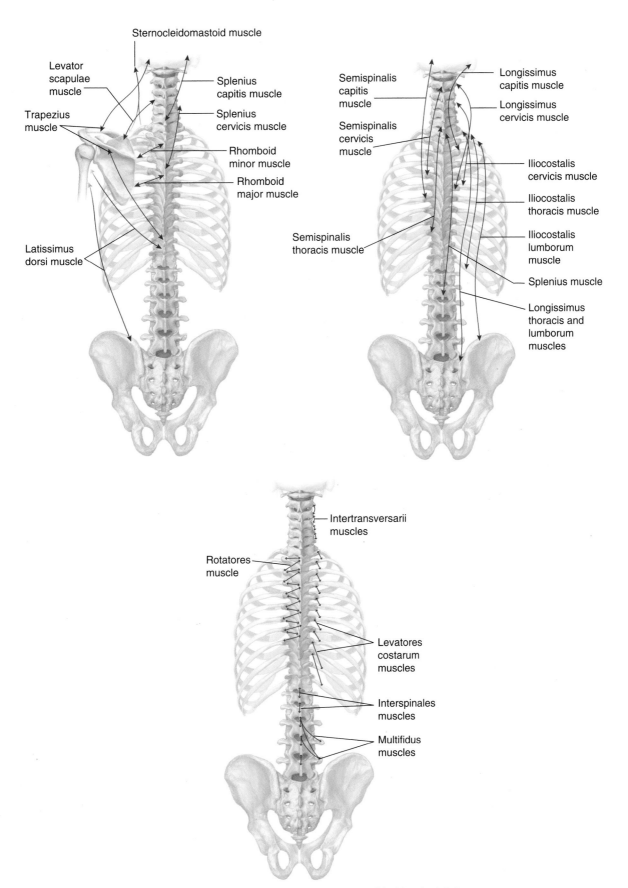

Figure 1.13. Muscles Producing Movements of the Vertebral Column

Spinal Meninges

I. General Comments (Fig. 1.14A,B)

A. **Spinal meninges:** membranes that surround, support, and protect the spinal cord and the spinal nerve roots
B. There are 3 layers of spinal meninges
   1. Dura mater
   2. Arachnoid mater
   3. Pia mater

II. Dura Mater

A. Outer layer of the 3 meninges
B. Dense, tough fibrous membrane (*dura mater* = tough mother)
C. Corresponds to the meningeal layer of the cranial dura mater
   1. Is attached to the margin of the foramen magnum of the skull
   2. Forms a sac containing the spinal cord and nerve roots
   3. Extends laterally around nerve roots and spinal nerves to fuse with the epineurium
   4. **Dural sac** ends at the S2 vertebral level
      a. Dura fuses with the filum terminale internum to form the **coccygeal ligament (filum terminale externum)**
      b. Coccygeal ligament attaches to the coccyx
D. **Epidural space**
   1. Space between the dural sac and the bones of the vertebral canal
   2. Contains fat and loose connective tissue
   3. Contains the veins of the internal vertebral venous plexus, which do not have valves

III. Arachnoid Mater

A. Middle layer of the meninges
B. Thin and delicate: "arachnoid" refers to the cobweb-like appearance of the arachnoid trabeculae
C. Lines the dural sac
D. Continuous with the cranial arachnoid mater
E. **Subdural space:** potential space between the dura mater and the arachnoid mater
F. **Subarachnoid space**
   1. Space surrounded by the arachnoid mater
   2. Continuous with the subarachnoid space of the cranium
   3. Contents
      a. Cerebrospinal fluid (20 to 35 mL)
      b. Arachnoid trabeculae: connect the arachnoid mater to the pia mater
      c. Spinal nerve roots
      d. Radicular vessels
      e. Denticulate ligaments and filum terminale internum
   4. Ends at the S2 vertebral level
   5. **Lumbar cistern**
      a. Extends from the conus medullaris (L2) to S2
      b. Contains spinal nerve roots (cauda equina)
      c. Location of lumbar puncture

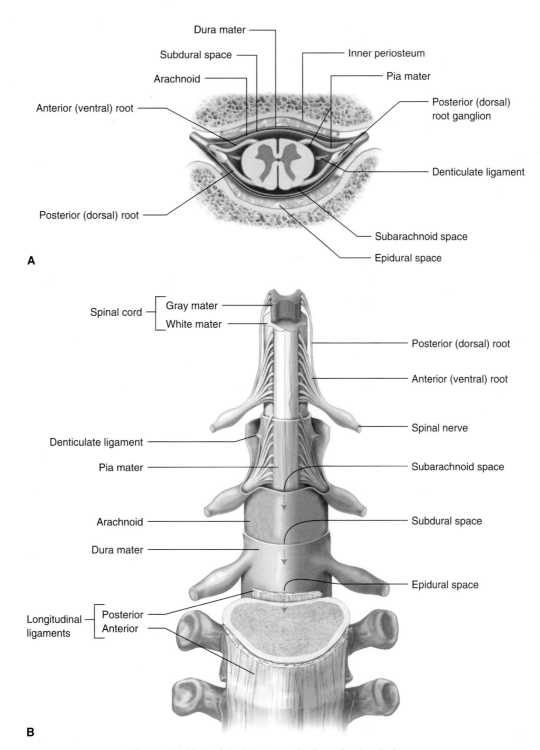

Figure 1.14A,B. Spinal Meninges. **A.** Cross Section. **B.** Spaces.

IV. Pia Mater (Fig. 1.14C,D)

A. Inner layer of the meninges
B. Delicate connective tissue
   1. Closely applied to spinal cord
   2. Highly vascular
C. Specializations
   1. Denticulate ligaments (bilateral)
     a. Lateral extension of the pia mater from the surface of the spinal cord
     b. Extends nearly the full length of the spinal cord
     c. Lies between the anterior and posterior nerve roots
     d. Denticulations
       i. 21 points of attachment of the pia mater to the dura mater
       ii. Attach between the exit points of the nerve roots
       iii. Anchor spinal cord laterally
   2. Filum terminale internum
     a. Extends inferiorly off the tip of the conus medullaris
     b. Enclosed within the coccygeal ligament where the dural sac ends at S2
     c. Anchors the spinal cord inferiorly
     d. Surrounded by cauda equina

V. Clinical Considerations

A. Visualization of the spinal cord and dural sac
   1. T2-weighted MRI will show cerebrospinal fluid (CSF) as white, contrasting with darker spinal cord and nerve rootlets; may reveal spinal stenosis or disc herniation
   2. Myelography involves radiography of the spine after injection of radiopaque dye into CSF
     a. Radiological procedure for examining the subarachnoid space
     b. Contrast medium is injected via lumbar puncture
B. Lumbar puncture (Fig. 1.14E–G)
   1. Used to sample CSF for diagnostic purposes
   2. Needle introduced into the subarachnoid space
   3. Usually performed at low lumbar levels (above or below the spine of L4)
   4. Spinal nerve roots are seldom damaged because they are suspended in CSF and move away from the needle point
   5. In the newborn, the spinal cord terminates at the lower border of L3, which makes lumbar puncture more risky
C. Spinal anesthesia
   1. Anesthetic agents injected into the subarachnoid space
   2. Needle punctures the dural sac between lumbar vertebrae
   3. Anesthetic mixes with CSF to anesthetize nerve roots
D. Epidural anesthesia
   1. Needle introduced into the epidural space
   2. Needle does not puncture the dural sac
   3. Anesthetic is injected into the fat that surrounds the dural sac
   4. Spinal nerves are anesthetized within the dural sleeves
E. Caudal anesthesia: epidural anesthesia performed by inserting a needle through the sacral hiatus
F. Meningitis
   1. Infection of the meninges
     a. Pachymeningitis: infection of the dura
     b. Leptomeningitis: infection of the arachnoid or pia
   2. Symptoms: headache; fever; mental confusion; neck stiffness; flexion at ankle, knee, and hip when the neck is bent; inability to extend the leg completely when in the sitting position or when lying with the thigh flexed upon the abdomen

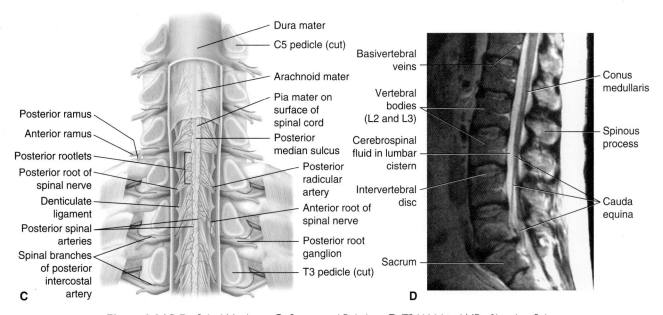

C

- Dura mater
- C5 pedicle (cut)
- Arachnoid mater
- Pia mater on surface of spinal cord
- Posterior median sulcus
- Posterior radicular artery
- Anterior root of spinal nerve
- Posterior root ganglion
- T3 pedicle (cut)

- Posterior ramus
- Anterior ramus
- Posterior rootlets
- Posterior root of spinal nerve
- Denticulate ligament
- Posterior spinal arteries
- Spinal branches of posterior intercostal artery

D

- Basivertebral veins
- Vertebral bodies (L2 and L3)
- Cerebrospinal fluid in lumbar cistern
- Intervertebral disc
- Sacrum
- Conus medullaris
- Spinous process
- Cauda equina

Figure 1.14C,D. Spinal Meninges. **C.** Spaces and Relations. **D.** T2-Weighted MR of Lumbar Spine

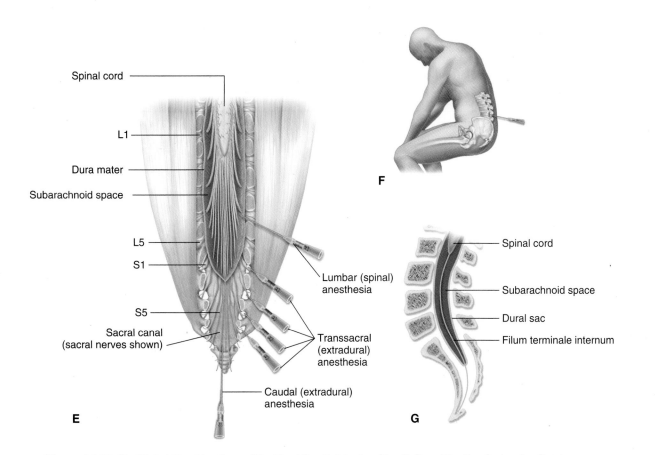

E

- Spinal cord
- L1
- Dura mater
- Subarachnoid space
- L5
- S1
- S5
- Sacral canal (sacral nerves shown)
- Lumbar (spinal) anesthesia
- Transsacral (extradural) anesthesia
- Caudal (extradural) anesthesia

F

G

- Spinal cord
- Subarachnoid space
- Dural sac
- Filum terminale internum

Figure 1.14E–G. Clinical Considerations of the Dural Sac. **E.** Injection Sites. **F.** Flexed Position for Lumbar Puncture. **G.** Lumbar Cistern

Spinal Cord

I. General Description (Fig. 1.15A)

A. Continuous with the lower end of the medulla oblongata at the foramen magnum
B. Length: 43 to 45 cm
C. Diameter varies at different levels
  1. Thoracic portion is approximately 1 cm in width
  2. **Cervical enlargement**
    a. Approximately 1.4 cm in width
    b. C5-T1 spinal cord segments
    c. C5-T1 vertebral levels
    d. Gives rise to nerves of the upper limb
  3. **Lumbosacral enlargement**
    a. Approximately 1.3 cm in width
    b. L1-S3 spinal cord segments
    c. T9-L1 vertebral levels
    d. Gives rise to nerves of the lower limb
D. Ends as **conus medullaris** at the level of the L1/2 intervertebral disc

II. External Appearance: Fissures and Sulci (Fig. 1.15B)

A. **Posterior median sulcus:** midline groove on the posterior surface
B. **Anterior median fissure**
  1. Midline groove on the anterior surface
  2. Anterior spinal artery lies in the anterior median fissure
C. **Posterolateral sulcus**
  1. Groove located just posterior to the line of attachment of the posterior nerve roots
  2. Represents the line of attachment of the posterior nerve roots
  3. Posterior spinal artery lies in the posterolateral sulcus
D. **Anterolateral sulcus:** represents the line of attachment of the anterior roots

III. Internal Structure

A. **Gray matter**
  1. Butterfly- (H-) shaped area of darker nervous tissue located centrally
  2. Contains bodies of neurons
  3. **Posterior horns**
    a. Narrow posterior projections
    b. Contain neurons that transmit afferent signals
  4. **Lateral horns**
    a. Lateral projections of the gray matter
    b. T1-L2 spinal cord segments
    c. Contain presynaptic sympathetic neurons
  5. **Anterior horns**
    a. Thick anterior projections
    b. Contain motor neurons
  6. **Gray commissure:** cross bar of the "H"
  7. **Central canal**
    a. Located within the gray commissure
    b. Continuous with the ventricular system of the brain
B. **White matter**
  1. Peripherally located nervous tissue made up of nerve fibers and glia
  2. **Posterior funiculus**
    a. Between posterior median sulcus and posterolateral sulcus
    b. Contains predominantly ascending tracts

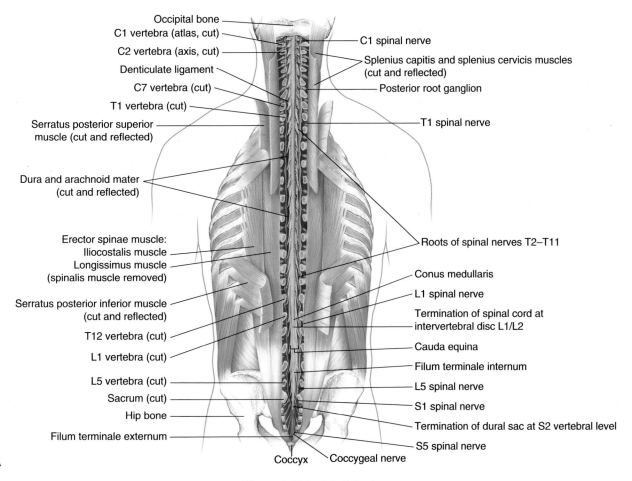

Occipital bone
C1 vertebra (atlas, cut)
C2 vertebra (axis, cut)
Denticulate ligament
C7 vertebra (cut)
T1 vertebra (cut)
Serratus posterior superior muscle (cut and reflected)
Dura and arachnoid mater (cut and reflected)
Erector spinae muscle:
Iliocostalis muscle
Longissimus muscle (spinalis muscle removed)
Serratus posterior inferior muscle (cut and reflected)
T12 vertebra (cut)
L1 vertebra (cut)
L5 vertebra (cut)
Sacrum (cut)
Hip bone
Filum terminale externum

C1 spinal nerve
Splenius capitis and splenius cervicis muscles (cut and reflected)
Posterior root ganglion
T1 spinal nerve
Roots of spinal nerves T2–T11
Conus medullaris
L1 spinal nerve
Termination of spinal cord at intervertebral disc L1/L2
Cauda equina
Filum terminale internum
L5 spinal nerve
S1 spinal nerve
Termination of dural sac at S2 vertebral level
S5 spinal nerve
Coccygeal nerve
Coccyx

A

Figure 1.15A. Spinal Cord

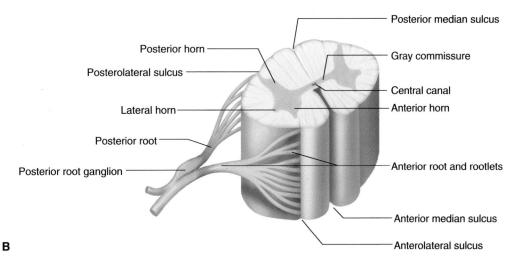

Posterior horn
Posterolateral sulcus
Lateral horn
Posterior root
Posterior root ganglion

Posterior median sulcus
Gray commissure
Central canal
Anterior horn
Anterior root and rootlets
Anterior median sulcus
Anterolateral sulcus

B

Figure 1.15B. Structure of the Spinal Cord

3. **Lateral funiculus**
   a. Between the emerging anterior rootlets and posterior rootlets
   b. Contains both ascending and descending tracts
4. **Anterior funiculus**
   a. Between anterior median fissure and the emerging anterior rootlets
   b. Contains predominately descending tracts

IV. Clinical Considerations

A. **Spina bifida**
   1. Failure of the neural arches to fuse during development
   2. Usually occurs in the lumbosacral region
   3. Several types are recognized
      a. **Spina bifida occulta**
         i. Defect in the neural arches that is covered by the skin
         ii. May result in no symptoms and may go undetected
         iii. May be present in 10% of otherwise normal people
      b. **Spina bifida cystica**
         i. Severe neural tube defect
         ii. Neural tube may form a cyst-like sac
         iii. There are 2 types:
            a) **Meningocele:** spinal cord develops normally and only the meninges protrude from the defect
            b) **Meningomyelocele:** both the meninges and the neural tissue protrude from the defect

B. **Syringomyelia**
   1. Enlargement of the central canal
   2. Places pressure on the spinal cord from within
   3. Destroys the function of the spinal cord

C. **Laminectomy**
   1. Surgical removal of the lamina of the vertebral arch
   2. Used to remove herniated nucleus pulposus and relieve pressure on neural structures from bony fragments, tumors, or hematomas

D. **Cordotomy**
   1. Surgical section of the spinal cord
   2. May be used to interrupt pain pathways (lateral spinothalamic tract) in cases of extreme, uncontrollable pain

Spinal Nerves and Their Branches <small>(Fig. 1.16A,B)</small>

I. Spinal Nerves

A. 31 pairs grouped regionally
  1. 8 cervical
  2. 12 thoracic
  3. 5 lumbar
  4. 5 sacral
  5. 1 coccygeal

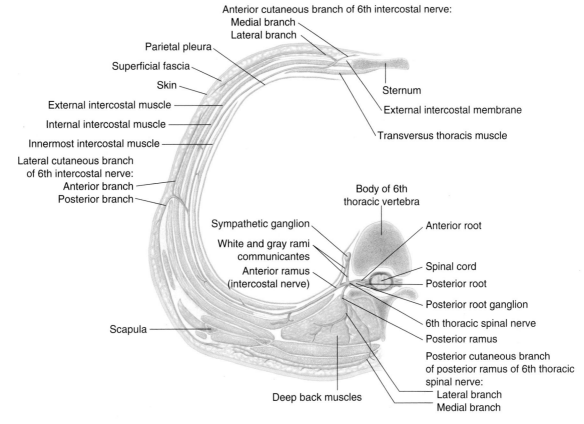

A

Figure 1.16A. Branching Pattern of a Typical Spinal Nerve

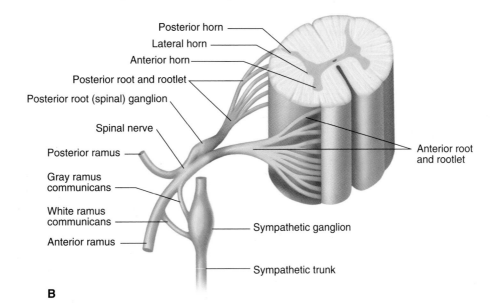

B

Figure 1.16B. Formation of a Typical Spinal Nerve

B. Origin from the spinal cord
   1. Posterior (dorsal) root
      a. Sensory (afferent)
      b. Arises from numerous rootlets adjacent to the posterolateral sulcus
      c. **Spinal (dorsal root) ganglion:** swelling composed of sensory nerve cell bodies
   2. Anterior (ventral) root
      a. Motor (efferent)
      b. Arises from numerous rootlets from the anterolateral sulcus
   3. Spinal cord segment: gives rise to rootlets that form 1 spinal nerve
C. Spinal nerve
   1. Formed by the joining of posterior and anterior roots
      a. Occurs just lateral to the spinal ganglion
      b. Point at which motor and sensory fibers intermingle to form mixed nerves
   2. In intervertebral foramen
   3. 1 to 2 mm in length
D. Branches of the spinal nerve
   1. Posterior ramus
      a. Travels posteriorly to innervate deep back muscles
      b. Continues as a cutaneous nerve branch to the skin of the back
   2. Anterior ramus
      a. Travels laterally to innervate the neck, trunk and limb muscles
      b. Supplies cutaneous nerve branches to the skin of the neck, trunk, and limbs
      c. Connections to the sympathetic trunk
         i. **White ramus communicans:** presynaptic sympathetic fibers passing from the anterior rami of spinal nerves T1-L2 to the sympathetic trunk
         ii. **Gray ramus communicans:** postsynaptic fibers passing from the sympathetic trunk to anterior rami of all spinal nerves (C1–coccygeal)

II. Relationship of Spinal Nerves to the Vertebral Column (Fig. 1.16C,D)

A. Cervical spinal nerves
   1. Roots run transversely toward intervertebral foramina
   2. 8 cervical spinal nerves but only 7 vertebrae
      a. Exit above the vertebra of the same number
      b. C8 exits below vertebra C7
B. Thoracic spinal nerves
   1. Roots run obliquely (inferolaterally) toward the intervertebral foramina
   2. 12 thoracic spinal nerves exit below the thoracic vertebrae of the same number
C. Lumbar, sacral, and coccygeal spinal nerves
   1. Roots descend nearly vertically toward the intervertebral foramina because the spinal cord ends at L1/2 intervertebral disc
   2. Lumbar spinal nerves exit below the vertebrae of the same number
   3. Branches of sacral spinal nerves exit through the sacral foramina (anterior and posterior) below the sacral segment of the same number

Spinal Nerve	Spinal Cord Segment at Vertebral Level	Spinal Nerve Exits Vertebral Canal
C1	C1	Above C1
C8	C7	Below C7
T1	T1	Below T1
T12	T8	Below T12
L2	T10	Below L2
L5	T12	Below L5
S3	L1	3rd sacral foramina (anterior and posterior)

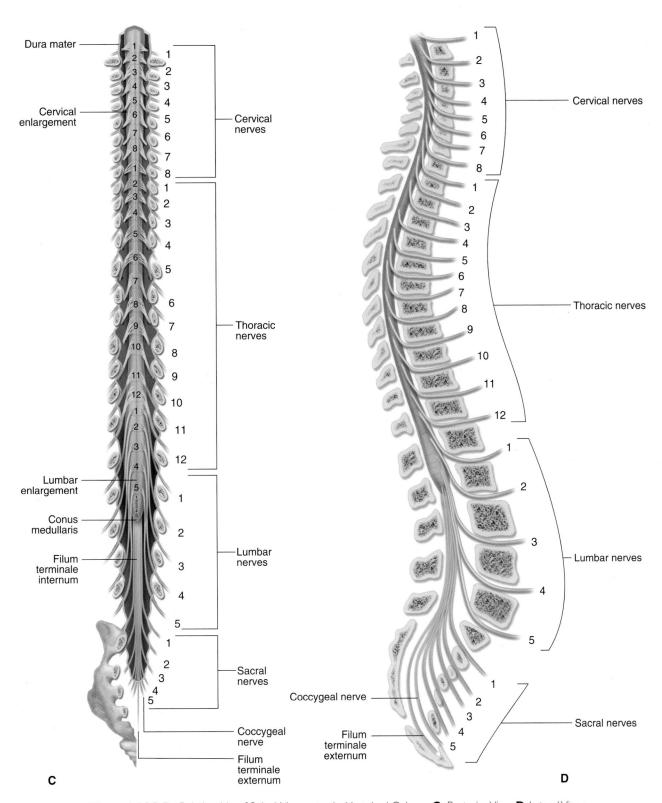

Dura mater

Cervical enlargement

Cervical nerves

Thoracic nerves

Lumbar enlargement

Conus medullaris

Filum terminale internum

Lumbar nerves

Sacral nerves

Coccygeal nerve

Filum terminale externum

C

Cervical nerves

Thoracic nerves

Lumbar nerves

Coccygeal nerve

Filum terminale externum

Sacral nerves

D

Figure 1.16C,D. Relationship of Spinal Nerves to the Vertebral Column. **C.** Posterior View. **D.** Lateral View

III. **Distribution of Anterior and Posterior Rami** (Fig. 1.16E)

A. Posterior rami
   1. All except C1, S4, S5, and coccygeal have lateral and medial branches
   2. Cervical
      a. C1: entire posterior ramus supplies suboccipital muscles
      b. C2: medial branch is a large cutaneous nerve (**greater occipital nerve**), lateral branch is muscular
      c. C3: medial branch is cutaneous to lower part of the back of the head; lateral branch is muscular
      d. C4 and C5: medial branches are muscular and cutaneous; lateral branch is muscular
      e. C5-8: both branches are muscular
   3. Thoracic
      a. T1-6: medial branches are cutaneous; lateral branches are muscular
      b. T7-12: medial branches are muscular; lateral branches are cutaneous
   4. Lumbar
      a. L1-3: medial branches are muscular; lateral branches go to the buttock as **superior cluneal nerves**
      b. L4: both branches are muscular
      c. L5: muscular
   5. Sacral and coccygeal
      a. S1-3: medial branches are muscular; lateral branches go to the skin on the buttock as **middle cluneal nerves**
      b. S4, S5, and coccygeal: cutaneous to the skin over the coccyx
B. Anterior rami
   1. Form plexuses
      a. **Cervical plexus:** C1-4
      b. **Brachial plexus:** C5-T1
      c. **Lumbar plexus:** L1-4
      d. **Sacral plexus:** L4-S3
   2. Thoracic nerves
      a. **Intercostal nerves:** T1-11
      b. **Subcostal nerve:** T12; below the 12th rib

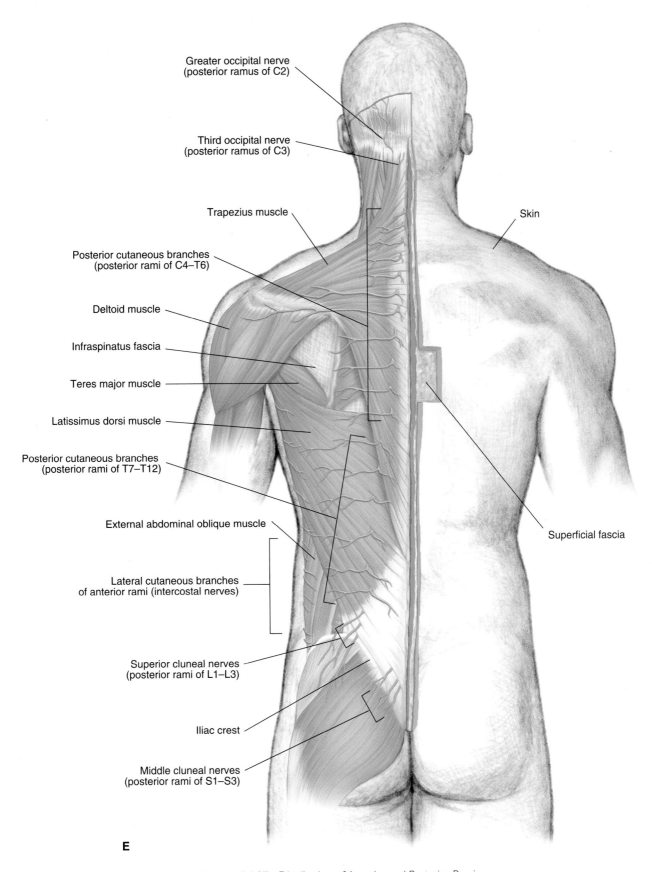

Greater occipital nerve
(posterior ramus of C2)

Third occipital nerve
(posterior ramus of C3)

Trapezius muscle

Posterior cutaneous branches
(posterior rami of C4–T6)

Deltoid muscle

Infraspinatus fascia

Teres major muscle

Latissimus dorsi muscle

Posterior cutaneous branches
(posterior rami of T7–T12)

External abdominal oblique muscle

Lateral cutaneous branches
of anterior rami (intercostal nerves)

Superior cluneal nerves
(posterior rami of L1–L3)

Iliac crest

Middle cluneal nerves
(posterior rami of S1–S3)

Skin

Superficial fascia

E

Figure 1.16E. Distribution of Anterior and Posterior Rami

Blood Supply of the Spinal Cord (Fig. 1.17)

I. Posterior Spinal Arteries

A. 1 on each side

B. Origin: fusion of multiple small branches from vertebral and posterior inferior cerebellar arteries with anastomoses with posterior radicular arteries throughout the length of the spinal cord

C. Course
   1. Descends through the foramen magnum to the spinal cord
   2. Descends in the posterolateral sulcus

D. Termination: on the conus medullaris

E. Distribution: supplies the posterior 1/3 of the spinal cord

II. Anterior Spinal Artery

A. Single artery in the midline of the spinal cord

B. Origin: midline fusion of the anterior spinal branches of the vertebral arteries with anastomoses with anterior radicular arteries throughout the length of the spinal cord

C. Course
   1. Descends through the foramen magnum
   2. Lies along the anterior median fissure

D. Termination: on the filum terminale internum

E. Distribution: supplies the anterior 2/3 of the spinal cord

III. Radicular Arteries

A. Origin: from spinal branches of
   1. Vertebral arteries
   2. Deep cervical arteries
   3. Ascending cervical arteries
   4. Inferior thyroid arteries
   5. Posterior intercostal arteries
   6. Lumbar arteries
   7. Lateral sacral arteries

B. Course
   1. Spinal branch passes through the intervertebral foramen to enter the dural sac
   2. Radicular arteries follow anterior and posterior roots to reach the spinal cord
      a. Anterior radicular artery
      b. Posterior radicular artery

C. Termination: anastomoses with anterior and posterior spinal arteries

D. Great radicular artery
   1. Arises from the spinal branch of a lower posterior intercostal, the subcostal, or an upper lumbar artery, usually on the left side
   2. Major contributor of blood to the anastomosis that supplies the lumbar and sacral segments of the spinal cord

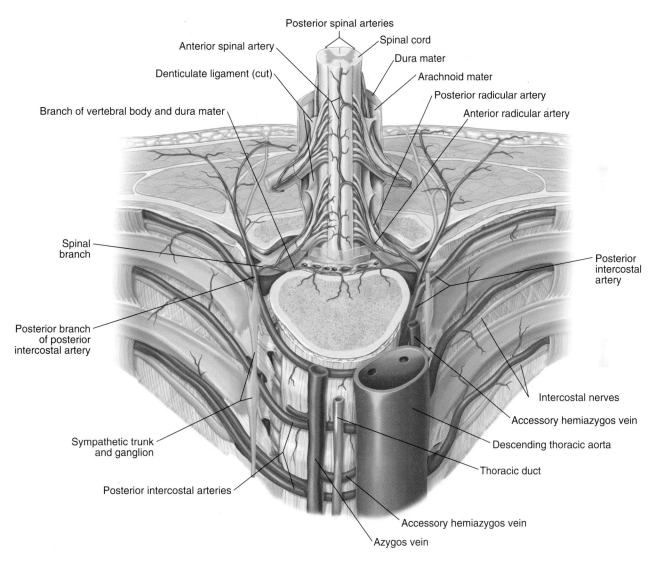

Posterior spinal arteries

Anterior spinal artery

Denticulate ligament (cut)

Branch of vertebral body and dura mater

Spinal cord

Dura mater

Arachnoid mater

Posterior radicular artery

Anterior radicular artery

Spinal branch

Posterior branch of posterior intercostal artery

Posterior intercostal artery

Intercostal nerves

Accessory hemiazygos vein

Descending thoracic aorta

Thoracic duct

Sympathetic trunk and ganglion

Posterior intercostal arteries

Accessory hemiazygos vein

Azygos vein

Figure 1.17. Blood Supply of the Spinal Cord

Veins of Spinal Cord and Vertebral Column

I. Veins of the Spinal Cord (Fig. 1.18A–C)

A. 6 longitudinal venous channels are located in the pia
  1. **Posterior median spinal vein:** along the posterior median sulcus
  2. **Anterior median spinal vein:** along the anterior median fissure
  3. **Posterior lateral spinal vein (2):** just posterior to each posterior root
  4. **Anterior lateral spinal vein (2):** just anterior to each anterior root

B. **Radicular veins**
  1. Travel laterally on nerve roots
  2. Drain into intervertebral veins

II. Veins of the Vertebral Column

A. Arranged in a plexus along the length of the vertebral column
B. 2 plexuses are described
  1. **External vertebral venous plexus**
    a. 2 freely anastomosing parts
      i. Anterior
        a) On the anterior surface of vertebral bodies
        b) Receive tributaries from vertebral bodies
      ii. Posterior: on the posterior surface of vertebral arches and processes
    b. Anastomose with internal vertebral venous plexus and intervertebral veins
  2. **Internal vertebral venous plexus**
    a. In vertebral canal embedded within the epidural fat (between dura mater and bone)
    b. Runs superoinferiorly
    c. Communicates with the dural venous sinuses in the skull
    d. Receives drainage from the bone and spinal cord
    e. 4 main channels
      i. Anterior (2)
        a) Lie on the posterior surface of vertebral bodies of the vertebrae, 1 on each side of the posterior longitudinal ligament
        b) Interconnected by transverse channels that receive **basivertebral veins**
      ii. Posterior (2): 1 on either side of the midline, anterior to vertebral arches and ligamenta flava
    f. Communications
      i. Posterior external vertebral venous plexus
      ii. Transverse channels at each vertebral level connect the internal plexuses
      iii. Radicular veins are tributary from spinal veins
      iv. Intervertebral veins
C. **Intervertebral veins**
  1. Course through the intervertebral foramina
  2. Drain the spinal cord via radicular veins
  3. Drain both internal and external vertebral venous plexuses
  4. Termination
    a. Vertebral veins
    b. Posterior intercostal veins
    c. Lumbar veins
    d. Lateral sacral veins

III. Clinical Considerations

A. Vertebral venous plexuses do not contain valves: blood can flow up or down the vertebral column depending on local blood pressure
B. Pelvic cancers (i.e., prostatic, uterine, ovarian) can metastasize to the vertebral column and cranial cavity

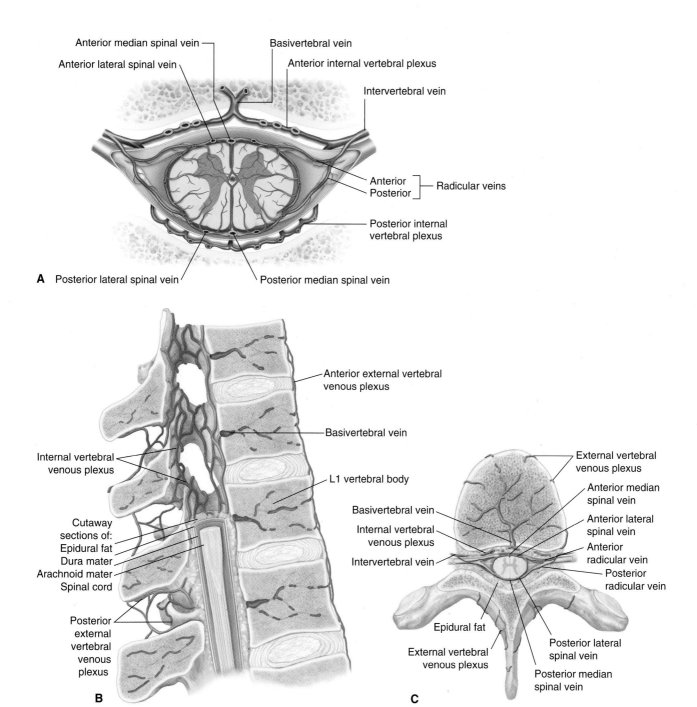

Anterior median spinal vein
Anterior lateral spinal vein
Basivertebral vein
Anterior internal vertebral plexus
Intervertebral vein
Anterior
Posterior ⎤ Radicular veins
Posterior internal vertebral plexus

A Posterior lateral spinal vein
Posterior median spinal vein

Anterior external vertebral venous plexus
Basivertebral vein
L1 vertebral body
Internal vertebral venous plexus
Cutaway sections of:
Epidural fat
Dura mater
Arachnoid mater
Spinal cord
Posterior external vertebral venous plexus

B

External vertebral venous plexus
Anterior median spinal vein
Anterior lateral spinal vein
Anterior radicular vein
Posterior radicular vein
Basivertebral vein
Internal vertebral venous plexus
Intervertebral vein
Epidural fat
External vertebral venous plexus
Posterior lateral spinal vein
Posterior median spinal vein

C

Figure 1.18. Veins of the Spinal Cord and Vertebral Column. **A.** Cross Section. **B.** Lateral View. **C.** Cross Section

Upper Limb

2.1	Introduction to the Upper Limb	64
2.2	Cutaneous Innervation of the Upper Limb	66
2.3	Superficial Veins and Deep Fascial Specializations of the Upper Limb	68
2.4	Lymphatics of the Upper Limb	70
2.5	Bones of the Pectoral (Shoulder) Girdle	72
2.6	Bone of the Arm: Humerus	74
2.7	Bones of the Forearm	76
2.8	Bones of the Wrist and Hand	79
2.9	Muscles of the Anterior Shoulder	82
2.10	Muscles of the Posterior Shoulder and the Rotator Cuff	84
2.11	Axilla and Brachial Plexus	87
2.12	Axillary Artery and Blood Supply to the Shoulder	92
2.13	Muscles of the Arm	95
2.14	Neurovasculature of the Arm	98
2.15	Muscles of the Anterior Forearm	100
2.16	Neurovasculature of the Anterior Forearm	103
2.17	Muscles of the Posterior Forearm	106
2.18	Neurovasculature of the Posterior Forearm	108
2.19	Dorsum of the Hand	110
2.20	Palm of the Hand, Superficial	114
2.21	Muscles of the Palmar Hand	119
2.22	Vessels of the Hand	123
2.23	Nerves of the Hand	126
2.24	Articulations of the Shoulder and Pectoral Girdle	129
2.25	Elbow Joint	133
2.26	Joints of the Wrist and Hand	136
2.27	Specific Nerve Injury: Median Nerve (C5-T1)	141
2.28	Specific Nerve Injury: Ulnar Nerve (C8,T1)	144
2.29	Specific Nerve Injury: Radial Nerve (C5-T1)	146

Introduction to the Upper Limb

I. Organ of Manipulation (*Manus* = Hand)

A. Joints, especially shoulder, emphasize mobility

II. General Organization (Fig. 2.1A–D)

A. Pectoral girdle (shoulder girdle)
   1. 2 bones: scapula and clavicle
   2. Connects via the clavicle to the manubrium of sternum
B. Axilla (armpit)
   1. Extends from the clavicle to the lower border of the pectoralis major and teres major
   2. Contains fat, brachial plexus, axillary vessels, and lymph nodes
C. Arm (brachium)
   1. Extends from the shoulder to the elbow
   2. 1 bone: humerus
   3. 3 compartments
      a. Anterior: flexor
      b. Posterior: extensor
      c. Neurovascular: brachial vessels and the median nerve
   4. Deltopectoral triangle: groove between the deltoid and the pectoralis major; contains the cephalic vein
D. Forearm (antebrachium)
   1. Extends from the elbow to the wrist
   2. 2 bones: radius (lateral) and ulna (medial)
   3. 2 compartments
      a. Anterior: flexor
      b. Posterior: extensor
   4. Cubital fossa: space anterior to elbow
E. Hand
   1. 8 carpal bones, 5 metacarpal bones, 14 phalanges
   2. Anatomical snuffbox: at the wrist at the base of the thumb dorsally; framed by the extensor pollicis longus (medially) and extensor pollicis brevis and the abductor pollicis longus (laterally) tendons

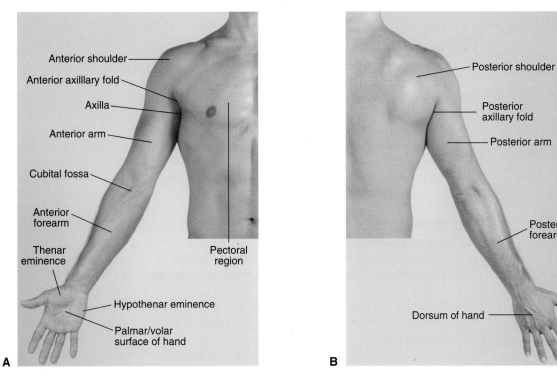

Figure 2.1A,B. Surface Anatomy of the Upper Limb. **A.** Anterior View. **B.** Posterior View.

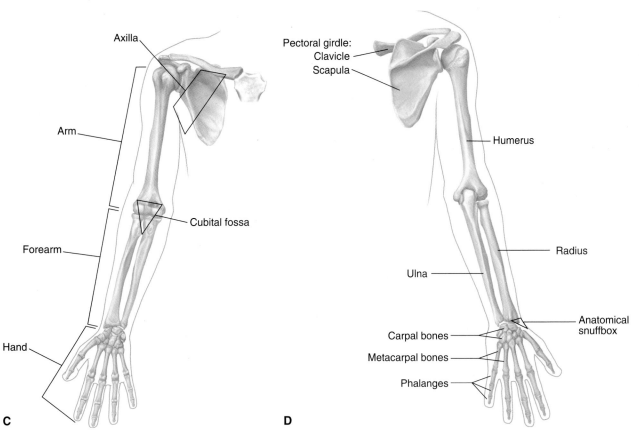

Figure 2.1C,D. Palpable Features of the Upper Limb. **C.** Anterior View. **D.** Posterior View.

Cutaneous Innervation of the Upper Limb

I. Dermatomes of the Upper Limb (Fig. 2.2A,B)

A. C4-T2 branches of anterior and posterior rami of spinal nerves
  1. Posterior rami C4-T6 branches distribute over the trapezius and scapula
  2. Anterior rami branches service the remainder
B. Helpful hints
  1. C6 along the lateral arm, forearm, and thumb
  2. C7 down posterior aspect of the arm, forearm, index, and middle fingers (remember, "peace sign" = C7)
  3. C8 along the medial arm, forearm, ring and little finger
  4. T2 near armpit

II. Cutaneous Nerves of the Upper Limb (Fig. 2.2C,D)

A. Shoulder and pectoral region
  1. Supraclavicular nerves (C3-4) to the skin at the root of the neck
    a. Lateral supraclavicular nerve to the skin over the point of the shoulder (acromion, lateral clavicle)
    b. Intermediate supraclavicular nerve passes over the middle of the clavicle
    c. Medial supraclavicular nerve to the skin over the medial clavicle and upper manubrium
  2. Posterior rami C4-T6 branches distribute over the trapezius and scapula
  3. Lateral and anterior cutaneous branches of intercostal nerves T1-5 to the skin over pectoral muscles
B. Arm
  1. Superior lateral brachial cutaneous nerve: from the axillary nerve (C5, C6)
  2. Inferior lateral brachial cutaneous nerve: from the radial nerve (C5, C6)
  3. Posterior brachial cutaneous nerve: from the radial nerve (C5-8)
  4. Medial brachial cutaneous nerve: from the medial cord of brachial plexus (C8, T1)
  5. Intercostobrachial nerve: lateral cutaneous branch of T2 (2nd intercostal)
    a. Communicates with the medial brachial cutaneous nerve
    b. May be injured during the axillary lymph node dissection
C. Forearm
  1. Lateral antebrachial cutaneous nerve: from the musculocutaneous nerve (C5, C6)
  2. Medial antebrachial cutaneous nerve: from the medial cord of brachial plexus (C8, T1)
  3. Posterior antebrachial cutaneous nerve: from the radial nerve (C5-8)
D. Hand
  1. Median nerve (C5-8)
    a. Palmar branch: lateral side of the palm
    b. Palmar digital branches: lateral 3½ digits (including nail bed)
  2. Ulnar nerve (C8, T1)
    a. Palmar branch: medial side of the palm
    b. Palmar branches: medial 1½ digits (including nail bed)
    c. Dorsal branch: provides dorsal digital branches to medial 2½ digits (excluding nail bed)
  3. Radial nerve (C6-8)
    a. Superficial branch: provides dorsal digital branches to lateral 2½ digits (excluding nail bed)

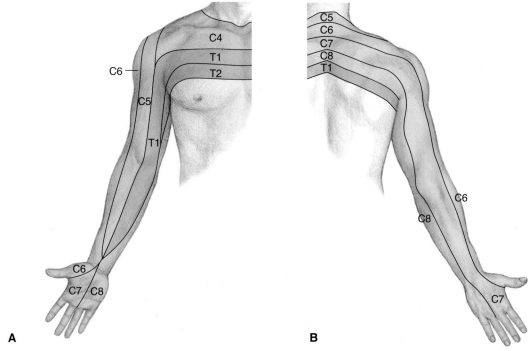

Figure 2.2A,B. Dermatomes of the Upper Limb. **A.** Anterior View. **B.** Posterior View.

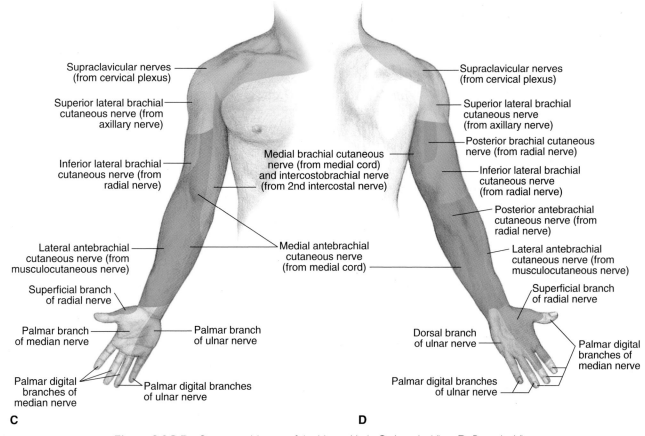

Figure 2.2C,D. Cutaneous Nerves of the Upper Limb. **C.** Anterior View. **D.** Posterior View.

Superficial Veins and Deep Fascial Specializations of the Upper Limb

I. Superficial Veins of the Upper Limb (Fig. 2.3A,B)

A. Cephalic vein
  1. Origin: lateral side of the dorsal venous network of hand
  2. Course: passes proximally along the anterolateral edge of the forearm, anterior to the lateral epicondyle, on biceps laterally; within the deltopectoral triangle, penetrates the clavipectoral fascia
  3. Termination: axillary vein

B. Basilic vein
  1. Origin: medial side of the dorsal venous network of hand
  2. Course: passes proximally along the anteromedial edge of the forearm, anterior to medial epicondyle, penetrates the brachial fascia at the midarm
  3. Termination: unites with paired brachial veins near the inferior border of teres major to form the axillary vein

C. Median cubital vein
  1. Origin: cephalic vein near the cubital fossa
  2. Course: passes medially across the cubital fossa, with the perforating vein communicating to brachial veins
  3. Termination: basilic vein

D. Median antebrachial vein (variable)
  1. Origin: palmar venous network
  2. Course: passes proximally on the anterior surface of the forearm
  3. Termination: median cubital vein

II. Clinical Considerations : Venipuncture

A. Access to veins for blood drawing and administration of drugs or fluids
B. Median cubital vein frequently used due to superficial location and tethering provided by perforating vein

III. Deep Fascial Specializations of the Upper Limb

A. Pectoralis fascia: invests the pectoralis major and continues inferiorly with the anterior abdominal wall fascia; laterally becomes the axillary fascia.
B. Axillary fascia: forms the floor of the axilla
C. Clavipectoral fascia
  1. Deep fascial sheet stretching from the clavicle to the axilla
  2. Thickened along inferior edge of the clavicle as costocoracoid ligament
  3. Envelopes pectoralis minor
  4. Extends from inferolateral edge of the pectoralis minor to the axillary fascia and the skin as suspensory ligament of axilla
D. Brachial fascia
  1. Investing fascia of the arm
  2. Surrounds 3 compartments of the arm
E. Antebrachial fascia
  1. Investing fascia of the forearm
  2. Surrounds 2 compartments of the forearm
  3. Thickens at the wrist to form the extensor retinaculum and palmar carpal ligament

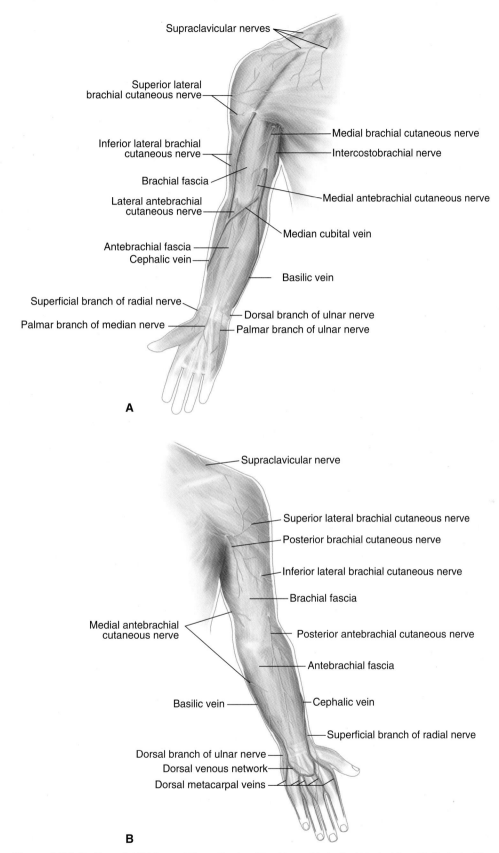

Supraclavicular nerves

Superior lateral brachial cutaneous nerve

Inferior lateral brachial cutaneous nerve

Brachial fascia

Lateral antebrachial cutaneous nerve

Antebrachial fascia

Cephalic vein

Superficial branch of radial nerve

Palmar branch of median nerve

Medial brachial cutaneous nerve

Intercostobrachial nerve

Medial antebrachial cutaneous nerve

Median cubital vein

Basilic vein

Dorsal branch of ulnar nerve

Palmar branch of ulnar nerve

A

Supraclavicular nerve

Superior lateral brachial cutaneous nerve

Posterior brachial cutaneous nerve

Inferior lateral brachial cutaneous nerve

Brachial fascia

Medial antebrachial cutaneous nerve

Posterior antebrachial cutaneous nerve

Antebrachial fascia

Cephalic vein

Basilic vein

Superficial branch of radial nerve

Dorsal branch of ulnar nerve

Dorsal venous network

Dorsal metacarpal veins

B

Figure 2.3A,B. Superficial Veins and Deep Fascia of the Upper Limb. **A.** Anterior View. **B.** Posterior View.

Lymphatics of the Upper Limb

I. Superficial Lymphatic Vessels (Fig. 2.4A)

A. Begin in the skin of the hand and ascend mostly with the superficial veins

B. Fine lymphatic channels; most dense on the palmar surface

C. Palmar digital lymph vessels pass primarily onto the dorsum near the base of the digit

D. Channels combine to form 2 primary channels draining along the radial and ulnar borders of the wrist

II. Lymphatics of the Forearm and Arm (Fig. 2.4B)

A. Radial and ulnar channels course onto the flexor surface of the forearm

B. Ulnar channel may have several cubital nodes located above the medial epicondyle

C. Ulnar channel follows the basilic vein to lateral axillary nodes

D. Radial channel follows the cephalic vein, and 10% have small deltopectoral nodes within deltopectoral triangle

III. Deep Lymphatics

A. Much less numerous than the superficial vessels

B. Drain the joint capsules, periosteum, tendons, nerves, and, to a lesser degree, muscles

C. Follow the major deep veins of the limb, along which lie small intercalated lymph nodes, and end in the lateral and central axillary nodes

IV. Axillary Lymph Nodes

A. 5 groups

  1. Lateral axillary (humeral) nodes

    a. Located adjacent to the distal end of the axillary vein

    b. Receive lymph from ulnar and deep lymph channels

  2. Anterior axillary (pectoral) nodes

    a. Located anterior to the axillary vein deep to the lateral border of the pectoralis major muscle

    b. Receive lymph from the breast (80%) and anterior chest wall

  3. Posterior axillary (subscapular) nodes

    a. Located posterior to the axillary vein and anterior to the subscapularis muscle

    b. Receive lymph from the posterior shoulder and the posterolateral chest wall

  4. Central axillary nodes

    a. Located adjacent to the axillary vein deep to the pectoralis minor muscle

    b. Receive lymph from anterior, lateral, and posterior axillary nodes

  5. Apical axillary nodes

    a. Located adjacent to the axillary vein superior to the upper border of pectoralis minor muscle

    b. Receive lymph from central axillary and deltopectoral nodes

B. Drain to supraclavicular nodes or the subclavian lymph trunk

  1. On the right side, the subclavian lymphatic trunk is usually joined by the jugular and bronchomediastinal trunks to form the right lymphatic duct, or it may enter the right venous angle independently

  2. On the left side, the subclavian trunk usually joins the thoracic duct

V. Clinical Considerations: Axillary Lymph Nodes

A. Patient with an infection or malignancy in the upper extremity may complain of tenderness and swelling in the axilla

B. This is due to involvement of the axillary nodes, especially the lateral group along the axillary vein, because these filter from much of the upper extremity

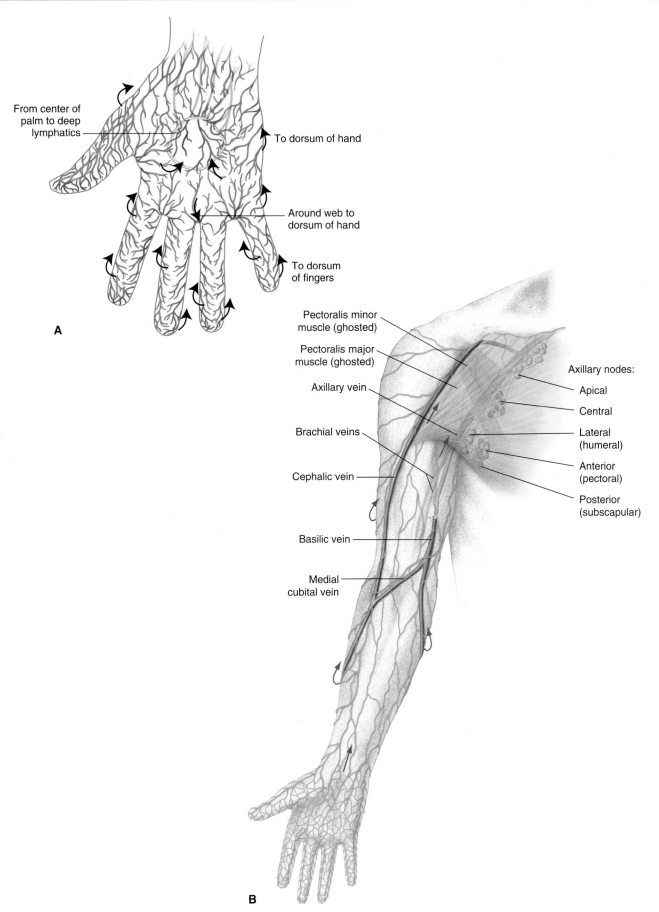

From center of
palm to deep
lymphatics

To dorsum of hand

Around web to
dorsum of hand

To dorsum
of fingers

A

Pectoralis minor
muscle (ghosted)

Pectoralis major
muscle (ghosted)

Axillary vein

Brachial veins

Cephalic vein

Basilic vein

Medial
cubital vein

Axillary nodes:

Apical

Central

Lateral
(humeral)

Anterior
(pectoral)

Posterior
(subscapular)

B

Figure 2.4A,B. A. Lymphatics of the Hand. Anterior View. **B.** Lymphatics of the Upper Limb. Anterior View.

Bones of the Pectoral (Shoulder) Girdle

I. Clavicle (Collar Bone) (Fig. 2.5A)

A. S-shaped "long" bone with body and sternal and acromial extremities
  1. Body
      a. Rounded medially, flattened laterally
      b. Convex anteriorly medially, concave anteriorly laterally
      c. Undersurface of the lateral part is marked by the conoid tubercle and the trapezoid line
      d. Undersurface of the medial part is marked by attachments of the costoclavicular ligament and the subclavius muscle
  2. Sternal end articulates with the sternum and the 1st costal cartilage
  3. Acromial end has smooth facet for articulation with the acromion

II. Scapula (Shoulder Blade) (Fig. 2.5B–D)

A. Flat and triangular with 2 surfaces, 3 angles, and 3 borders
  1. Surfaces
      a. Anterior (costal): concave subscapular fossa
      b. Posterior: divided by the spine into supraspinous and infraspinous fossae
  2. Angles
      a. Lateral: glenoid cavity rests on the neck of the scapula, with supraglenoid and infraglenoid tubercles
      b. Superior: attachment of the levator scapulae muscle
      c. Inferior: attachment of latissimus dorsi muscle fibers (variable)
  3. Borders
      a. Lateral: thickened; the neck extends from the superior end, whereas the inferior angle lies at the inferior end
      b. Medial: relatively thin
      c. Superior: thin; the coracoid process extends superiorly immediately medial to the scapular neck, with the scapular notch located medial to the coracoid process

III. Ossification

A. Clavicle, from 3 centers (earliest bone to ossify)

Location	Appears	Fuses
Medial (in body)	5th–6th fetal week	By 25th year
Lateral (in body)	5th–6th fetal week	By 25th year
Sternal end	18th–20th year	By 25th year

B. Scapula, from 7 or more centers

Location	Appears	Fuses
Body	8th fetal week	15th year
Middle coracoid	15th–18th month	15th year
Upper glenoid	10th year	16th–18th year
Root of coracoid	14th–20th year	By 25th year
Base of acromion	14th–20th year	By 25th year
Inferior angle	14th–20th year	By 25th year
End of acromion	14th–20th year	By 25th year
Vertebral border	14th–20th year	By 25th year

IV. Clinical Considerations: Clavicle Fractures

A. Most frequently broken bone
B. Usually breaks in the medial portion, with downward displacement of the lateral fragment

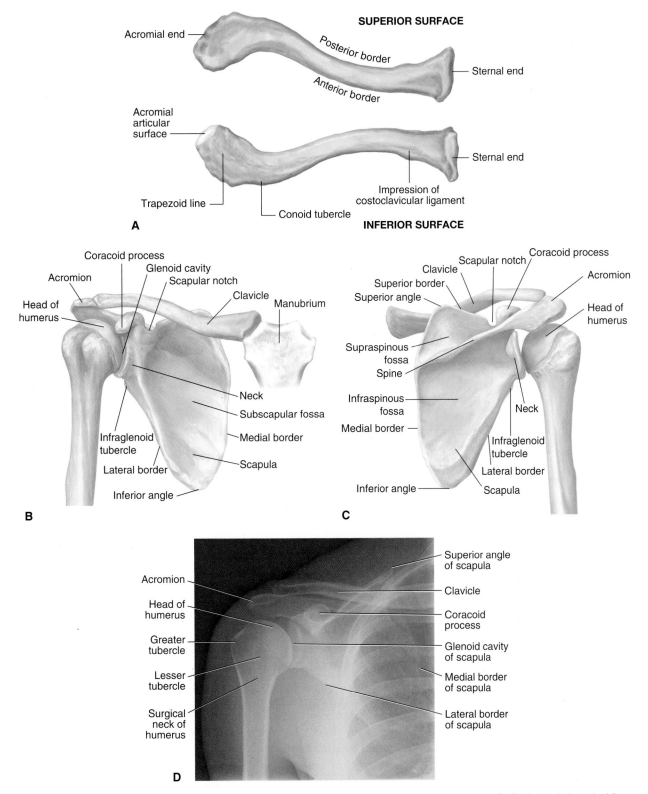

Figure 2.5A–D. Bones of the Pectoral Girdle. **A.** Right Clavicle. **B.** Anterior View. **C.** Posterior View. **D.** Radiograph, Anterior View.

Bone of the Arm: Humerus

I. Parts (Fig. 2.6A,B)

A. Proximal end
1. Head: articulates with the scapula at the glenoid cavity
2. Anatomical neck: where the smooth articular surface of the head meets the shaft
3. Surgical neck: tapers into the fairly rounded upper shaft
4. Greater tubercle: lateral prominence with attachments for supraspinatus, infraspinatus, and teres minor muscles
5. Lesser tubercle: medial prominence; attachment for the subscapularis muscle
6. Intertubercular (bicipital) groove: occupied by round tendon of the long head of the biceps brachii muscle; lies between the greater and lesser tubercles and the crests distal to them

B. Shaft
1. Flattens anteroposteriorly distally
2. Deltoid tuberosity: lateral prominence near the midshaft; attachment for the deltoid muscle
3. Radial groove (sulcus): shallow groove descending inferolaterally on the posterior surface; occupied by the radial nerve and deep brachial vessels
4. Lateral supracondylar ridge: laterally flared flattened crest for attachment of brachioradialis and extensor carpi radialis longus muscles
5. Medial supracondylar ridge: medially flared flattened crest above the medial epicondyle

C. Distal end
1. Medial epicondyle: attachment for the common flexor tendon; grooved posteriorly by the ulnar nerve
2. Lateral epicondyle: attachment for the common extensor tendon
3. Trochlea: spool-shaped smooth surface that lies within the trochlear notch of the ulna
4. Capitulum: smaller spool-shaped smooth area for articulation with the radial head
5. Coronoid fossa: anterior fossa to accommodate the coronoid process of the ulna
6. Olecranon fossa: posterior fossa to accommodate the olecranon of the ulna
7. Radial fossa: a shallow fossa superior to the capitulum anteriorly to accommodate the head of the radius when the forearm is fully flexed

II. Ossification (From 8 Centers)

Location	Appears	Fuses
Body	8th fetal week	16th–17th year
Head	1st year	16th–17th year
Greater tubercle	3rd year	16th–17th year
Lesser tubercle	5th year	16th–17th year
Capitulum	2nd year	16th–17th year
Trochlea	12th year	16th–17th year
Lateral eipcondyle	13th year	16th–17th year
Medial epicondyle	5th year	18th year

III. Blood Supply

A. Proximal end: anterior and posterior humeral circumflex arteries
B. Body: nutrient artery from the brachial or the deep brachial artery
C. Distal end: ulnar and radial collateral arteries

IV. Clinical Considerations

A. Surgical neck fracture: common site; may damage the axillary nerve and the posterior humeral circumflex artery
B. Humeral shaft fracture: may damage the radial nerve and the deep brachial artery
C. Medial epicondyle fracture or trauma: may damage the ulnar nerve
D. Traumatic separation of the proximal epiphysis of the humerus: possible until 18 (female) or 20 (male) years of age

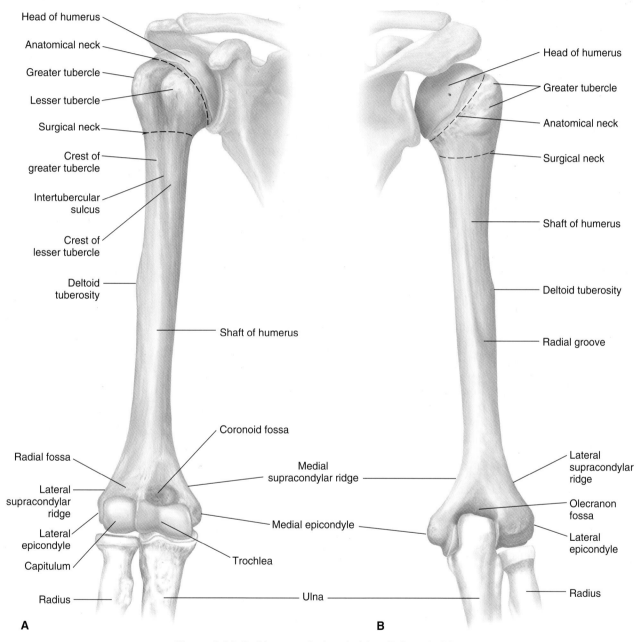

Figure 2.6A,B. Humerus. **A.** Anterior View. **B.** Posterior View.

Bones of the Forearm

I. Ulna: Medial Bone of the Forearm (Fig. 2.7A–C)

A. Proximal end
1. Olecranon: attachment of the triceps brachii
2. Trochlear notch: fits the trochlea of the humerus
3. Coronoid process: projection at the distal edge of the trochlear notch
4. Radial notch: shallow depression laterally distal to the trochlear notch for the head of the radius
5. Ulnar tuberosity: on the distal portion of the coronoid process; attachment of the brachialis muscle

B. Shaft
1. Sharp flattened interosseous border faces laterally
2. Slightly concave anteriorly

C. Distal end
1. Head: relatively small, cylindrical; pivots within the ulnar notch of the radius during pronation/supination
2. Styloid process: thin projection; anchors the radioulnar articular disc

II. Radius: Lateral Bone of the Forearm

A. Proximal end
1. Head: cylindrical; pivots within the radial notch of the ulna during pronation/supination
2. Neck: constriction distal to the head
3. Radial tuberosity: anteromedial projection; attachment of the biceps brachii muscle

B. Shaft
1. Sharp, flattened interosseous border faces medially
2. Slightly concave anteriorly

C. Distal end
1. Ulnar notch: medial, for the ulnar head
2. Carpal articular surface: for trapezium and lunate
3. Dorsal radial tubercle: on the dorsal surface; wrapped by the tendon of the extensor pollicis longus
4. Styloid process: triangular distal projection; attachment for the brachioradialis muscle

III. Ossification

A. Ulna

Location	Appears	Fuses
Proximal (olecranon)	10th year	16th year
Shaft	8th fetal week	
Distal (head)	4th year	20th year

B. Radius

Location	Appears	Fuses
1. Proximal (head)	5th year	17th–18th year
2. Shaft	8th fetal week	
3. Distal end	2nd year	20th year

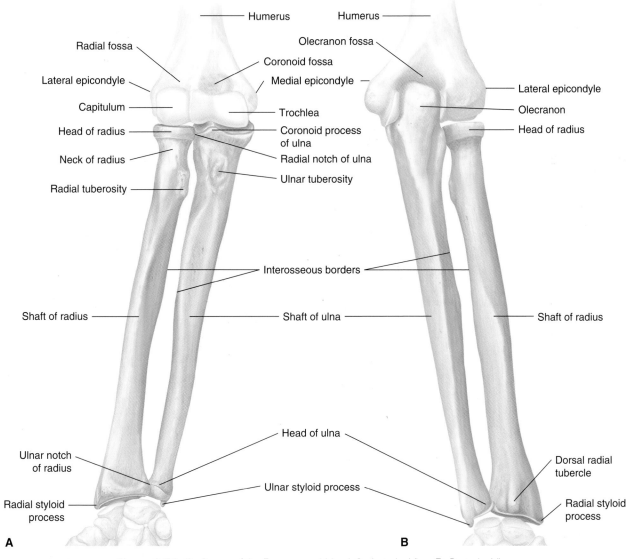

Humerus

Humerus

Radial fossa

Olecranon fossa

Coronoid fossa

Lateral epicondyle

Medial epicondyle

Lateral epicondyle

Capitulum

Trochlea

Olecranon

Head of radius

Coronoid process
of ulna

Head of radius

Neck of radius

Radial notch of ulna

Radial tuberosity

Ulnar tuberosity

Interosseous borders

Shaft of radius

Shaft of ulna

Shaft of radius

Head of ulna

Ulnar notch
of radius

Dorsal radial
tubercle

Radial styloid
process

Ulnar styloid process

Radial styloid
process

A

B

Figure 2.7A–B. Bones of the Forearm and Hand. **A.** Anterior View. **B.** Posterior View.

IV. Clinical Considerations

A. Ulna more likely fractured by elbow trauma; the radius more likely fractured by fall on the outstretched hand

B. Colles fracture: the distal end of the radius, displaced dorsally; may cause "dinner fork" deformity

C. Distal radial epiphyseal separation: may occur up to 20th year and may be confused with Colles fracture

D. Smith fracture: the distal end of the radius displaced ventrally; from fall on the flexed wrist

E. Positioning of the elbow and hand varies according to the site of the radial fracture: the elbow should be flexed, and the forearm supinated if the fracture is proximal to insertion of the pronator teres or midpronated if the fracture is distal

F. Radial styloid process lies approximately 1 cm distal to the ulnar styloid, important for diagnosis of wrist injuries

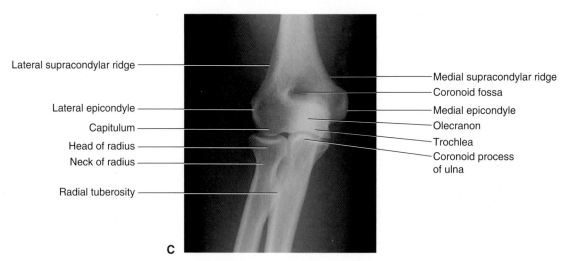

Figure 2.7C. Bones of the Forearm and Hand. Radiograph, Anterior View.

Bones of the Wrist and Hand

I. Carpal Bones (Wrist Bones): 8 Bones Arranged in 2 Rows (Fig. 2.8A–C)

A. Proximal row
   1. Scaphoid: boat-shaped; most frequently fractured carpal bone; has tubercle for attachment of the flexor retinaculum
   2. Lunate: crescent-shaped; most frequently dislocated carpal bone
   3. Triquetrum: pyramidal-shaped; has oval articular facet on the palmar surface for the pisiform bone
   4. Pisiform: small, pea-shaped; sesamoid bone within the tendon of the flexor carpi ulnaris

B. Distal row
   1. Trapezium: has saddle-shaped facet for the 1st metacarpal and tubercle for attachment of the flexor retinaculum
   2. Trapezoid: wedge-shaped
   3. Capitate: the largest carpal bone; first to ossify
   4. Hamate: a hook-like process (hamulus) from the palmar surface

II. Metacarpals

A. 5 bones numbered from the lateral to the medial
B. Common characteristics: base articulates with the carpal bones, shaft, rounded head

III. Phalanges

A. 14 bones
   1. 2 in thumb (proximal and distal)
   2. 3 in digits 2 to 5 (proximal, middle, and distal)

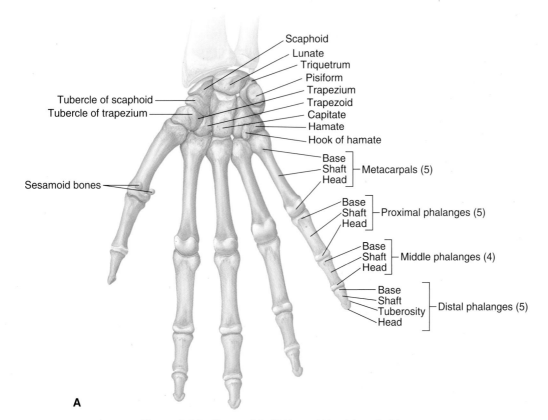

Figure 2.8A. Bones of the Wrist and Hand. Anterior View.

  B. Common characteristics: base, shaft (rounded dorsally, flattened ventrally), distal end

   1. Proximal phalanges have concave base; middle and distal phalanges have bases with the central parasagittal ridge

   2. Distal ends of proximal and middle phalanges have 2 condyles separated by the shallow groove

IV. Ossification

 A. Carpals: from 1 center in each, which appear as follows:

   1. Capitate and hamate, 1st year

   2. Triquetrum, 3rd year

   3. Lunate and trapezium, 5th year

   4. Scaphoid, 6th year

   5. Trapezoid, 8th year

   6. Pisiform, 12th year

 B. Metacarpals: from 2 centers, the body and the distal end, which appear and close as follows:

   1. Body, 8th and 9th fetal week

   2. Distal end, 3rd year

   3. They join in the 20th year: the 1st metacarpal has the center in the body and the base, which for the body appears in the 8th to 9th fetal week; the base appears in the 3rd year, and they join in the 20th year

 C. Phalanges: from 2 centers, the body and the base; which appear as follows:

   1. Body, 8th week

   2. Base at 3 to 4 years in the proximal row; later in distal rows

   3. They unite in the 20th year

V. Clinical Considerations

 A. Ossification centers: appearance and closure is important medicolegally and in radiologic examination of the young

 B. Fractures: 70% to 75% of fractures of the carpus include the scaphoid; in 10% to 15%, avascular necrosis occurs in the proximal part

 C. In the proximal row of carpal bones, only the scaphoid and lunate articulate with the radius; thus, they transmit the entire force of a fall on the hand to the forearm

 D. Except for the pisiform, no muscles attach to the proximal row of carpal bones

 E. The capitate forms the "keystone" of the carpal arch (carpal tunnel); a fall on the base of the palm forces the head of the capitate upward into the concave waist of the scaphoid, accounting for the frequency of fractures of the latter bone from a fall on the hand

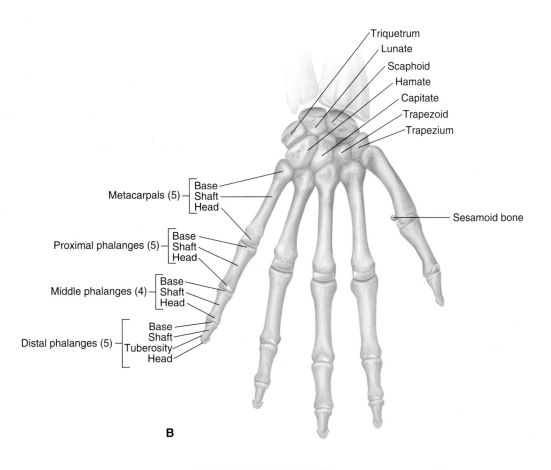

Triquetrum
Lunate
Scaphoid
Hamate
Capitate
Trapezoid
Trapezium

Sesamoid bone

Metacarpals (5) — Base
Shaft
Head

Proximal phalanges (5) — Base
Shaft
Head

Middle phalanges (4) — Base
Shaft
Head

Distal phalanges (5) — Base
Shaft
Tuberosity
Head

B

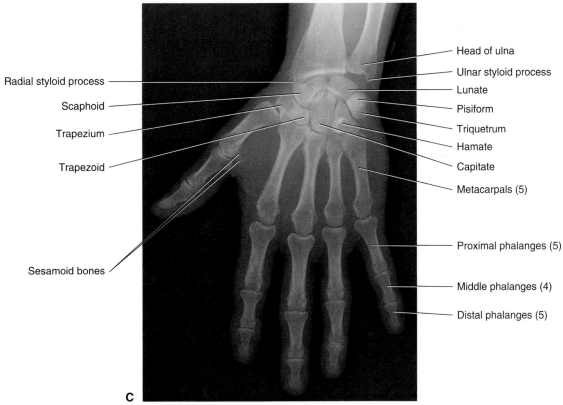

Radial styloid process

Scaphoid

Trapezium

Trapezoid

Sesamoid bones

Head of ulna
Ulnar styloid process
Lunate
Pisiform
Triquetrum
Hamate
Capitate
Metacarpals (5)

Proximal phalanges (5)

Middle phalanges (4)

Distal phalanges (5)

C

Figure 2.8B,C. Bones of the wrist and hand **B.** Posterior View. **C.** Radiograph, Anterior View.

Muscles of the Anterior Shoulder

I. Muscles of the Anterior Shoulder (Fig. 2.9A,B)

Muscle	Origin	Insertion	Action	Nerve
Pectoralis major	Medial clavicle, the anterolateral sternum to the 7th costal cartilage, costal cartilages 2–6, aponeurosis of the external abdominal oblique	Crest of the greater tubercle of the humerus	Flexes, adducts, and rotates the arm medially	Medial and lateral pectoral Clavicular head (C5-6) Sternocostal head (C7-8,T1)
Pectoralis minor	Upper outer surface of ribs 3–5	Coracoid process of the scapula	Draws the scapula down and forward	Medial pectoral (C6-8)
Subclavius	1st rib cartilage	Subclavian groove of the clavicle	Draws the clavicle down and forward	Nerve to subclavius (C5-6)
Serratus anterior	Outer surface of ribs 1–8	Medial border of the scapula	Rotates the scapula, raising the point of the shoulder; protracts the scapula (draws the scapula forward)	Long thoracic (C5-7)
Deltoid	Lateral 1/3 of the clavicle, the acromion, the lower lip of the crest of the spine of the scapula	Deltoid tuberosity of the humerus	Abducts the arm; anterior fibers flex and medially rotate the arm; posterior fibers extend and laterally rotate the arm	Axillary nerve (C5-6)

II. Special Features

A. The action of the serratus anterior and trapezius in the rotation of the scapula makes it possible to abduct the arm more than 90°

B. When the hands are fixed, as in gripping an object over the head, the pectoralis major helps to draw the body toward the hands

C. Pectoralis minor is useful as a landmark for axillary structures, because, with the coracoid process, it forms an arch deep to which pass the vessels and nerves to the upper limb

D. Deltoid is the principle abductor of the arm, but, due to poor mechanical advantage, it cannot initiate this action; supraspinatus initiates abduction of the arm

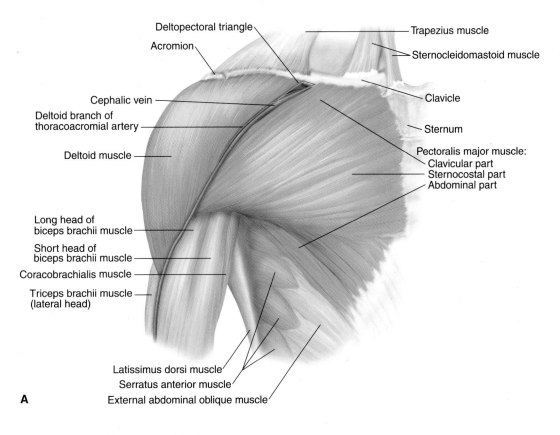

Deltopectoral triangle

Acromion

Cephalic vein

Deltoid branch of
thoracoacromial artery

Deltoid muscle

Long head of
biceps brachii muscle

Short head of
biceps brachii muscle

Coracobrachialis muscle

Triceps brachii muscle
(lateral head)

Trapezius muscle

Sternocleidomastoid muscle

Clavicle

Sternum

Pectoralis major muscle:
Clavicular part
Sternocostal part
Abdominal part

Latissimus dorsi muscle

Serratus anterior muscle

External abdominal oblique muscle

A

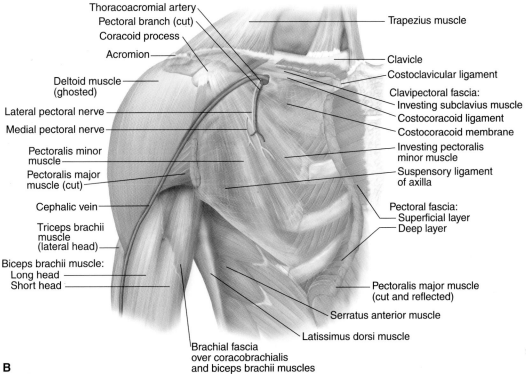

Thoracoacromial artery

Pectoral branch (cut)

Coracoid process

Acromion

Deltoid muscle
(ghosted)

Lateral pectoral nerve

Medial pectoral nerve

Pectoralis minor
muscle

Pectoralis major
muscle (cut)

Cephalic vein

Triceps brachii
muscle
(lateral head)

Biceps brachii muscle:
Long head
Short head

Trapezius muscle

Clavicle

Costoclavicular ligament

Clavipectoral fascia:
Investing subclavius muscle
Costocoracoid ligament
Costocoracoid membrane

Investing pectoralis
minor muscle

Suspensory ligament
of axilla

Pectoral fascia:
Superficial layer
Deep layer

Pectoralis major muscle
(cut and reflected)

Serratus anterior muscle

Latissimus dorsi muscle

Brachial fascia
over coracobrachialis
and biceps brachii muscles

B

Figure 2.9A,B. Muscles of the Shoulder Region. **A.** Anterior view. **B.** Anterior view.

Muscles of the Posterior Shoulder and the Rotator Cuff

I. Muscles of the Posterior Shoulder and the Rotator Cuff (Fig. 2.10A–E)

Muscle	Origin	Insertion	Action	Nerve
Deltoid	Lateral 1/3 of the clavicle, the acromion, the lower lip of the crest of the spine of the scapula	Deltoid tuberosity of the humerus	Abducts the arm; anterior fibers flex and medially rotate the arm; posterior fibers extend and laterally rotate the arm	Axillary (C5-6)
Teres major	Dorsal surface of the inferior angle of the scapula	Crest of the lesser tubercle of the humerus	Adducts, extends, and rotates the arm medially	Lower subscapular (C5-6)
Supraspinatus	Supraspinatus fossa	Greater tubercle of the humerus (highest facet)	Abduct the arm (initiate abduction)	Suprascapular (C4-6)
Infraspinatus	Infraspinatus fossa	Greater tubercle of the humerus (middle facet)	Laterally rotates the arm	Suprascapular (C5-6)
Teres minor	Upper 2/3 of the lateral border of the scapula	Greater tubercle of the humerus (lowest facet)	Laterally rotates the arm	Axillary (C5-6)
Subscapularis	Subscapular fossa, the medial part	Lesser tubercle of the humerus	Rotates the arm medially	Upper and lower subscapular (C5-7)

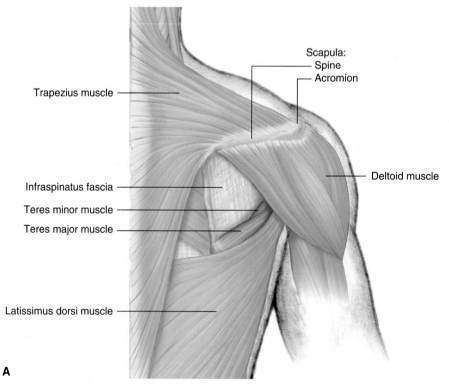

Figure 2.10A. Muscles of the Shoulder Region. Posterior View, Superficial.

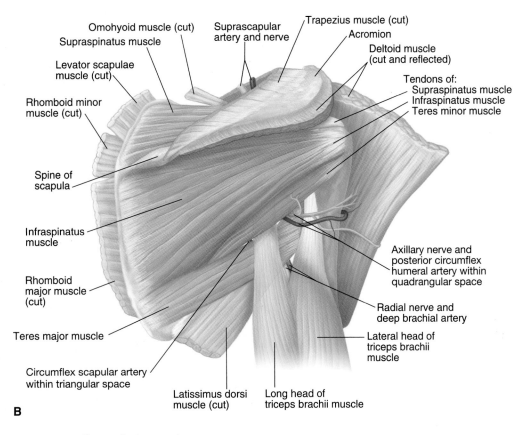

Omohyoid muscle (cut)

Suprascapular artery and nerve

Trapezius muscle (cut)

Acromion

Supraspinatus muscle

Deltoid muscle (cut and reflected)

Levator scapulae muscle (cut)

Tendons of:
Supraspinatus muscle
Infraspinatus muscle
Teres minor muscle

Rhomboid minor muscle (cut)

Spine of scapula

Infraspinatus muscle

Axillary nerve and posterior circumflex humeral artery within quadrangular space

Rhomboid major muscle (cut)

Radial nerve and deep brachial artery

Teres major muscle

Lateral head of triceps brachii muscle

Circumflex scapular artery within triangular space

Latissimus dorsi muscle (cut)

Long head of triceps brachii muscle

B

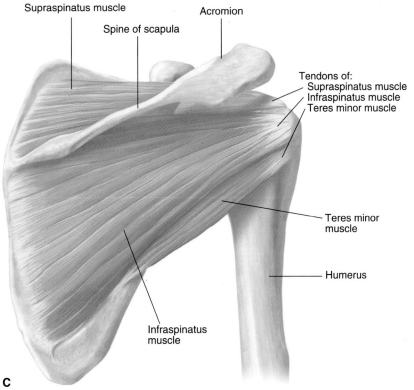

Supraspinatus muscle

Spine of scapula

Acromion

Tendons of:
Supraspinatus muscle
Infraspinatus muscle
Teres minor muscle

Teres minor muscle

Humerus

Infraspinatus muscle

C

Figure 2.10B,C. B. Muscles of the Shoulder Region. Posterior View, Deep. **C.** Muscles of the Rotator Cuff. Posterior View.

II. Special Features

A. Rotator cuff muscles (4): supraspinatus, infraspinatus, teres minor, and subscapularis

B. Supraspinatus does not rotate the humerus; instead, it initiates abduction of the arm, which is completed by deltoid

C. Rotator cuff muscles fix the head of the humerus in the glenoid cavity during abduction and flexion of the arm

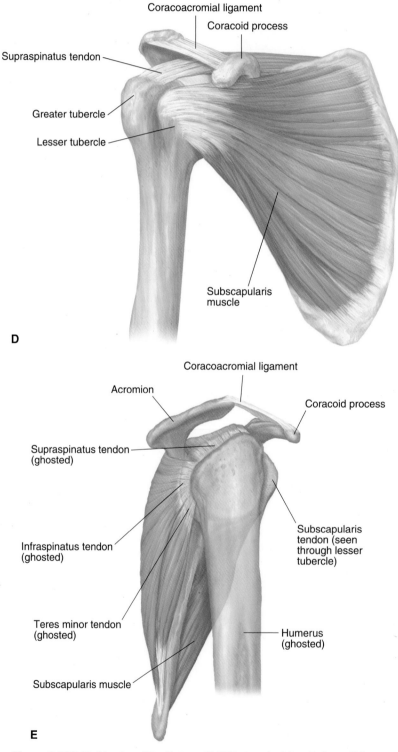

Figure 2.10D,E. Muscles of the Rotator Cuff. **D.** Anterior View. **E.** Lateral View.

Axilla and Brachial Plexus

I. Axilla: Space of the Armpit

A. Boundaries:
1. Superiorly by the clavicle, the scapula, and the 1st rib
2. Inferiorly by the skin at the lower borders of the pectoralis major and the teres major/latissimus dorsi
3. Anteriorly by pectoral muscles
4. Posteriorly by the subscapularis
5. Medially by the serratus anterior
6. Laterally by the humerus

B. Contents
1. Brachial plexus
2. Axillary fat and fascia
3. Axillary vessels and branches
4. Axillary lymph nodes

II. Brachial Plexus (Fig. 2.11A,B)

A. Components: roots, trunks, divisions, cords, and branches

B. Formation
1. Roots: anterior rami of C5-8 and T1
   a. Branches:
      i. C5 provides small contribution to the phrenic nerve
      ii. Dorsal scapular nerve: from the posterior aspect of C5 root; innervates the lower portion of the levator scapulae and the rhomboideus minor and major
      iii. Long thoracic nerve: from C5-7
      iv. Direct branches to scalenes (C5-6)
2. Trunks: formed near the lateral border of the scalene muscles in the posterior triangle of the neck
   a. Upper trunk: formed by union of C5 and C6
      i. Only trunk to have branches
      ii. Suprascapular nerve: innervates supraspinatus and infraspinatus
      iii. Nerve to subclavius
   b. Middle trunk: continuation of C7
   c. Lower trunk: formed by union of C8 and T1
3. Divisions: trunks are short and split into anterior and posterior divisions
4. Cords:
   a. Lateral cord: formed by union of the anterior divisions of the upper and middle trunks
   b. Medial cord: formed by the anterior division of the lower trunk
   c. Posterior cord: union of all 3 posterior divisions
5. Branches: other than those noted from roots or trunks
   a. Lateral cord (3 branches)
      i. Lateral pectoral nerve (C5-7)
      ii. Musculocutaneous (C5-7)
      iii. Lateral contribution to the median nerve (C6-7)
   b. Medial cord (5 branches)
      i. Medial pectoral (C8, T1)
      ii. Medial brachial cutaneous (C8, T1)
      iii. Medial antebrachial cutaneous (C8, T1)
      iv. Ulnar (C8, T1)
      v. Medial contribution to the median nerve (C8)
   c. Posterior cord (5 branches)
      i. Upper subscapular (C5)
      ii. Thoracodorsal (middle subscapular) (C6-8)

      iii. Lower subscapular (C6)

      iv. Axillary (C5-6)

      v. Radial (C5-8, T1)

C. Special features

  1. 2 roots of the brachial plexus (C5-6) lie above and 2 below (C8, T1) the level of the cricoid cartilage

  2. Trunks of the plexus lie between the scalene muscles, medial to the midpoint of the clavicle

  3. Divisions of the plexus lie posterior to the midpoint of the clavicle, adjacent to the 3rd part of the subclavian artery and the beginning of the axillary artery

  4. Cords of the plexus extend laterally from the midpoint of the clavicle to the inferomedial aspect of the coracoid process of the scapula

---

III. Clinical Considerations

A. Introduction to brachial plexus injuries

  1. Brachial plexus can be injured by stretching, wounding, and by disease in the neck and axilla

  2. Injury may involve roots, trunks, divisions, cords, or cord branches and result in loss of muscle movement (paralysis) as well as loss of cutaneous sensation or feeling (anesthesia); paralysis can be complete (no movement) or incomplete (weak movement)

B. Upper brachial plexus injuries (**Erb** or **Erb-Duchenne palsy**)

  1. Generally result from marked separation of the neck and shoulder as a result of a blow to the region or a birth injury due to stretching of the nerves at delivery

  2. Anterior and posterior roots of spinal nerves C5-6 may be pulled out of the spinal cord, resulting in

    a. Loss of function of the posterior axial muscles over the area of the back supplied by posterior primary rami

    b. Loss of sensation in the upper limb related to the anterior rami and paralysis of muscles of the shoulder and arm, particularly deltoid, supraspinatus, infraspinatus, teres minor, biceps brachii, brachioradialis, and supinator

      i. Deltoid and supraspinatus paralysis: the arm cannot be abducted from side

      ii. Flexors of elbow are paralyzed

      iii. Loss of biceps and supinator: supination of forearm is greatly weakened

      iv. Weakness of the pectoralis major (lateral pectoral nerves, C5-7) and latissimus dorsi (C6-8) and loss of the infraspinatus (C5-6) lead to the medial shoulder rotation

  3. If upper trunk is torn or severed as it emerges between the anterior and middle scalene muscles, loss of flexion, abduction, and lateral rotation of the shoulder joint as well as loss of the elbow joint flexion occurs

    a. Limb hangs by the side in the medial rotation at the shoulder with the forearm pronated, in the so-called "waiter's tip" position

    b. Also anesthesia over an area on the lateral side of the arm results

  4. If lesion is confined to C5, no sensory change occurs; if both C5 and C6 are involved, loss of sensation occurs on the lateral upper limb

(Continued on page 90)

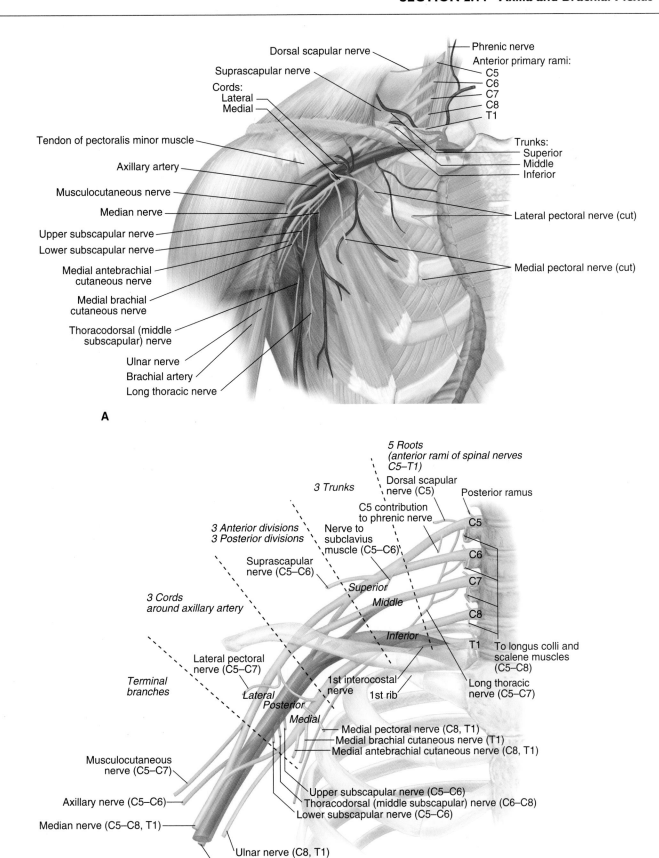

Figure 2.11A,B. A. Axilla and Brachial Plexus. Anterior View. **B.** Brachial Plexus Schema. Anterior View.

III. Clinical Considerations

    5. Incorrect use of crutches (**crutch palsy**) may compress axillary structures, particularly the posterior cord: the radial nerve is predominantly affected, leading to paralysis of the triceps, anconeus, and wrist extensors, with the inability to extend the elbow, wrist joint, and fingers, resulting in a **wrist drop**

C. Lower brachial plexus injuries

    1. Not as common as upper plexus injuries

    2. Result from a sudden upward pull of the shoulder (at birth and in adult injuries), which injures the lower trunk (C8-T1), with paralysis and anesthesia generally affecting the area supplied by the ulnar nerve

    3. **Klumpke palsy** (paralysis, Dejerine-Klumpke syndrome): atrophic paralysis of the forearm and small muscles of the hand with paralysis of the cervical sympathetic system; predominantly occurs with a birth injury due to arm being forcibly abducted over the head

        a. Paralysis of small muscles of hand and weakness of the flexors of the fingers and thumb, with reduced sensation along the ulnar side of the arm, forearm, and hand

        b. Similar to ulnar nerve paralysis plus addition of paralysis of thenar muscles and flexors of the digits

D. Cervical rib syndrome

    1. Cervical rib exerts pressure on the lower trunk of the plexus and compresses nerves as well as blood vessels supplying them (anoxia of the axons)

    2. Tingling and numbness occur in the upper extremity, which are relieved when the pressure is removed

E. Cervical cord neuropraxia (transient quadriplegia): the transient neurologic condition characterized by temporary loss of motor or sensory function (or both), secondary to the central cord contusion (injury) with or without associated ischemia

F. Injuries to brachial plexus branches

    1. Dorsal scapular nerve (C5)

        a. Innervates rhomboids and the lower portion of the levator scapulae

        b. Injury leads to impairment of scapular retraction and downward rotation

    2. Long thoracic nerve (C5-7)

        a. Innervates the serratus anterior muscle

        b. Injury leads to paralysis of the serratus anterior muscle, resulting in a **winged scapula**, in which the vertebral border and inferior angle of the scapula become very prominent, because the scapula is no longer held tightly against the chest wall; this effect is accentuated when the patient pushes against a wall with both hands

        c. In addition, flexing or abducting the arm above 45° from the body is difficult because the muscle also helps to protract and upwardly rotate the scapula, enabling the glenoid cavity to face superiorly in these motions

    3. Suprascapular nerve (C5-6)

        a. Innervates supraspinatus and infraspinatus muscles and shoulder joint

        b. Injury hinders initiation of abduction at the shoulder (somewhat questionable) as well as weakens lateral rotation at the shoulder

    4. Pectoral nerves

        a. Lateral pectoral from C5 to C7 to the pectoralis major muscle

        b. Medial pectoral from C8 to T1 to pectoralis minor and part of major muscles

        c. Injury results in severe loss of flexion of the shoulder joint

III. Clinical Considerations

5. Nerve to subclavius muscle (C5)
   a. Injury not easily detected
   b. May see loss of cutaneous sensation (anesthesia) over area just below the clavicle
6. Upper subscapular (C5-6) to the subscapularis muscle and lower subscapular (C5-6) to the subscapularis and teres major muscles
   a. Injury may impair the shoulder joint function due to loss of muscles that help hold the head of the humerus to the glenoid cavity
   b. Loss of the teres major weakens the shoulder extension as well
7. Thoracodorsal (C6-8)
   a. Injury paralyzes latissimus dorsi and weakens the actions of extension, adduction, and medial rotation of the shoulder
   b. Injury would particularly affect the shoulder extension
8. Axillary nerve (C5-6)
   a. Innervates the deltoid and teres minor muscles
   b. Paralysis leads to an impaired ability to abduct the arm from the side more than ±30° (some abduction is possible via the supraspinatus muscle), and there is weakness of flexion and extension of the shoulder
   c. Loss of shoulder roundness due to atrophy of the deltoid muscle
   d. Loss of sensation is over lateral side of the proximal arm (deltoid area)
9. Musculocutaneous nerve (C5-7)
   a. Innervates the biceps brachii, coracobrachialis, and brachialis muscles
   b. Injury causes great loss of flexion of the elbow, which is not complete, because the brachioradialis and flexor muscles of the forearm (arising from the 2 epicondyles) are still intact
   c. The branches to the brachialis by the radial nerve are thought to be sensory; thus, if the musculocutaneous nerve is cut, the muscle is usually completely paralyzed
   d. Supination of the forearm is weakened by the loss of the biceps brachii, which becomes wasted and atrophic
   e. Flexion at the shoulder is slightly involved due to loss of the coracobrachialis and biceps brachii
   f. Sensory loss on the lateral aspect of the forearm (lateral antebrachial cutaneous nerve), which depends on the extent of overlapping of adjacent nerves

Axillary Artery and Blood Supply to the Shoulder

I. Axillary Artery (Fig. 2.12A,B)

A. Origin: subclavian artery becomes the axillary artery at the lateral border of the 1st rib

B. Termination: becomes brachial artery at the lower border of the teres major muscle

C. Parts: determined by relationship with pectoralis minor

   1. 1st part: from the 1st rib to the upper border of the pectoralis minor muscle

   2. 2nd part: lies behind the pectoralis minor muscle

   3. 3rd part: from the lower border of the pectoralis minor muscle to the lower border of the tendon of the teres major muscle

D. Branches: 1 from the 1st part, 2 from the 2nd part, 3 from the 3rd part

   1. Superior thoracic: from the 1st part; supplies a small area of the upper lateral chest wall

   2. Thoracoacromial: from the 2nd part; supplies pectoral muscles and the shoulder joint with 4 types of branches

      a. pectoral: supplies the pectoralis major and minor

      b. clavicular: supplies the subclavius muscle

      c. deltoid: into deltopectoral groove; supplies the anterior deltoid and upper pectoralis major

      d. acromial: laterally beneath the acromion, supplies the deltoid and shoulder joint

   3. Lateral thoracic: from the 2nd part, supplies the serratus anterior

   4. Anterior circumflex humeral: from the 3rd part; supplies anterior arm muscles

   5. Posterior circumflex humeral: from the 3rd part; supplies posterior arm muscles and the humeral head

   6. Subscapular: from the 3rd part; 2 major branches supply the latissimus dorsi, teres major, teres minor, and infraspinatus

      a. Thoracodorsal: accompanies the nerve to the latissimus dorsi

      b. Circumflex scapular: wraps the lateral border of the scapula to supply the teres minor and infraspinatus

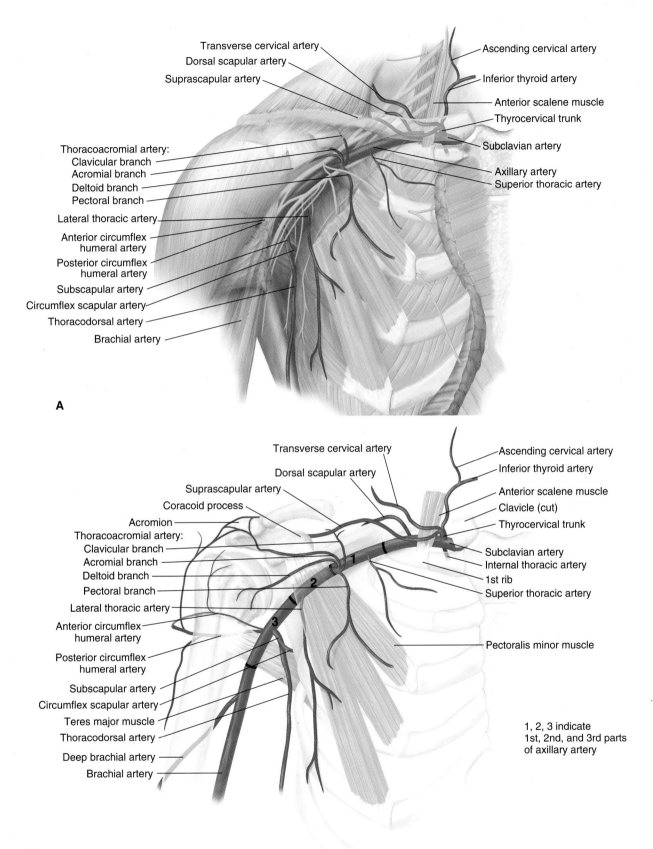

Transverse cervical artery

Dorsal scapular artery

Suprascapular artery

Ascending cervical artery

Inferior thyroid artery

Anterior scalene muscle

Thyrocervical trunk

Subclavian artery

Thoracoacromial artery:

Clavicular branch

Acromial branch

Deltoid branch

Pectoral branch

Lateral thoracic artery

Anterior circumflex humeral artery

Posterior circumflex humeral artery

Subscapular artery

Circumflex scapular artery

Thoracodorsal artery

Brachial artery

Axillary artery

Superior thoracic artery

A

Transverse cervical artery

Dorsal scapular artery

Suprascapular artery

Coracoid process

Acromion

Thoracoacromial artery:

Clavicular branch

Acromial branch

Deltoid branch

Pectoral branch

Lateral thoracic artery

Anterior circumflex humeral artery

Posterior circumflex humeral artery

Subscapular artery

Circumflex scapular artery

Teres major muscle

Thoracodorsal artery

Deep brachial artery

Brachial artery

Ascending cervical artery

Inferior thyroid artery

Anterior scalene muscle

Clavicle (cut)

Thyrocervical trunk

Subclavian artery

Internal thoracic artery

1st rib

Superior thoracic artery

Pectoralis minor muscle

1, 2, 3 indicate
1st, 2nd, and 3rd parts
of axillary artery

B

Figure 2.12A,B. Axillary Artery and Brachial Plexus. **A.** Anterior View. **B.** Axillary Artery Schema. Anterior View.

II. Collateral Circulation of the Shoulder (Fig. 2.12C)

A. All moveable joints possess collateral channels to compensate for potential vessel constriction during joint motion

B. Collateral channels of the shoulder come from subclavian and axillary arteries

  1. Suprascapular: from the thyrocervical trunk from the subclavian; passes over the superior transverse scapular ligament and around the notch of the scapular spine to anastomose with the circumflex scapular

  2. Dorsal scapular: from subclavian; passes along the medial scapular border

  3. Circumflex scapular: from the subscapular from the axillary; passes around the lateral scapular border and anastomoses with the suprascapular artery deep to infraspinatus

  4. Anterior and posterior circumflex humeral: from the axillary; encircle the surgical neck of the humerus and anastomose with each other and with the deep brachial artery

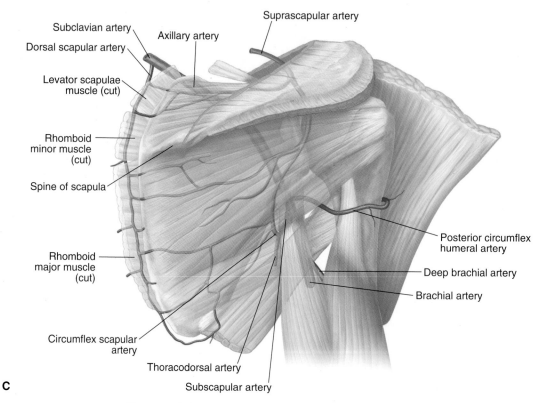

Figure 2.12C. Blood Supply to the Shoulder. Posterior View.

Muscles of the Arm

I. Muscles of the Arm (Fig. 2.13A–D)

Muscle	Origin	Insertion	Action	Innervation
Coracobrachialis	Apex of the coracoid process of the scapula	Middle shaft of the humerus	Flexes and adducts the arm	Musculocutaneous (C5-7)
Biceps				
Long head	Supraglenoid tubercle	Radial tuberosity; bicipital aponeurosis to the fascia of the forearm	Flexes the arm and the forearm; supinates the hand	Musculocutaneous (C5-7)
Short head	Apex of the coracoid process of the scapula			
Brachialis	Lower half of the anterior surface of the humerus	Ulnar tuberosity	Flexes the forearm	Musculocutaneous (C5-6)
Triceps				
Long head	Infraglenoid tubercle of the scapula	Olecranon	Extends the forearm; long head only: extends and adducts the arm	Radial (C6-8)
Lateral head	Posterior humerus above the radial groove			
Medial head	Posterior humerus below the radial groove			

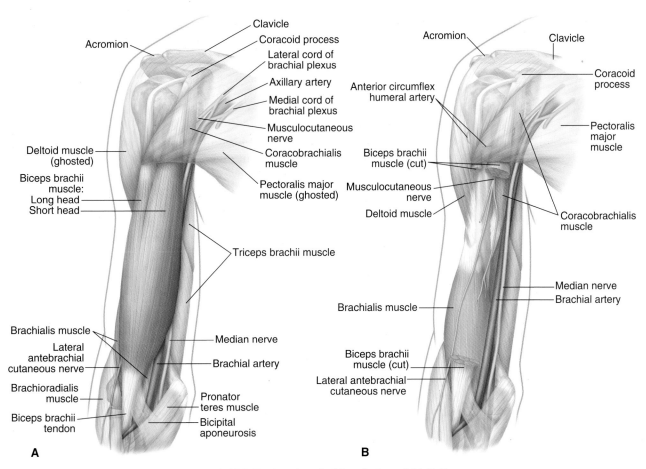

Figure 2.13A,B. Arm, Anterior View. **A.** Superficial. **B.** Deep.

II. Special Features

A. Tendon of origin of the long head of the biceps runs over the head of the humerus, surrounded by a synovial sheath that follows the tendon as far as the surgical neck of the humerus; the tendon is held in the intertubercular groove by the transverse humeral ligament and the tendon of the pectoralis major muscle

B. The bicipital aponeurosis overlies the brachial artery, thereby protecting it; further, it supports the median cubital vein, making it easier to introduce a needle

III. Clinical Considerations

A. Fractures of humerus: displacement of bone fragments after fracture may be determined by muscle attachments; for example, after fracture through the surgical neck:

  1. Proximal fragment
     a. Both medial and lateral rotators are attached to the proximal fragment; therefore, it is not rotated, because they are balanced
     b. The supraspinatus muscle is attached to the proximal piece and is unopposed; therefore, the proximal fragment is abducted
  2. Distal fragment
     a. This part has no lateral rotators attached to it but does have medial rotators, resulting in medial rotation
     b. The distal part also has the large and powerful adductors, latissimus dorsi and pectoralis major, attached to it, causing adduction
  3. Additionally, the ends of the 2 pieces will override each other, because of the pull of biceps, triceps, and coracobrachialis muscles

B. The biceps reflex is routinely tested during physical examination

  1. Limb is relaxed and passively pronated and partially extended at the elbow
  2. Examiner places thumb firmly on the biceps tendon and taps the reflex hammer at the base of the thumb's nail bed
  3. A normal response is immediate involuntary contraction of the biceps, which confirms the integrity of the musculocutaneous nerve and C5 and C6 spinal cord segments

C. Rupture of the tendon of the long head of the biceps brachii

  1. Results from wear and tear of an inflamed tendon moving back and forth through the intertubercular groove of the humerus
  2. Usually occurs as a sudden "snap" or "pop" in people older than 35 years of age
  3. The detached muscle belly forms a ball near the center of the distal portion of the anterior aspect of the arm (**Popeye deformity**)

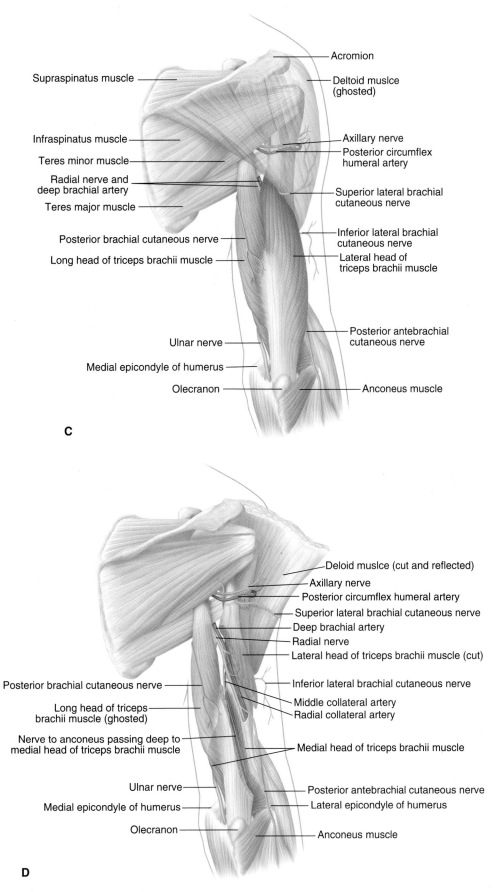

Acromion

Deltoid muslce (ghosted)

Supraspinatus muscle

Infraspinatus muscle

Teres minor muscle

Radial nerve and deep brachial artery

Teres major muscle

Axillary nerve

Posterior circumflex humeral artery

Superior lateral brachial cutaneous nerve

Posterior brachial cutaneous nerve

Long head of triceps brachii muscle

Inferior lateral brachial cutaneous nerve

Lateral head of triceps brachii muscle

Posterior antebrachial cutaneous nerve

Ulnar nerve

Medial epicondyle of humerus

Olecranon

Anconeus muscle

C

Deloid muslce (cut and reflected)

Axillary nerve

Posterior circumflex humeral artery

Superior lateral brachial cutaneous nerve

Deep brachial artery

Radial nerve

Lateral head of triceps brachii muscle (cut)

Posterior brachial cutaneous nerve

Long head of triceps brachii muscle (ghosted)

Inferior lateral brachial cutaneous nerve

Middle collateral artery

Radial collateral artery

Nerve to anconeus passing deep to medial head of triceps brachii muscle

Medial head of triceps brachii muscle

Ulnar nerve

Medial epicondyle of humerus

Olecranon

Posterior antebrachial cutaneous nerve

Lateral epicondyle of humerus

Anconeus muscle

D

Figure 2.13C,D. Arm. **C.** Posterior View, Superficial. **D.** Posterior View, Deep.

Neurovasculature of the Arm

I. Brachial Artery (Fig. 2.14A)

A. Continuation of the axillary artery at the inferior border of the teres major muscle; terminates in the cubital fossa, where it divides into radial and ulnar arteries

B. Branches in arm
   1. Deep brachial: enters the radial groove behind the humerus; terminates as radial collateral and middle collateral arteries
   2. Superior ulnar collateral: runs with the ulnar nerve behind the medial intermuscular septum
   3. Inferior ulnar collateral: descends to the back of the elbow

II. Nerves (Fig. 2.14B)

A. Median
   1. 1st lateral to, then crosses, and, finally, is medial to the brachial artery
   2. No branches in the arm

B. Musculocutaneous
   1. Pierces the coracobrachialis muscle, sending branches to it, biceps, and brachialis muscles
   2. Continues as the lateral antebrachial cutaneous nerve

C. Radial
   1. Passes in the radial groove on the back of the humerus with the deep brachial artery, pierces the lateral intermuscular septum, and divides into superficial and deep branches in front of the lateral epicondyle
   2. In the arm, gives branches to triceps and to the skin (posterior brachial, inferior lateral brachial, and posterior antebrachial cutaneous nerves)

D. Ulnar
   1. Medial to axillary and brachial arteries to the middle of the arm, pierces the medial intermuscular septum, and runs with the superior ulnar collateral artery to a groove behind the medial epicondyle of the humerus
   2. No branches in the arm

III. Special Features

A. Brachial artery lies successively on 3 muscles, gives 3 main branches, is in contact with 3 important nerves, and is associated with 3 veins
   1. 3 muscles constitute the floor on which the artery runs (from above downward): are the long head of the triceps, coracobrachialis, and brachialis
   2. 3 main branches: deep brachial, the superior ulnar collateral, and inferior ulnar collateral
   3. 3 important nerves associated with the artery: radial, ulnar, and median
   4. 3 veins associated with the artery: 2 venae comitantes (brachial veins) and basilic

B. Bifurcation is not constant and may take place at a high level in the arm

C. Brachial artery lies anterior to triceps and brachialis; its pulsations can be felt throughout its course

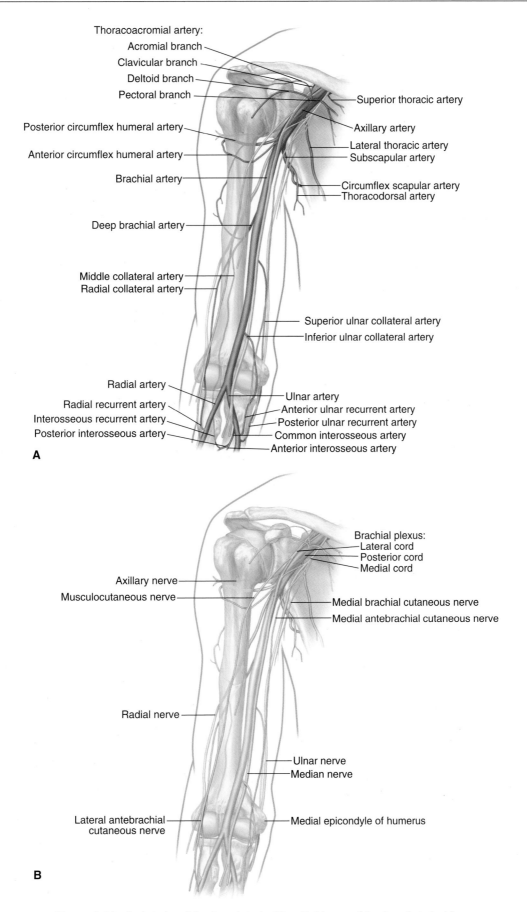

Figure 2.14. A. Arteries of the Arm. Anterior View. **B.** Nerves of the Arm. Anterior View.

Muscles of the Anterior Forearm

I. Superficial Group (Fig. 2.15A)

Muscle	Origin	Insertion	Action	Nerve
Pronator teres	Common flexor tendon and (deep or ulnar head) from the medial side of the coronoid process of the ulna	Midpoint of the lateral side of the shaft of the radius	Pronates and flexes the forearm	Median (C6-7)
Flexor carpi radialis	Common flexor tendon from the medial epicondyle of the humerus	Base of the 2nd and 3rd metacarpals	Flexes the wrist; abducts the hand	Median (C6-7)
Palmaris longus	Medial epicondyle of the humerus	Distal half of the flexor retinaculum and palmaris aponeurosis	Flexes the hand (at wrist) and tightens the palmar aponeurosis	Median (C8)
Flexor carpi ulnaris	Common flexor tendon and (ulnar head) from the medial border of the olecranon and the upper 2/3 of the posterior border of the ulna	Pisiform, hook of the hamate, and the base of the 5th metacarpal	Flexes the wrist; adducts hand	Ulnar (C7-8)

II. Intermediate Group (Fig. 2.15B)

Muscle	Origin	Insertion	Action	Nerve
Flexor digitorum superficialis	Humeroulnar head: common flexor tendon; Radial head: the middle 1/3 of the radius	Shafts of the middle phalanges of digits 2–5	Flexes the metacarpophalangeal and proximal interphalangeal joints	Median (C7-8,T1)

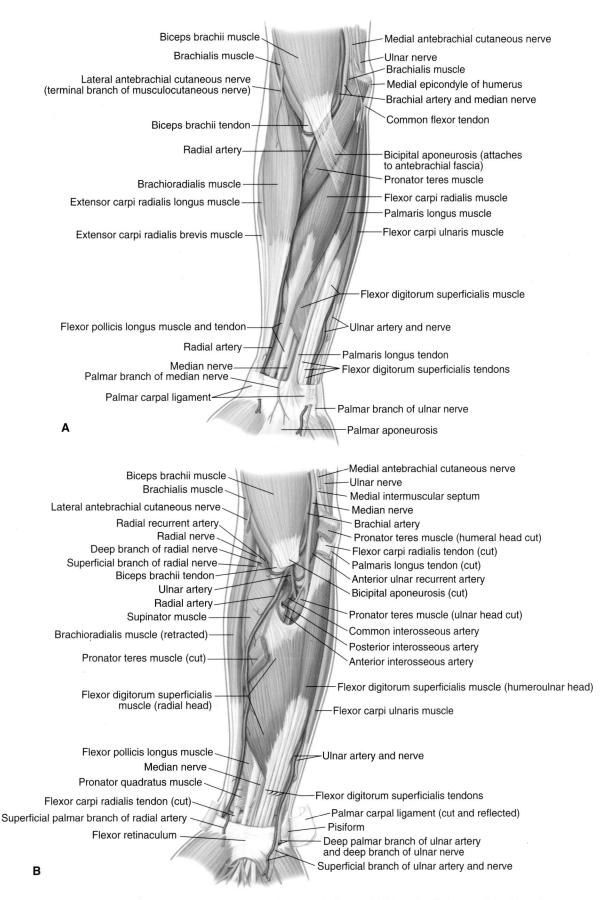

Biceps brachii muscle
Brachialis muscle
Lateral antebrachial cutaneous nerve
(terminal branch of musculocutaneous nerve)
Biceps brachii tendon
Radial artery
Brachioradialis muscle
Extensor carpi radialis longus muscle
Extensor carpi radialis brevis muscle

Medial antebrachial cutaneous nerve
Ulnar nerve
Brachialis muscle
Medial epicondyle of humerus
Brachial artery and median nerve
Common flexor tendon
Bicipital aponeurosis (attaches to antebrachial fascia)
Pronator teres muscle
Flexor carpi radialis muscle
Palmaris longus muscle
Flexor carpi ulnaris muscle

Flexor digitorum superficialis muscle

Flexor pollicis longus muscle and tendon
Radial artery
Median nerve
Palmar branch of median nerve
Palmar carpal ligament

Ulnar artery and nerve
Palmaris longus tendon
Flexor digitorum superficialis tendons

Palmar branch of ulnar nerve
Palmar aponeurosis

A

Biceps brachii muscle
Brachialis muscle
Lateral antebrachial cutaneous nerve
Radial recurrent artery
Radial nerve
Deep branch of radial nerve
Superficial branch of radial nerve
Biceps brachii tendon
Ulnar artery
Radial artery
Supinator muscle
Brachioradialis muscle (retracted)
Pronator teres muscle (cut)

Medial antebrachial cutaneous nerve
Ulnar nerve
Medial intermuscular septum
Median nerve
Brachial artery
Pronator teres muscle (humeral head cut)
Flexor carpi radialis tendon (cut)
Palmaris longus tendon (cut)
Anterior ulnar recurrent artery
Bicipital aponeurosis (cut)
Pronator teres muscle (ulnar head cut)
Common interosseous artery
Posterior interosseous artery
Anterior interosseous artery

Flexor digitorum superficialis
muscle (radial head)

Flexor digitorum superficialis muscle (humeroulnar head)
Flexor carpi ulnaris muscle

Flexor pollicis longus muscle
Median nerve
Pronator quadratus muscle
Flexor carpi radialis tendon (cut)
Superficial palmar branch of radial artery
Flexor retinaculum

Ulnar artery and nerve

Flexor digitorum superficialis tendons
Palmar carpal ligament (cut and reflected)
Pisiform
Deep palmar branch of ulnar artery
and deep branch of ulnar nerve
Superficial branch of ulnar artery and nerve

B

Figure 2.15A,B. Muscles of the Anterior Forearm. **A.** Superficial Dissection. **B.** Intermediate Dissection.

III. Deep Group (Fig. 2.15C)

Muscle	Origin	Insertion	Action	Nerve
Flexor digitorum profundus	Posterior border of the ulna, the proximal 2/3 of the medial border of the ulna, the interosseous membrane	Base of the distal phalanx of digits 2–5	Flexes the metacarpophalangeal, proximal interphalangeal and distal interphalangeal joints	Anterior interosseous of the median; ulnar (C8,T1)
Flexor pollicis longus	Anterior surface of the radius and interosseous membrane	Base of the distal phalanx of the thumb	Flexes the metacarpophalangeal and interphalangeal joints of the thumb	Anterior interosseous of the median (C8,T1)
Pronator quadratus	Medial side of the anterior surface of the distal 1/4 of the ulna	Anterior surface of the distal 1/4 of the radius	Pronates the forearm	Anterior interosseous of the median (C8,T1)

IV. Special Features

A. The muscles of the anterior forearm are concerned with pronation of the forearm, flexion and abduction at the wrist, and with flexion of the digits

B. The most common variation among this group of muscles is the absence of the palmaris longus muscle (about 12%)

C. In the "power grip," the wrist is extended and slightly adducted, while the powerful long flexors of the digits contract

D. The superficial and intermediate muscles cross the elbow joint, whereas the deep muscles do not

E. Brachioradialis muscle is a flexor of the forearm but is found in the posterior (extensor) compartment of the forearm and is, thus, supplied by the radial nerve (it is an exception to the fact that the radial nerve supplies only extensor muscles and that all flexors are located in the anterior (flexor) compartment)

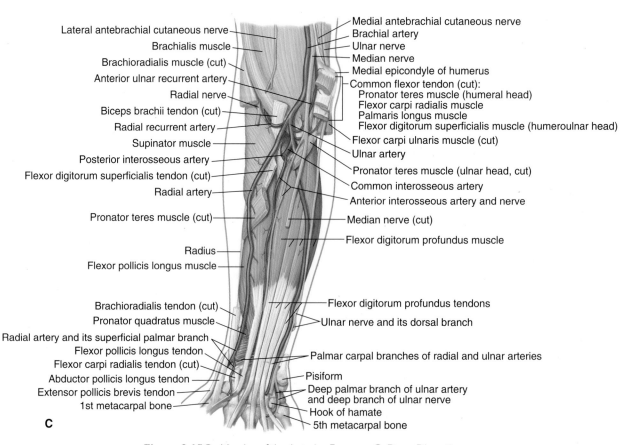

C

Figure 2.15C. Muscles of the Anterior Forearm. **C.** Deep Dissection.

Neurovasculature of the Anterior Forearm

I. Radial Artery (Fig. 2.16A,B)

A. Extends from the neck of the radius to the medial side of the radial styloid process
B. Relations

	Anterior	
	Skin and fascia, brachioradialis muscle	
Lateral	**Radial Artery**	**Medial**
Brachioradialis muscle, superficial radial nerve		Pronator teres and flexor carpi radialis muscles
	Posterior	
	Biceps tendon, supinator, flexor digitorum superficialis, pronator teres, flexor pollicis longus and pronator quadratus muscles, radius	

C. Branches: radial recurrent, muscular, palmar carpal, and superficial palmar

II. Ulnar Artery

A. Extends from the neck of radius to the flexor retinaculum at the wrist
B. Relations

	Anterior	
	Skin and fascia, superficial flexor muscles, median nerve	
Lateral	**Ulnar Artery**	**Medial**
Flexor digitorum superficialis muscle		Flexor carpi ulnaris muscle and ulnar nerve
	Posterior	
	Brachialis and flexor digitorum profundus muscles	

C. Branches: anterior and posterior ulnar recurrent, common interosseous, and muscular

III. Common Interosseous Artery

A. Trunk arising from the ulnar artery below the radial tuberosity to the upper interosseous membrane
B. Divides into:
  1. Posterior interosseous: passes through the interosseous membrane to supply the posterior forearm
  2. Anterior interosseous
     a. Travels down the forearm on the interosseous membrane to the upper border of the pronator quadratus muscle, where it sends a branch through the interosseous membrane to the dorsum to join the posterior interosseous artery, and a small branch continues under the pronator quadratus muscle to the palmar carpal network
     b. Gives muscular and nutrient (radius and ulna) branches and a branch to the median nerve

IV. Median Nerve (Fig. 2.16C,D)

A. Passes between heads of the pronator teres muscle; lies between flexor digitorum superficialis and profundus muscles; near the wrist is more superficial, between tendons of flexor digitorum superficialis and flexor carpi radialis muscles; and then passes the deep and medial to the tendon of the palmaris longus muscle

B. Branches to all superficial muscles except the flexor carpi ulnaris
   1. Anterior interosseous branch accompanies the anterior interosseous artery on the interosseous membrane to supply the flexor pollicis longus, the pronator quadratus, and the radial half of flexor digitorum profundus muscles
   2. Palmar branch to the skin of the palm

V. Ulnar Nerve

A. From behind medial epicondyle, enters the forearm through the flexor carpi ulnaris muscle, continues between this and the flexor digitorum profundus, and, in the lower half of the forearm, the ulnar artery lies close to its medial side; both artery and nerve are covered by the skin and the fascia lateral to the flexor carpi ulnaris muscle

B. Branches to the flexor carpi ulnaris and the medial half of the flexor digitorum profundus muscles
   1. Dorsal branch to the dorsum of hand and ulnar 2½ digits
   2. Palmar cutaneous to the medial side of the palm

VI. Radial Nerve

A. Divides into superficial and deep branches as it lies between brachialis and brachioradialis muscles

B. Superficial branch: runs beneath the brachioradialis muscle just lateral to the radial artery
   1. In the lower 3rd of the forearm, crosses to the dorsum
   2. Cutaneous to the dorsum of the hand and radial 2½ digits

C. Deep branch: passes through the supinator to innervate posterior forearm extensor muscles

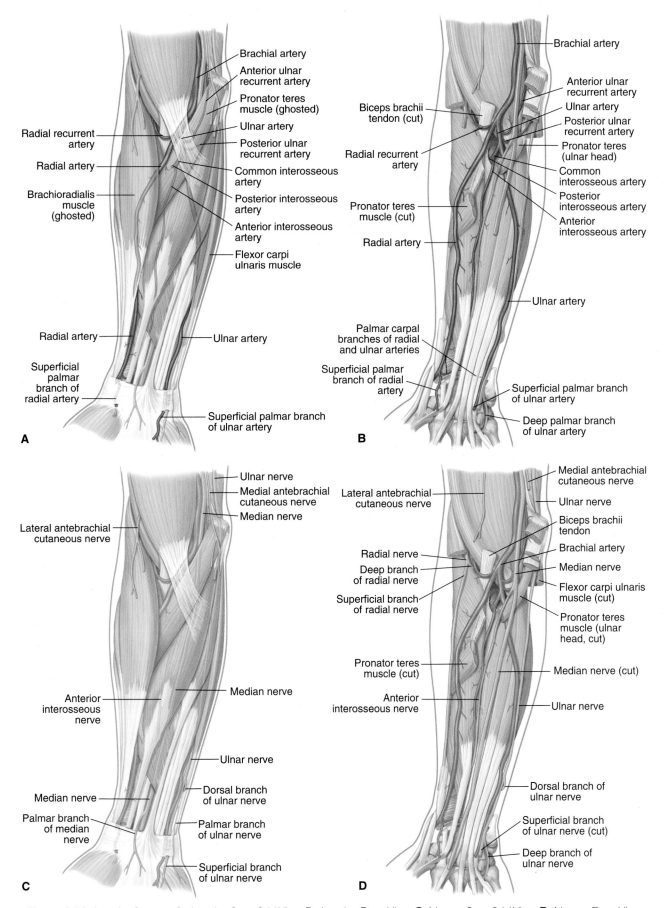

Figure 2.16 Anterior forearm. **A.** Arteries. Superficial View. **B.** Arteries. Deep View. **C.** Nerves. Superficial View. **D.** Nerves. Deep View.

Muscles of the Posterior Forearm

I. Muscles of the Posterior Forearm

A. Superficial group (Fig. 2.17A)

Muscle	Origin	Insertion	Action	Nerve
Brachioradialis	Upper 2/3 of the lateral supracondylar ridge of the humerus	Lateral side of the base of the styloid process of the radius	Flexes the elbow; assists in pronation and supination	Radial (C5-7)
Extensor carpi radials longus	Lower 1/3 of the lateral supracondylar ridge of the humerus	Dorsum of the 2nd metacarpal bone (base)	Extends the wrist; abducts the hand	Radial (C6-7)
Extensor carpi radialis brevis	Common extensor tendon (the lateral epicondyle of the humerus)	Dorsum of the 3rd metacarpal bone (base)	Extends the wrist; abducts the hand	Radial (C7-8)
Extensor digitorum	Common extensor tendon (the lateral epicondyle of the humerus)	Extensor expansion of digits 2–5	Extends the metacarpophalangeal, proximal interphalangeal and distal interphalangeal joints of digits 2–5; extends the wrist	Deep radial (C7-8)
Extensor digiti minimi	Common extensor tendon (the lateral epicondyle of the humerus)	Joins the extensor digitorum tendon to the 5th digit and inserts into the extensor expansion	Extends the metacarpophalangeal, proximal interphalangeal, and distal interphalangeal joints of the 5th digit	Deep radial (C7-8)
Extensor carpi ulnaris	Common extensor tendon and the middle 1/2 of the posterior border of the ulna	Medial side of the base of the 5th metacarpal	Extends the wrist; adducts the hand	Deep radial (C7-8)
Anconeus	Lateral epicondyle of the humerus	Lateral side of the olecranon and the upper 1/4 of the ulna	Extends the forearm	Radial (C7-8, T1)

B. Deep group (Fig. 2.17B)

Muscle	Origin	Insertion	Action	Nerve
Supinator	Lateral epicondyle of the humerus, supinator crest, and fossa of the ulna, radial collateral ligament, and anular ligament	Lateral side of the proximal 1/3 of the radius	Supinates the forearm	Deep radial (C5-6)
Abductor pollicis longus	Middle 1/3 of the posterior surface of the radius, interosseous membrane, and the midportion of the posterolateral ulna	Radial side of the base of the 1st metacarpal	Abducts and extends the thumb at the carpometacarpal joint	Deep radial (C7-8)
Extensor pollicis brevis	Interosseous membrane and the posterior surface of the distal radius	Base of the proximal phalanx of the thumb	Extends the thumb at the metacarpophalangeal joint	Deep radial (C7-8)
Extensor pollicis longus	Interosseous membrane and the middle part of the posterolateral surface of the ulna	Base of the distal phalanx of the thumb	Extends the thumb at the interphalangeal joint	Deep radial (C7-8)
Extensor indicis	Interosseous membrane and the posterolateral surface of the distal ulna	Joins the tendon of the extensor digitorum to the 2nd digit; both tendons insert into the extensor expansion	Extends the index finger at the metacarpophalangeal, proximal interphalangeal, and distal interphalangeal joints	Deep radial (C7-8)

C. Special features: deep radial nerve passes between 2 heads of the supinator muscle

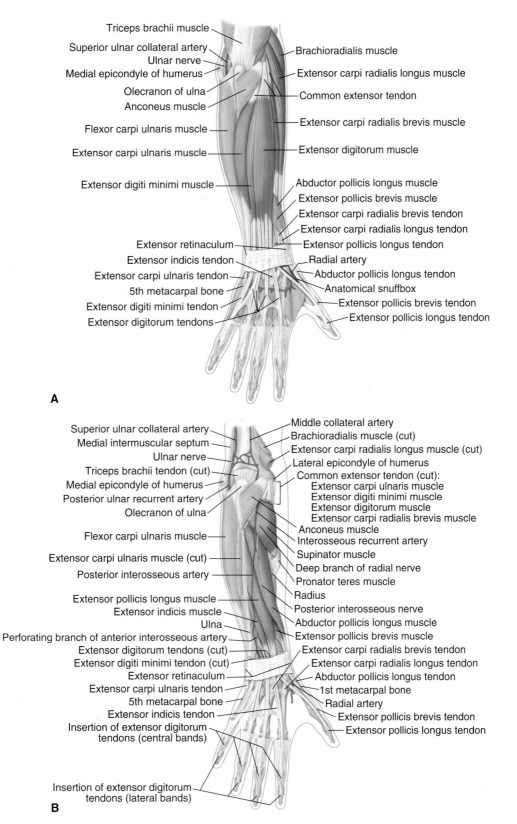

Triceps brachii muscle
Superior ulnar collateral artery
Ulnar nerve
Medial epicondyle of humerus
Olecranon of ulna
Anconeus muscle
Flexor carpi ulnaris muscle
Extensor carpi ulnaris muscle
Extensor digiti minimi muscle
Extensor retinaculum
Extensor indicis tendon
Extensor carpi ulnaris tendon
5th metacarpal bone
Extensor digiti minimi tendon
Extensor digitorum tendons

Brachioradialis muscle
Extensor carpi radialis longus muscle
Common extensor tendon
Extensor carpi radialis brevis muscle
Extensor digitorum muscle
Abductor pollicis longus muscle
Extensor pollicis brevis muscle
Extensor carpi radialis brevis tendon
Extensor carpi radialis longus tendon
Extensor pollicis longus tendon
Radial artery
Abductor pollicis longus tendon
Anatomical snuffbox
Extensor pollicis brevis tendon
Extensor pollicis longus tendon

A

Superior ulnar collateral artery
Medial intermuscular septum
Ulnar nerve
Triceps brachii tendon (cut)
Medial epicondyle of humerus
Posterior ulnar recurrent artery
Olecranon of ulna
Flexor carpi ulnaris muscle
Extensor carpi ulnaris muscle (cut)
Posterior interosseous artery
Extensor pollicis longus muscle
Extensor indicis muscle
Ulna
Perforating branch of anterior interosseous artery
Extensor digitorum tendons (cut)
Extensor digiti minimi tendon (cut)
Extensor retinaculum
Extensor carpi ulnaris tendon
5th metacarpal bone
Extensor indicis tendon
Insertion of extensor digitorum tendons (central bands)
Insertion of extensor digitorum tendons (lateral bands)

Middle collateral artery
Brachioradialis muscle (cut)
Extensor carpi radialis longus muscle (cut)
Lateral epicondyle of humerus
Common extensor tendon (cut):
Extensor carpi ulnaris muscle
Extensor digiti minimi muscle
Extensor digitorum muscle
Extensor carpi radialis brevis muscle
Anconeus muscle
Interosseous recurrent artery
Supinator muscle
Deep branch of radial nerve
Pronator teres muscle
Radius
Posterior interosseous nerve
Abductor pollicis longus muscle
Extensor pollicis brevis muscle
Extensor carpi radialis brevis tendon
Extensor carpi radialis longus tendon
Abductor pollicis longus tendon
1st metacarpal bone
Radial artery
Extensor pollicis brevis tendon
Extensor pollicis longus tendon

B

Figure 2.17A,B. Muscles of the Posterior Forearm. **A.** Superficial View. **B.** Deep View.

Neurovasculature of the Posterior Forearm

I. Vessels: Posterior Interosseous Artery (Fig. 2.18)

A. Arises from the common interosseous artery at the upper border of interosseous membrane over which it passes, comes through between the borders of supinator and abductor pollicis longus muscles, and descends through the forearm between superficial and deep layers; in the lower forearm is joined by one of the terminal branches of the anterior interosseous artery and enters the dorsal carpal network

B. Branches: muscular; interosseous recurrent artery, which ascends between the olecranon and the lateral epicondyle under anconeus muscle to anastomose with the middle collateral artery, the inferior ulnar collateral artery, and the posterior ulnar recurrent artery

II. Nerves: Radial Nerve

A. Pierces the lateral intermuscular septum of arm, runs between brachialis and brachioradialis muscles, and branches in front of the lateral epicondyle

B. Branches

1. Superficial branch: cutaneous to the dorsum of the hand and radial 2½ digits
2. Deep branch: curves around the lateral border of radius within the supinator muscle, continues between superficial and deep layers of muscles to the midforearm; then, as the posterior interosseous nerve, it lies between the interosseous membrane and the extensor pollicis longus muscle
   a. Continues to the posterior of the carpus, giving branches to extensor muscles
   b. Sensory to the wrist joint

III. Clinical Considerations

A. Damage to the radial nerve
1. Above the elbow
   a. Leads to **wrist drop**, the inability to extend the hand at the wrist
   b. Extension of the metacarpophalangeal joints is also impossible
   c. Sensation on the lateral side of the back of the hand is also lost
   d. Because of the shortness of the extensor muscles of the digits, however, a person with wrist drop can passively extend the wrist by tightly clenching the fingers
2. Lesions of the deep branch of the radial may have varying effects, but complete loss abolishes extension at the metacarpophalangeal joints of the digits, while allowing extension of the wrist through the radial extensors
3. All the extensor muscles are innervated through the radial nerve
   a. The brachioradialis and extensor carpi radialis longus receive their innervation from the radial nerve before it divides (while it lies anterior to the lateral epicondyle)
   b. The rest (supinator, extensor carpi radialis brevis, extensor digitorum, extensor digiti minimi, extensor carpi ulnaris, abductor pollicis longus, extensor pollicis brevis, extensor pollicis longus, and extensor indicis) receive their innervation from the deep branch of the radial nerve
   c. Typically the brachioradialis receives fibers from the 5th and 6th cervical nerves; the radial extensors from about C6 and C7; the extensor digitorum and extensor digiti minimi from C6, C7, and C8; and the ulnar extensor from these or C7 and C8 only

III. Clinical Considerations

   B. The insertion of the extensor carpi radialis brevis tendon into the base of the 3rd metacarpal bone is a common site for a cystic swelling (**ganglion cyst**) of the tendon sheath

   C. Tennis elbow (lateral epicondylitis)

     1. Characterized by pain and joint tenderness at or just distal to the lateral epicondyle of the humerus

     2. Due to premature degeneration of the common extensor origin of the superficial extensor muscles of the forearm, it is not confined to tennis players but may develop after an elbow injury or be due to "overactivity" of the superficial extensor muscles (e.g., lifting and throwing snow with a shovel)

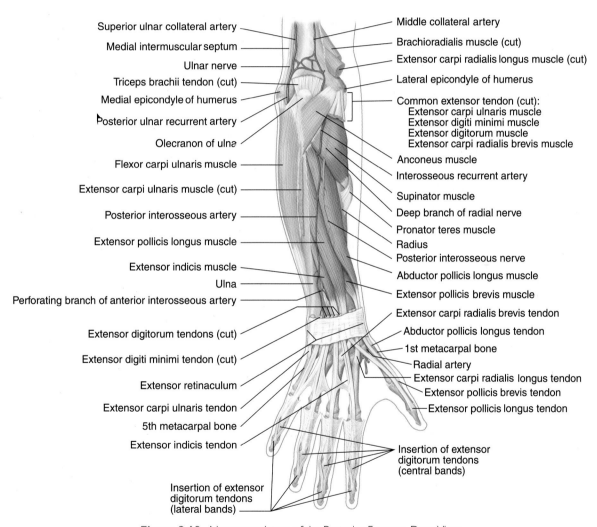

Figure 2.18. Neurovasculature of the Posterior Forearm. Deep View.

Dorsum of the Hand

I. Skin of the Dorsum of the Hand (Fig. 2.19A,B)

A. Characteristics
   1. Thin and loose in contrast with the tight relationship of the skin of the palm and its underlying fascia and palmar aponeurosis
   2. Tissue is so lax that a fold of the skin can be grasped and elevated several centimeters off the underlying deep fascia
B. Dorsal subcutaneous space
   1. Lies between the skin and the deep fascia over the extensor tendons and is due to looseness of the areolar tissue
   2. Sensory nerves, veins, and lymphatics course through this loose areolar layer

II. Cutaneous Nerves of the Dorsum of the Hand

A. Superficial branch of the radial nerve: its dorsal digital branches innervate the dorsum of the hand radially and the radial 2½ digits
B. Dorsal cutaneous branch of the ulnar nerve: its dorsal digital branches innervate the dorsum of the hand medially and the ulnar 2½ digits
C. Distribution of dorsal digital branches of the superficial radial and the dorsal cutaneous branch of the ulnar is variable
D. Branches of palmar digital branches of median and ulnar nerves innervate the skin over the dorsal distal phalanx (nail bed)

III. Vessels of the Dorsum of the Hand

A. Radial artery
   1. Dorsal carpal arch: primarily from the radial, with anastomosis with the branch of the ulnar artery
      a. Dorsal metacarpal arteries: from the dorsal carpal arch branch into dorsal digital arteries
      b. 1st dorsal metacarpal artery: directly from the radial artery
   2. After passing through anatomical snuffbox, the radial artery passes through the 1st dorsal interosseous muscle to become major contribution to the deep palmar arch
B. Dorsal venous network: drains dorsal digital and dorsal metacarpal veins into the cephalic vein on the radial side and the basilic vein on the ulnar side

IV. Lymphatics of the Dorsum of the Hand

A. Most of the lymph from the palmar aspects of the fingers, web areas, and hypothenar and thenar eminences flows into the lymph channels and lacunae found in the loose areolar layer on the dorsum of the hand
B. Accounts for lymphedematous swelling seen on the back of the hand even when the infection is on the palmar surface of fingers, web space, or hypothenar or thenar areas

V. Extensor Retinaculum and Extensor Expansions (Fig. 2.19C–F)

A. Extensor retinaculum
   1. Holds extensor tendons in place in the wrist region, preventing "bowstringing" of the tendons when the hand is extended at the wrist
   2. Synovial tendon sheaths are present as the tendons pass over the dorsum of the wrist, which reduce friction for the extensor tendons as they pass through the osseofibrous tunnel formed by the attachments of the extensor retinaculum to the distal ulna and radius
B. Extensor expansions
   1. Over the metacarpophalangeal joint, each extensor tendon flares laterally and medially to form an extensor expansion.
   2. Over the proximal interphalangeal joint, the extensor expansion splits into 3 slips: the middle going to the base of the middle phalanx, and the 2 collateral slips going to the base of the distal phalanx

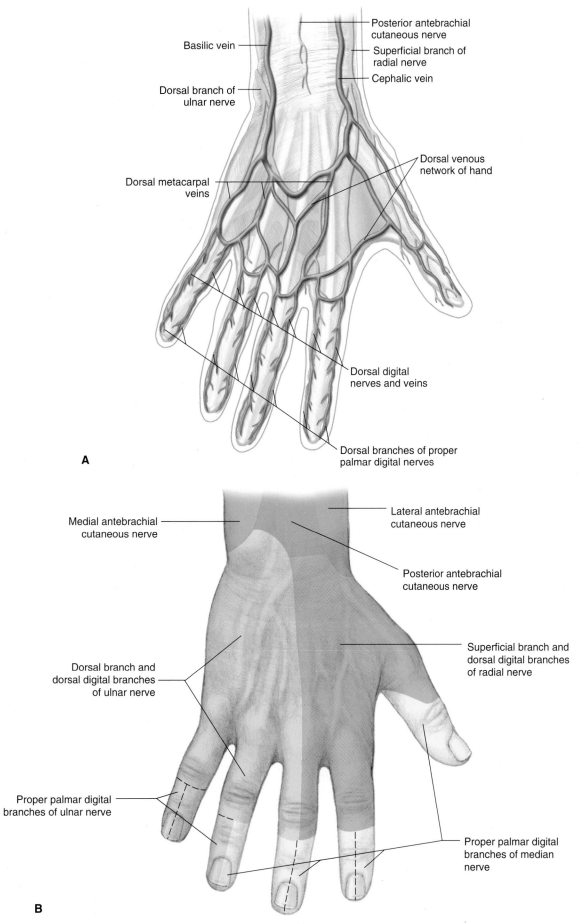

Posterior antebrachial
cutaneous nerve

Basilic vein

Superficial branch of
radial nerve

Cephalic vein

Dorsal branch of
ulnar nerve

Dorsal venous
network of hand

Dorsal metacarpal
veins

Dorsal digital
nerves and veins

A

Dorsal branches of proper
palmar digital nerves

Medial antebrachial
cutaneous nerve

Lateral antebrachial
cutaneous nerve

Posterior antebrachial
cutaneous nerve

Superficial branch and
dorsal digital branches
of radial nerve

Dorsal branch and
dorsal digital branches
of ulnar nerve

Proper palmar digital
branches of ulnar nerve

Proper palmar digital
branches of median
nerve

B

Figure 2.19A,B. Cutaneous Nerves of the Hand. Posterior View. **A.** Dissection. **B.** Nerve Territories.

VI. Special Features

A. Dorsal subaponeurotic space
 1. Lies between the fused deep dorsal fascia and extensor tendons, which form its roof, and the interossei muscles and metacarpal bones, which form its floor
 2. The latter structures form a barrier to the palm; thus, this space is infrequently involved in hand infections

B. Anatomical snuffbox
 1. Bounded by the tendons of the abductor pollicis longus and the extensor pollicis brevis laterally and the extensor pollicis longus medially
 2. Crossed superficially by branches of the superficial branch of the radial nerve
 3. Contains the radial artery lying against the scaphoid bone
 4. Scaphoid fracture may be palpated within the anatomical snuffbox

C. Extensor tendons stand out clearly (to about knuckles) when the wrist is extended and fingers are abducted

D. Knuckles: visible when the hand is made into a fist; represent the heads of the metacarpal bones

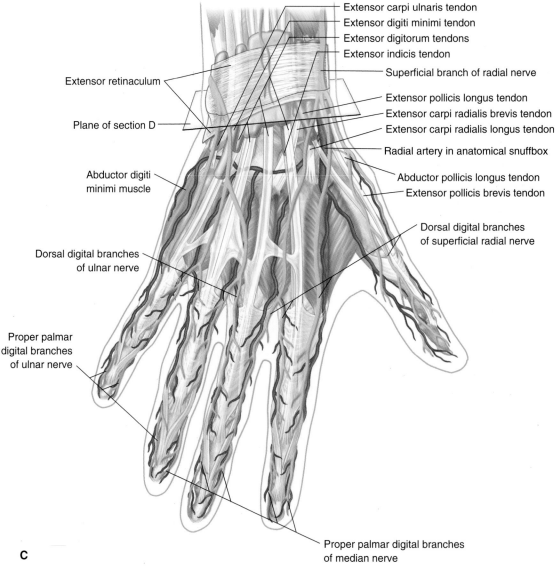

C

Figure 2.19C. Hand. Posterior View, Superficial Dissection.

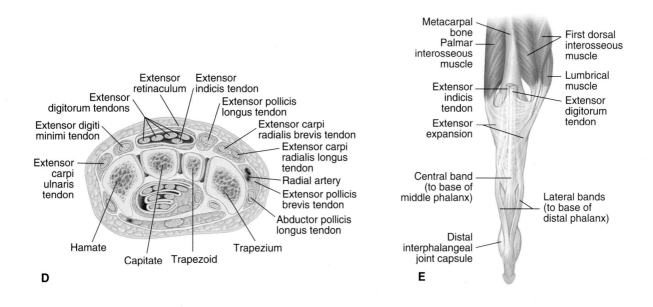

D.

E.

Extensor retinaculum
Extensor indicis tendon
Extensor digitorum tendons
Extensor digiti minimi tendon
Extensor carpi ulnaris tendon
Hamate
Capitate
Trapezoid
Trapezium
Extensor pollicis longus tendon
Extensor carpi radialis brevis tendon
Extensor carpi radialis longus tendon
Radial artery
Extensor pollicis brevis tendon
Abductor pollicis longus tendon

Metacarpal bone
Palmar interosseous muscle
Extensor indicis tendon
Extensor expansion
Central band (to base of middle phalanx)
Distal interphalangeal joint capsule
First dorsal interosseous muscle
Lumbrical muscle
Extensor digitorum tendon
Lateral bands (to base of distal phalanx)

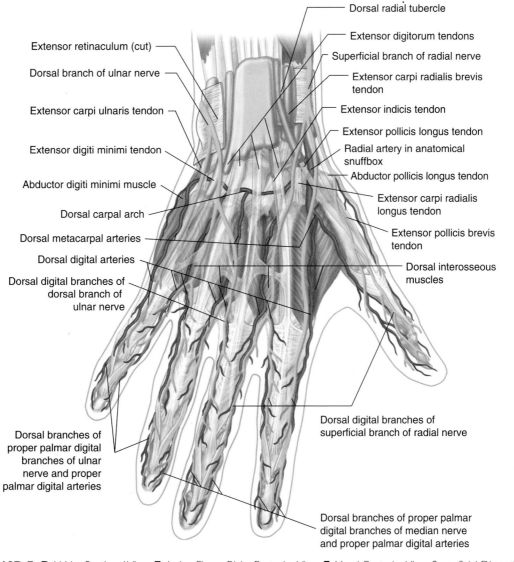

F.

Extensor retinaculum (cut)
Dorsal branch of ulnar nerve
Extensor carpi ulnaris tendon
Extensor digiti minimi tendon
Abductor digiti minimi muscle
Dorsal carpal arch
Dorsal metacarpal arteries
Dorsal digital arteries
Dorsal digital branches of dorsal branch of ulnar nerve
Dorsal branches of proper palmar digital branches of ulnar nerve and proper palmar digital arteries

Dorsal radial tubercle
Extensor digitorum tendons
Superficial branch of radial nerve
Extensor carpi radialis brevis tendon
Extensor indicis tendon
Extensor pollicis longus tendon
Radial artery in anatomical snuffbox
Abductor pollicis longus tendon
Extensor carpi radialis longus tendon
Extensor pollicis brevis tendon
Dorsal interosseous muscles
Dorsal digital branches of superficial branch of radial nerve
Dorsal branches of proper palmar digital branches of median nerve and proper palmar digital arteries

Figure 2.19D-F. D. Wrist, Sectional View. **E.** Index Finger, Right, Posterior View. **F.** Hand. Posterior View, Superficial Dissection.

Palm of the Hand, Superficial

I. Skin of the Palm

A. Characteristics
1. Thick, coarse, and more vascular than on the dorsum
2. Contains no hair or sebaceous glands, but sweat glands are numerous
B. Bound to the palmar aponeurosis by fibrous septa or fasciculi between which is found granular fat

II. Palmar Flexion Creases (Fig. 2.20A)

A. Radial longitudinal (vertical) partially encircles the thenar eminence; for movement of opposition of the thumb (formed by the short muscle of the thumb)
B. Midpalmar begins at the distal transverse crease and ends on the hypothenar eminence (formed by the short muscles of the 5th digit)
C. Proximal transverse begins on the radial border of the palm, in common with the radial longitudinal crease and superficial to the head of the 2nd metacarpal bone
1. Extends medially and slightly proximally across the palm, superficial to shafts of 3rd, 4th, and 5th metacarpals
2. Useful for movement of the index finger
3. Marks convexity of the superficial palmar arterial arch
D. Distal transverse
1. Begins near the cleft between index and middle fingers and crosses the palm superficial to heads of 2nd, 3rd, and 4th metacarpals
2. Useful in movement of medial 3 digits (marks metacarpal heads)

III. Digital Flexion Creases (Fig. 2.20B)

A. Each of the medial 4 digits usually has 3 transverse flexion creases; all deepen with flexion of the digits
1. Proximal: at the root of the finger, about 2 cm distal to the metacarpophalangeal joint
2. Distal: lies proximal to the distal interphalangeal joint
3. Middle: lies over the proximal interphalangeal joint
B. The thumb has only 2 flexion creases
1. The proximal crosses the thumb obliquely, proximal to the 1st metacarpophalangeal joint
2. The distal lies proximal to the interphalangeal joint

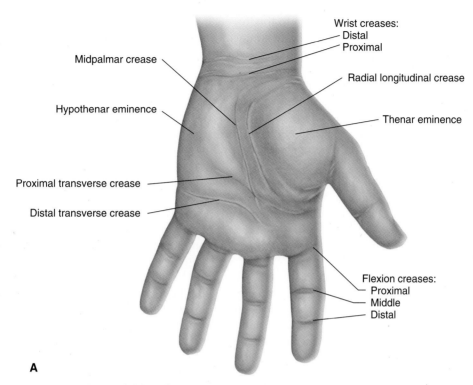

Figure 2.20A. Cutaneous Features of the Palm of the Hand. Right.

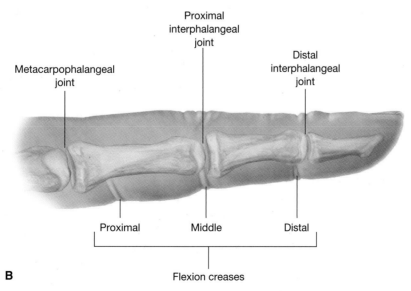

Figure 2.20B. Flexion Creases of the Fingers.

IV. Deep Palmar Fascia (Fig. 2.20C)

A. Continuous proximally with the antebrachial fascia and at the borders of the palm with the fascia on the dorsum of the hand

    1. Thin over the thenar and hypothenar eminences, but thick in the palm, where it forms the **palmar aponeurosis**

    2. Continues distally onto the fingers by helping to form the **fibrous digital sheaths**

B. Palmar fascia is in intimate contact with the thenar and hypothenar muscles, which helps prevent the formation of a space over the muscles within which pus could accumulate

C. Palmar aponeurosis

    1. Strong, heavy, dense, well-defined triangular layer of the deep fascia in the middle of the palm

    2. Apex (proximally) is anchored to the **flexor retinaculum (transverse carpal ligament)**, and its base (distally) ends opposite the metacarpophalangeal joints, where it divides at the roots of the fingers as 4 heavy, longitudinal bands or fiber slips, which fuse with the fibrous digital sheaths.

    3. Consists of 2 layers: the longitudinal and the transverse

        a. Longitudinal layer

            i. More superficial and represents an extension of the tendon of the palmaris longus to the fingers

            ii. Forms bands distally over the long flexor tendons and fuses to the fibrous digital sheaths

        b. Transverse layer

            i. Lies deeper and is attached to the flexor retinaculum

            ii. These fibers are especially prominent between the diverging longitudinal bands and extend as far distally as the heads of the metacarpals to form the **superficial transverse metacarpal ligament**

    4. Covers the long tendons of the digital muscles as they pass through the hand and also covers the arteries and nerves destined for the fingers: vessels and nerves escape from the aponeurosis to proceed to the web between each 2 digits before dividing to reach contiguous sides of the 2 digits

    5. Septa

        a. Extend from the deep aspect of the palmar aponeurosis in the distal part of the palm

        b. Form the sides of the anular fibrous canals for passage of the ensheathed flexor tendons and lumbrical muscles as well as the blood vessels and nerves

        c. Appear unattached on their deep aspect, but just distal to the ends of the midpalmar and thenar spaces; they actually attach to the deep transverse metacarpal ligament

        d. A particular septum, from the aponeurosis to the 3rd metacarpal bone, separates the **thenar space** (bursa) from the **midpalmar space** (bursa)

    6. Lateral edges of the palmar aponeurosis meet the deep fascia surrounding the thenar and hypothenar muscles

V. Cutaneous Nerves of the Palm of the Hand (Fig. 2.20D)

A. Median nerve (C5-8)

    1. Palmar branch: lateral side of the palm

    2. Palmar digital branches: lateral 3½ digits (including nail bed)

B. Ulnar nerve (C8, T1)

    1. Palmar branch: medial side of the palm

    2. Palmar branches: medial 1½ digits (including nail bed)

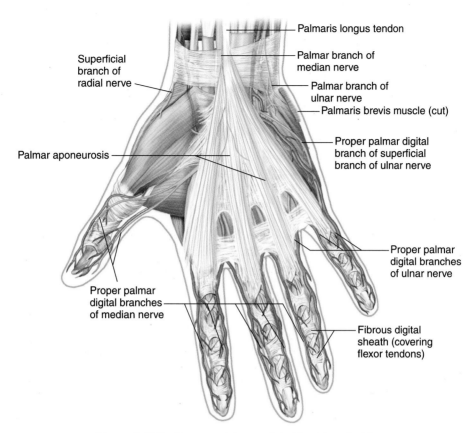

Palmaris longus tendon

Palmar branch of median nerve

Palmar branch of ulnar nerve

Palmaris brevis muscle (cut)

Proper palmar digital branch of superficial branch of ulnar nerve

Superficial branch of radial nerve

Palmar aponeurosis

Proper palmar digital branches of ulnar nerve

Proper palmar digital branches of median nerve

Fibrous digital sheath (covering flexor tendons)

Figure 2.20C. Cutaneous Nerves of the Hand. Anterior View.

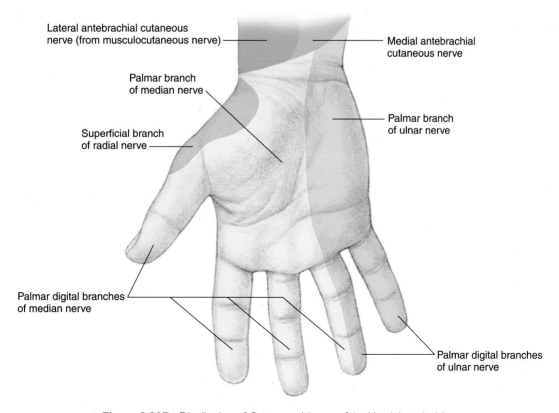

Lateral antebrachial cutaneous nerve (from musculocutaneous nerve)

Medial antebrachial cutaneous nerve

Palmar branch of median nerve

Palmar branch of ulnar nerve

Superficial branch of radial nerve

Palmar digital branches of median nerve

Palmar digital branches of ulnar nerve

Figure 2.20D. Distribution of Cutaneous Nerves of the Hand. Anterior View.

VI. Clinical Considerations

A. Simian crease is the single transverse palmar crease seen in the hand of people with Down syndrome

B. The skin is firmly bound to the underlying connective tissue and structures deep to it at the skin creases

   1. Thus, these are to be avoided in surgical incisions on the palmar surface of fingers

   2. In addition, scar tissue in the area of the creases may limit the range of motion (ROM)

C. The great majority of hand infections, excluding those of the fingers, are found in the hollow of the palm between or distal to the hypothenar and thenar eminences

D. Palmar aponeurosis

   1. Dupuytren contracture

      a. Often familial disease of unknown origin but with hereditary predisposition apparently involving many genetic factors

      b. Manifests as a progressive fibrosis, which typically produces abnormal bands of fibrous tissue that extend from the aponeurosis to the bases of the phalanges and pull 1 or more digits into marked flexion at the metacarpophalangeal joints so that they cannot be straightened

      c. May cause surprisingly little disability, but if the middle and index fingers are affected, the hand is virtually useless

   2. Thickness of the palmar aponeurosis prevents excessive swelling in the palm of the hand when the palmar spaces are filled with pus; instead, marked edema is evident in the loose subcutaneous tissue of the dorsum of the hand

Muscles of the Palmar Hand

I. Muscles of the Hand (Fig. 2.21A,B)

A. 1 muscle in the superficial palmar space; all others arranged in 4 compartments: thenar, hypothenar. central, and adductor-interosseous

B. Superficial palmar space (not within a compartment)

Muscle	Origin	Insertion	Action	Nerve
Palmaris brevis	Fascia overlying the hypothenar eminence	Skin of the palm near the ulnar border of the hand	Draws the skin of the ulnar side of the hand toward the center of the palm	Superficial ulnar (C8,T1)

C. Thenar compartment (muscles of the thumb)

Muscle	Origin	Insertion	Action	Nerve
Abductor pollicis brevis	Flexor retinaculum, scaphoid, trapezium	Base of the proximal phalanx of the 1st digit	Abducts thumb	Recurrent branch of the median (C8,T1)
Flexor pollicis brevis	Flexor retinaculum, trapezium	Proximal phalanx of the 1st digit	Flexes the carpometacarpal and metacarpophalangeal joints of the thumb	Recurrent branch of the median (C8,T1)
Opponens pollicis	Flexor retinaculum, trapezium	Shaft of the 1st metacarpal	Opposes the thumb	Recurrent branch of the median (C8,T1)

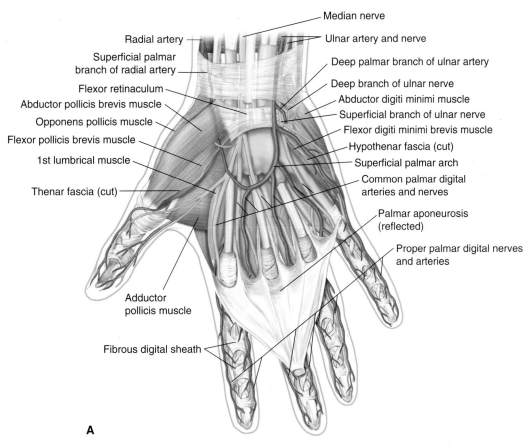

Figure 2.21A. Hand. Anterior View, Superficial Dissection.

D. Hypothenar compartment

Muscle	Origin	Insertion	Action	Nerve
Abductor digiti minimi	Pisiform	Base of the proximal phalanx of the 5th digit on its ulnar side	Abducts the 5th digit	Deep ulnar (C8,T1)
Flexor digiti minimi brevis	Hook of the hamate and the flexor retinaculum	Proximal phalanx of the 5th digit	Flexes the carpometacarpal and metacarpophalangeal joints of the 5th digit	Deep ulnar (C8,T1)
Opponens digiti minimi	Hook of the hamate and the flexor retinaculum	Shaft of the 5th metacarpal	Opposes the 5th digit	Deep ulnar (C8,T1)

E. Central compartment

Muscle	Origin	Insertion	Action	Nerve
Lumbricals 1 and 2	Radial side of flexor digitorum profundus tendons of digits 2–3	Extensor expansion on the radial side of the proximal phalanx of digits 2–3	Flex the metacarpophalangeal joints; extend the proximal and distal interphalangeal joints of digits 2–3	Median (C8,T1)
Lumbricals 3 and 4	Adjoining sides of flexor digitorum profundus tendons of digits 4–5	Extensor expansion on the radial side of the proximal phalanx of digits 4–5	Flex the metacarpophalangeal joints; extend the proximal and distal interphalangeal joints of digits 4–5	Deep ulnar (C8,T1)

F. Adductor-interosseous compartment (**Fig. 2.21C**)

Muscle	Origin	Insertion	Action	Nerve
Adductor pollicis	Oblique head: the capitate and the base of the 2nd and 3rd metacarpals Transverse the head: the shaft of the 3rd metacarpal	Base of the proximal phalanx of the thumb	Adducts the thumb	Deep ulnar (C8,T1)
Palmar interossei	3 muscles, arising from the palmar surface of the shafts of metacarpals 2, 4, and 5 (the palmar interosseous of the thumb is usually fused with the adductor pollicis muscle)	Base of the proximal phalanx and extensor expansion of the medial side of digit 2 and lateral side of digits 4 and 5	Flexes the metacarpophalangeal; extends proximal and distal interphalangeal joints and adducts digits 2, 4, and 5 (adduction of the digits of the hand is in reference to the midline of the 3rd digit)	Deep ulnar (C8,T1)
Dorsal interossei	4 muscles, each arising from 2 adjacent metacarpal shafts	Base of the proximal phalanx and the extensor expansion on lateral side of the 2nd digit, lateral and medial sides of the 3rd digit, and medial side of the 4th digit	Flex the metacarpophalangeal joint, extend the proximal and distal interphalangeal joints of digits 2–4; abduct digits 2–4 (abduction of digits in the hand is defined as movement away from the midline of the 3rd digit)	Deep ulnar (C8,T1)

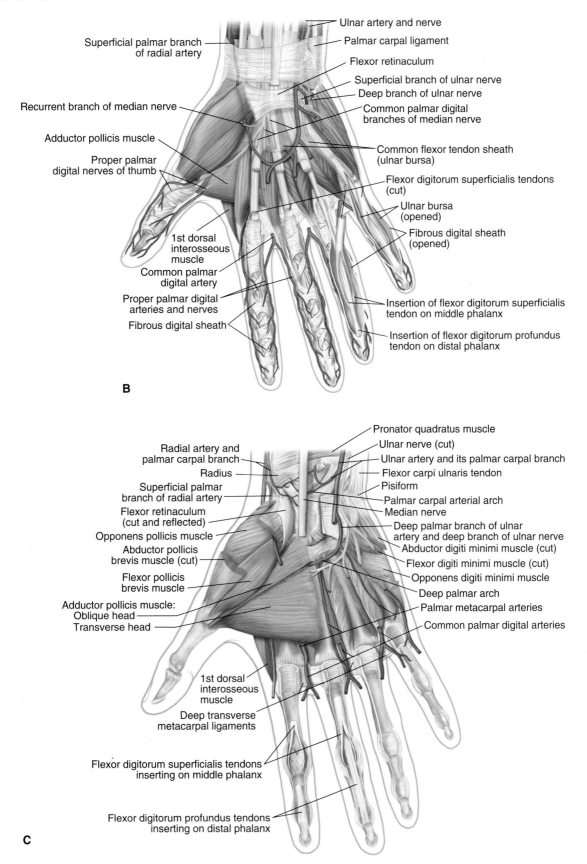

Figure 2.21 B,C. Hand. Anterior View. **B.** Intermediate Dissection. **C.** Deep Dissection.

II. Special Features (Fig. 2.21D–F)

A. Palmar interossei muscles adduct (member PAD) and dorsal interossei muscles abduct (member DAB) the digits, or they can flex the metacarpophalangeal joints and extend the interphalangeal joints, but they cannot do both at the same time

B. Lumbricals and interossei muscles are important in movements related to fine movements of the digits, such as typing, writing, and playing piano

III. Clinical Considerations

A. Recurrent branch of the median nerve supplies thenar muscles and lies quite superficial; thus, it can be severed by minor lacerations of the palm near the thenar eminence, making the thumb almost useless

B. An intact abductor pollicis longus and adductor pollicis can combine to imitate opposition if the median nerve is severed at the wrist

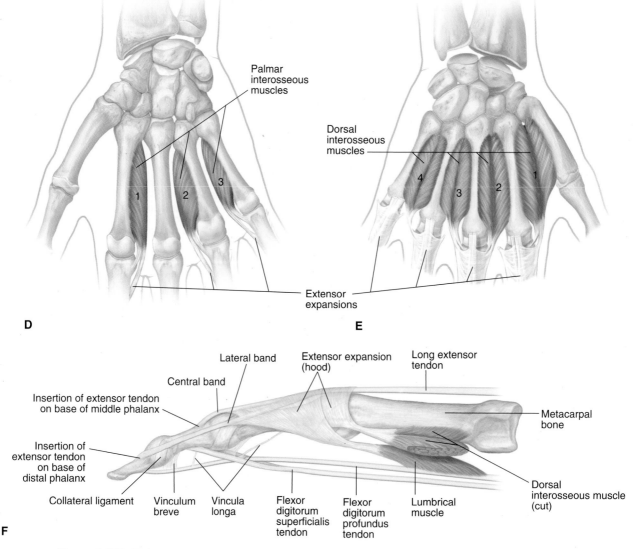

Figure 2.21D–F. Interosseous Muscles. **D.** Anterior View. **E.** Posterior View **F.** Extensor Expansion, Lateral View.

Vessels of the Hand

I. Ulnar Artery (Fig. 2.22A–C)

A. Passes anterior to the flexor retinaculum and terminates by dividing into deep and superficial branches near the hook of the hamate

B. Wrist branches of the ulnar artery

1. Dorsal carpal: passes deep to the flexor carpi ulnaris muscle, crosses the ulnar side of the wrist joint, and continues in a plane deep to the extensor carpi ulnaris to join a similar branch of the radial artery to form the **dorsal carpal arch**

2. Palmar carpal: joins with that of the radial to form the **palmar carpal arch**

3. Proper palmar digital: passes along the medial border of the 5th digit

4. Deep branch: passes between abductor digiti minimi and flexor digiti minimi muscles and then deep to the opponens digiti minimi to join the deep palmar arch

5. Superficial palmar arch

   a. Direct continuation of the ulnar artery

   b. Lies superficial to the tendons in the hand as well as lumbricals and distal to the deep palmar arch

   c. Branches of the ulnar and median nerves are deep to it

   d. Its branches are 3 **common palmar digital arteries**, which pass between the long flexor tendons and, at the finger webs, divide into 2 branches, the *proper palmar digital arteries*, 1 for each of the contiguous sides of the fingers

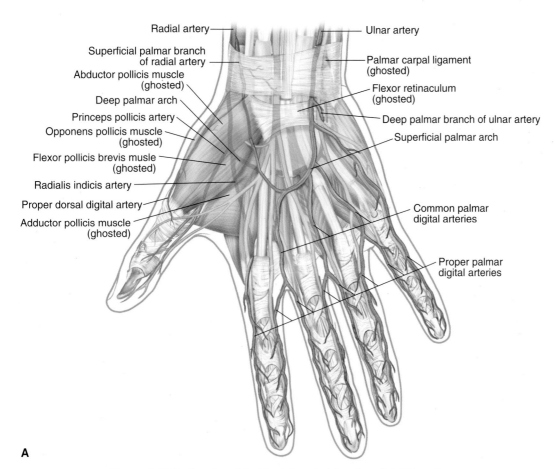

A

Figure 2.22A. Arteries of the Hand. Anterior View, Superficial Dissection.

II. Radial Artery

A. Crosses the distal end of the radius at the wrist and winds around trapezium and the 1st metacarpal bone to reach the dorsal surface; here it pierces the 1st dorsal interosseus muscle to reach the space between the 1st and 2nd metacarpal bones where it enters the palm between the oblique and transverse heads of the adductor pollicis muscle to become the **deep palmar arch** by joining a smaller deep branch of the ulnar artery

B. Wrist and hand branches of the radial artery
1. Palmar carpal: runs deep to flexor tendons and forms the anterior carpal arch by joining a similar branch from the ulnar artery
2. Superficial palmar: crosses the wrist through or superficial to the thenar muscles to terminate by helping to form the **superficial palmar arch**
3. Dorsal carpal: crosses the wrist and helps form the dorsal carpal arch with branches from ulnar and anterior interosseous arteries
   a. 3 dorsal metacarpal arteries arise from this network, course down on the 2nd, 3rd, and 4th interosseus muscles and then bifurcate into the dorsal digital branches of the middle, ring, and little fingers.
   b. These arteries communicate with palmar digital branches of the superficial palmar arch
4. 1st dorsal metacarpal:
   a. Arises before the radial enters the 1st dorsal interosseus muscle
   b. Divides into 2 dorsal digital branches to supply adjacent sides of the thumb and index finger
5. Princeps pollicis:
   a. Arises after the radial penetrates the 1st dorsal interosseous muscle
   b. Sends 2 branches to thumb on either side of the flexor pollicis longus tendon
6. Radialis indicis:
   a. Arises after the radial penetrates the 1st dorsal interosseous muscle
   b. Passes between the 1st dorsal interosseus and the transverse head of the adductor pollicis to supply the radial side of the index finger
7. Deep palmar arch:
   a. The continuation of the radial artery in the hand is the deep palmar arch
   b. It is joined by the deep branch of the ulnar artery
   c. 2 types of branches
      i. Recurrent branches: pass over the front of the wrist joint to anastomose with the palmar carpal arch
      ii. Palmar metacarpal branches (3): lie on the interosseous muscles of medial 3 spaces; each has perforating branches that pass through spaces between metacarpals to join dorsal metacarpal arteries and communicating branches that join the common palmar digital branches of the superficial arch before they bifurcate into proper palmar digital arteries

III. Veins

A. Venae comitantes accompany all arteries
B. Superficial and deep venous palmar arches associated with the superficial and deep palmar arterial arches drain into the deep veins of the forearm
C. Palmar and dorsal digital veins drain primarily to dorsal metacarpal veins, which drain into the dorsal venous network (arch), draining into cephalic and basilic veins

IV. Clinical Considerations

A. In cases of hand wounds involving arteries, extensive anastomoses make ligation of both ends of severed vessels necessary
B. Allen test: test for patency of radial and ulnar arteries or collateral circulation between them
1. Patient makes a tight fist, expressing the blood from the hand
2. Examiner then compresses either the radial or the ulnar artery and then has patient open the hand
   a. If the hand turns pinkish, the connection between and both vessels are patent
   b. If, on opening the hand blood fails to return to palm and fingers, the noncompressed artery is occluded or insufficient, and there is no collateral circulation between the two

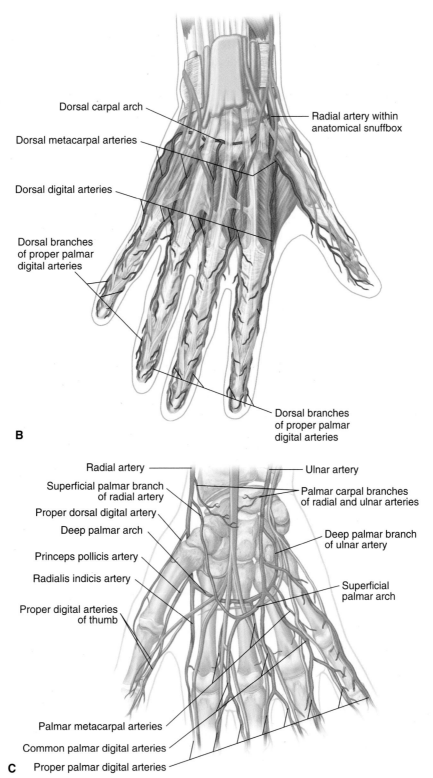

Dorsal carpal arch

Dorsal metacarpal arteries

Dorsal digital arteries

Dorsal branches of proper palmar digital arteries

Radial artery within anatomical snuffbox

Dorsal branches of proper palmar digital arteries

B

Radial artery

Superficial palmar branch of radial artery

Proper dorsal digital artery

Deep palmar arch

Princeps pollicis artery

Radialis indicis artery

Proper digital arteries of thumb

Ulnar artery

Palmar carpal branches of radial and ulnar arteries

Deep palmar branch of ulnar artery

Superficial palmar arch

Palmar metacarpal arteries

Common palmar digital arteries

C Proper palmar digital arteries

Figure 2.22B,C. Arteries of the Hand. **B.** Posterior View, Deep Dissection. **C.** Anterior View, Deep Dissection.

Nerves of the Hand

I. Median Nerve (C5-T1) (Fig. 2.23A)

A. Proximal to flexor retinaculum: gives the palmar cutaneous branch to the radial palm and then descends into the hand deep to the flexor retinaculum

B. Beneath flexor retinaculum: divides into a recurrent branch and 3 common palmar digital branches, which appear in the palm of the hand superficial to the tendons but deep to the superficial palmar arch

    1. Recurrent branch: motor to the 3 thenar eminence muscles (abductor pollicis brevis, flexor pollicis brevis, and opponens pollicis)

    2. Common palmar digital nerves

        a. 1st (radial-most) common palmar digital nerve passes on the anterior surface of the adductor pollicis muscle to trifurcate into proper digital branches for both sides of the palmar surface of the thumb as well as the radial surface of the index finger and the 1st lumbrical muscle

        b. 2nd and 3rd **common palmar digital nerves** pass on the surface of the 2nd and 3rd lumbrical muscles

            i. Supply the 2nd lumbrical muscle

            ii. Each of the **common palmar digitals** divides into 2 proper digital branches, which supply contiguous sides of the index and middle fingers and of the middle and ring fingers

II. Ulnar Nerve (C8,T1)

A. Proximal to the flexor retinaculum: gives the **dorsal cutaneous branch** to the back of the hand on the ulnar side and the **palmar cutaneous branch** to the palm and then enters the palm lateral to the pisiform and medial to the hook of the hamate on the anterior surface of the flexor retinaculum

B. On the flexor retinaculum: divides into superficial and deep branches

    1. Superficial branch: innervates the palmaris brevis muscle and then passes distally, where it divides into a proper and a common palmar digital branch

        a. Proper palmar digital branch supplies the medial (ulnar) side of the little finger

        b. Common palmar digital branch follows the 4th lumbrical muscle to the web between the ring and little fingers, where it divides into **proper digital branches** for contiguous sides of those fingers

    2. Deep branch: follows the deep branch of the ulnar artery between the abductor digiti minimi and flexor digiti minimi and deep to the opponens digiti minimi

        a. Supplies these muscles and crosses the palm with the deep palmar arch

        b. Gives branches to all interosseus muscles, 3rd and 4th lumbrical muscles, and joints and bones of the hand and terminates by supplying the oblique and transverse heads of the adductor pollicis muscle

III. Nerves of the Dorsum of the Hand: Sensory Only (Fig. 2.23B,C)

A. Superficial branch of the radial nerve

    1. Dorsum of the wrist and hand on the radial side

    2. Small portion of the thenar eminence

    3. Dorsal digital branches supply radial 2½ digits

B. Dorsal branch of the ulnar nerve

    1. Dorsum of the wrist and hand on the ulnar side

    2. Dorsal digital branches supply ulnar 2½ digits

C. Nail bed (dorsum over the distal phalanx): supplied by the proper palmar digital nerve

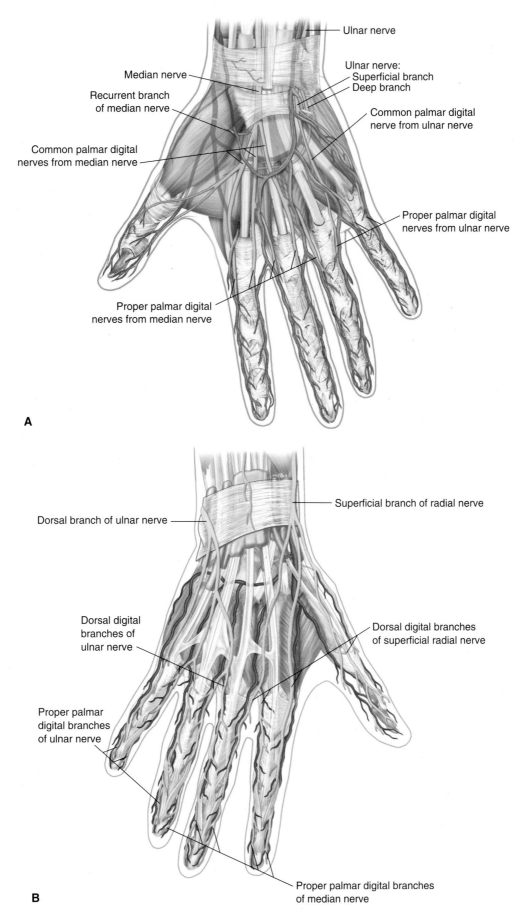

Ulnar nerve

Median nerve

Recurrent branch of median nerve

Ulnar nerve:
Superficial branch
Deep branch

Common palmar digital nerve from ulnar nerve

Common palmar digital nerves from median nerve

Proper palmar digital nerves from ulnar nerve

Proper palmar digital nerves from median nerve

A

Superficial branch of radial nerve

Dorsal branch of ulnar nerve

Dorsal digital branches of ulnar nerve

Dorsal digital branches of superficial radial nerve

Proper palmar digital branches of ulnar nerve

Proper palmar digital branches of median nerve

B

Figure 2.23A,B. Nerves of the Hand. **A.** Anterior View. **B.** Posterior View.

IV. Clinical Considerations

A. Knowledge of position of the proper digital nerves makes adequate nerve blocks possible for surgery of the digits

B. Recurrent branch of the median nerve usually arises just distal to the flexor retinaculum but may penetrate this ligament

C. Median nerve injury frequently occurs just proximal to the flexor retinaculum, the common site for suicide attempts

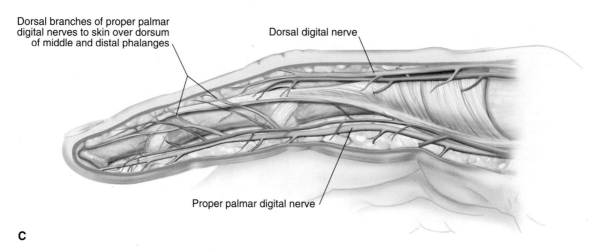

Dorsal branches of proper palmar digital nerves to skin over dorsum of middle and distal phalanges

Dorsal digital nerve

Proper palmar digital nerve

C

Figure 2.23C. Nerves of the Hand. **C.** Nerves of the Digits, Lateral View.

Articulations of the Shoulder and Pectoral Girdle

I. Pectoral (Shoulder) Girdle

A. Bones through which the upper extremity is attached to the trunk

B. Comprises 2 bones, the clavicle and scapula, joined to the axial skeleton (trunk) at the sternoclavicular joint and to each other via the acromioclavicular joint

C. Shoulder joint is between the scapula (glenoid cavity) and the head of the humerus

II. Articulations (Fig. 2.24A–C)

A. Acromioclavicular joint

   1. Type: arthrodial, plane type of synovial joint

   2. Bones: acromion of the scapula with the clavicle

   3. Movement: gliding, rotation of the scapula on the clavicle

   4. Ligaments

      a. Articular capsule completely surrounds articular areas

      b. Superior acromioclavicular covers joint superiorly

      c. Inferior acromioclavicular covers joint inferiorly

      d. Articular disc frequently absent or incomplete

      e. Coracoclavicular not part of joint but keeps the clavicle against the acromion

         i. Trapezoid from upper surface of the coracoid process to the trapezoid line on the inferior surface of the clavicle; limits rotation of the scapula

         ii. Conoid from the base of the coracoid process to the conoid tubercle on the inferior surface of the clavicle; limits the rotation of the scapula

B. Sternoclavicular joint

   1. Type: arthrodial, saddle type of synovial joint

   2. Bones: clavicle with the manubrium of sternum and cartilage of the 1st rib

   3. Movements: gliding, with some motion in almost any direction

   4. Ligaments

      a. Articular capsule surrounds articulation

      b. Anterior sternoclavicular: from the clavicle to the anterior surface of manubrium

      c. Posterior sternoclavicular: between posterior surfaces of the clavicle and the manubrium

      d. Interclavicular: joins the superior surface of the 2 clavicles across the sternal notch and limits depression of the shoulder

      e. Costoclavicular: from the 1st costal cartilage to the costal tuberosity on the inferior surface of the clavicle; limits elevation of the shoulder

      f. Articular disc: between the sternum and the clavicle and attached to the clavicle and sternum; helps limit depression of the shoulder

C. Glenohumeral joint (shoulder joint)

   1. Type: enarthrodial (ball and socket)

   2. Bones: spherical head of the humerus and the glenoid cavity of the scapula

   3. Movements: flexion, extension, abduction, adduction, medial rotation, lateral rotation, and circumduction

   4. Ligaments

      a. Articular capsule:

         i. From edge of the glenoid cavity and the glenoid labrum to the anatomical neck of the humerus

         ii. Strengthened by muscle tendons and glenohumeral bands or ligaments: anteriorly, the subscapular muscle; posteriorly, the infraspinatus and teres minor muscle; above, the supraspinatus muscle; below, the long head of the triceps

      b. Coracohumeral: from the coracoid to the greater tubercle

    c. Glenohumeral: usually 3 bands or ligaments representing thickenings of the anterior portion of the articular capsule
       i. From the medial side of the glenoid cavity to the lower part of the lesser tubercle
       ii. From the lower edge of the glenoid cavity to the lower anatomical neck
       iii. From above the glenoid rim near the root of the coracoid process along the medial side of biceps tendon to a depression above the lesser tubercle of the humerus
    d. Transverse humeral: bridges the intertubercular sulcus (groove)
    e. Glenoid labrum: fibrocartilage attached to edges of the glenoid cavity to deepen it and protect the bony margin; above, biceps tendon (long head) attaches to it
  5. Synovial membrane
    a. From the glenoid cavity over the labrum
    b. Lines inside of the capsule and is reflected on the anatomical neck to the articular cartilage
    c. Encloses the tendon of the long head of the biceps muscle in a tubular sheath, the intertubercular synovial sheath

III. Muscles Acting on the Shoulder Girdle

Elevation	Depression	Protraction[a]	Retraction[b]	Upward Rotation	Downward Rotation
Upper trapezius, levator scapulae, sternocleidomastoid, rhomboids	Subclavius, pectoralis minor, lower trapezius	Serratus anterior, pectoralis minor	Rhomboids, middle and lower trapezius	Upper and lower trapezius, serratus anterior	Levator scapulae, rhomboids, pectoralis major and minor, latissimus dorsi

[a]Protraction: drawing forward or anterior.
[b]Retraction: drawing backward or posterior.

IV. Muscles Acting on the Shoulder Joint

Flexion	Extension	Abduction	Adduction	Medial Rotation	Lateral Rotation
Pectoralis major (clavicular head)	Latissimus dorsi, teres major	Deltoid (as whole)	Pectoralis major (as whole)	Pectoralis major (as whole)	Infraspinatus, teres minor
Deltoid (anterior fibers), coracobrachialis, biceps	Deltoid (posterior fibers), triceps (long head)	Supraspinatus	Latissimus dorsi, teres major, subscapularis, triceps (long head)	Latissimus dorsi, teres major, subscapularis, deltoid (anterior fibers)	Deltoid (posterior fibers)

V. Pectoral Girdle and Shoulder: ROM

A. Sternoclavicular joint:
  1. Very stable and the only joint between the shoulder girdle and the axial skeleton
  2. Permits only a few degrees of movement in only 2 directions:
    a. The clavicle can be **flexed**, with its lateral end moving anteriorly as one reaches for an object
    b. The lateral end of the clavicle can be **elevated**, as with shrugging the shoulders
B. Acromioclavicular joint: is small and allows the scapula to move on the lateral end of the clavicle by rotating on 2 axes
  1. A **vertical axis,** whereby the glenoid cavity faces further forward (the reverse movement allows the glenoid to face laterally)
  2. A **horizontal axis,** allowing the glenoid to face upwards laterally (the reverse movement returns the glenoid back to normal, facing laterally and slightly forwards)

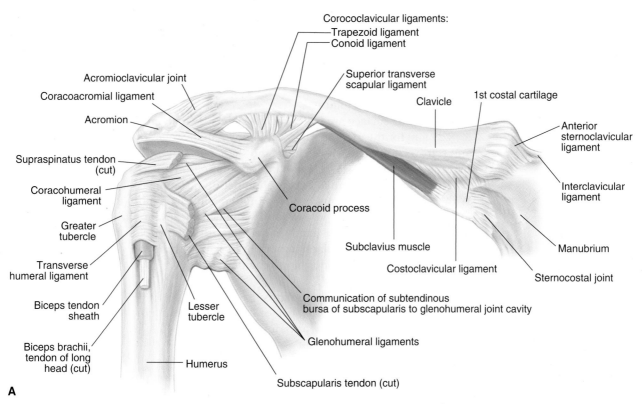

Figure 2.24A. Articulations of the Shoulder and Pectoral Girdle. Anterior View.

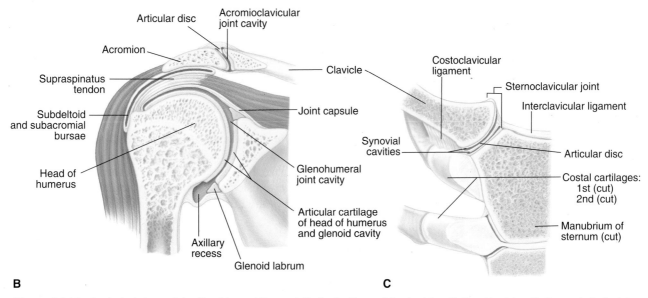

Figure 2.24A–C. Articulations of the Shoulder and Pectoral Girdle. **A.** Coronal Section View. **B.** Shoulder Joint. **C.** Sternoclavicular Joint

C. Shoulder (glenohumeral) joint ROM

Abduction[a]	Adduction	Flexion[a]	Extension	Internal Rotation	External Rotation	Circumduction
180°	45°–60°	180°	45°–50°	30°–90°	60°–90°	360°

[a]**Abduction and flexion:** are the result of glenohumeral motion (120°) in the early stage, and scapular rotation of 60° in the later stage: a 2:1 ratio. Acromioclavicular joint movement is responsible for the early portion of scapular rotation, and sternoclavicular movement is responsible for the later part.

D. Essentials of ROM: The shoulder
  1. Stability of the shoulder joint:
    a. Limited by the surface area of the humeral head, which measures 48 × 45 mm versus 35 × 25 mm for the glenoid cavity, and bony stability relies on the inclination of 125° and retroversion of 25° of the head and slight back-tilt of the glenoid cavity
    b. Associated ligaments (middle and inferior glenohumeral as well as the rotator cuff) are predominantly essential for the shoulder joint stability
    c. With extensive movements at the shoulder joint: ligaments that set a fixed limit to movement contribute little to joint stability; instead, muscles provide stability by keeping the humeral head firmly in contact with the glenoid cavity, in all positions
    d. The rotator cuff is particularly important in stability function
  2. Major muscle forces in shoulder biomechanics:
    a. Glenohumeral joint:
      i. Abduction: deltoid; supraspinatus
      ii. Adduction: latissimus dorsi, pectoralis major, teres major
      iii. Flexion: pectoralis major, anterior deltoid, biceps
      iv. Extension: latissimus dorsi
      v. Internal (medial) rotation: subscapularis, teres major
      vi. External (lateral) rotation: infraspinatus, teres minor, posterior deltoid
    b. Scapular motions:
      i. Rotation: upward: upper and lower trapezius, serratus anterior; downward: levator scapulae, rhomboids, pectoralis minor,
      ii. Retraction: trapezius, rhomboids, latissimus dorsi
      iii. Protraction: serratus anterior, pectoralis minor

VI. Clinical Considerations

A. Separated shoulder: disruption of the acromioclavicular joint
  1. Occurs with force exerted on the upper limb or acromion (the acromion usually passes inferior to the lateral end of the clavicle)
  2. May also stretch or rupture the coracoclavicular ligaments
B. Shoulder dislocation: displacement of the humeral head from the glenoid cavity
  1. Most of the strength of the glenohumeral joint is provided by the rotator cuff muscle tendons (supraspinatus, infraspinatus, teres minor, and subscapularis) that run above, behind, and in front of the capsule
  2. Weakest part is below, where dislocation is easier, especially when the arm is abducted; in this position, the humeral head breaks through the capsule below the glenoid cavity
C. Painful arc syndrome:
  1. Supraspinatus tendon is separated from the overlying acromion, the coracoacromial ligament, and the upper part of the deltoid muscle by the **subacromial bursa** (there may be a lateral subdeltoid bursa, but the two are usually fused)
  2. Calcium deposits in the tendinous floor of the bursa may cause disability of the shoulder, provoking a **bursitis**, which makes movements painful

Elbow Joint

I. Humeroulnar Joint (Fig. 2.25A–C)

A. Type: ginglymus (hinge)

B. Bones: trochlea of the humerus with the trochlear notch of the ulna, the capitulum of the humerus with the radial head

C. Movements: flexion and extension

D. Ligaments

1. Articular capsule
   a. In front: extends from the medial epicondyle and the front of the humerus above the coronoid and radial fossae to the anterior coronoid process, the anular ligament, and the collateral ligaments
   b. Behind: it extends from the humerus (behind capitulum) and the medial side of trochlea to the margins of the olecranon, the posterior part of ulna, and the anular ligament
2. Ulnar collateral extends from the front and back of the medial epicondyle to the medial side of the coronoid process and olecranon
3. Radial collateral extends from below the lateral epicondyle to the anular ligament and the lateral margin of the ulna

E. Synovial membrane: very extensive

1. Extends from margins of articular areas of the humerus
2. Lines the 3 fossae of the humerus and the inside of the capsule
   a. 3 fat pads exist between the synovia and the capsule: over the olecranon fossa, over the coronoid fossa, and over the radial fossa
   b. The former is pressed by the triceps muscle into the fossa during flexion
   c. The other 2 are pressed by the brachialis muscle into their fossae in extension of the forearm
3. Forms a sac between the head of the radius, the radial notch, and the anular ligament.

F. Muscles acting on the joint

Flexion	Extension
Biceps	Triceps
Brachialis	Anconeus
Brachioradialis	Extensor carpi radialis longus and brevis
Pronator teres	Extensor digitorum
Flexor carpi radialis and ulnaris	Extensor digiti minimi
Palmaris longus	Extensor carpi ulnaris
Flexor digitorum superficialis	Supinator

II. Radioulnar Joint

A. Proximal

1. Type: trochoid (pivot)
2. Bones: head of the radius and the radial notch of ulna
3. Movements: pronation and supination of the forearm
4. Ligaments
   a. Anular encircles the radial head, attached to ends of the radial notch
   b. Quadrate between the neck of the radius and the lower part of the radial notch of the ulna

B. Muscles acting on the proximal radioulnar joint

Supination	Pronation
Biceps and supinator	Pronator teres
Extensors of the thumb	Pronator quadratus

III. Elbow Joint

A. ROM (between the trochlea and the capitulum of the humerus and the notch of the ulna and the head of the radius)

Flexion	Extension	Pronation	Supination
135°ᵃ	0°–5°ᵃ	75°–90°ᵇ	80°–90°ᵇ

ᵃHyperflexion: 150°; hyperextension: 10°; functional ROM: 30° to 130°; axis of rotation is the center of the trochlea. Flexion and extension occurs essentially at the humeroulnar joint. Flexion is limited by contact between the forearm and arm; extension is limited by contact between the olecranon process and the floor of the olecranon fossa.
ᵇFunctional pronation and supination: 50°; axis of movement (defines a cone) is a line from the capitulum through the radial head and to the distal ulna. Pronation and supination occurs essentially at the superior radioulnar joint.

B. Essentials of the elbow joint ROM
1. The **carrying angle:** is normally "valgus" (angulation is away from the midline of the body, i.e., "bent out" at the elbow), due to the fact that the medial margin of the trochlea extends further distally than the capitulum, requiring the forearm to deviate slightly to the lateral side.
   a. Angle is approximately 7° in the male and 13° in the female (Note: the carrying angle decreases with flexion)
   b. The radial head provides about 30% of valgus stability and is more important in 0% to 30% of flexion and pronation
2. The elbow joint is a very stable joint: dislocation of the joint usually takes place in association with adjacent fractures
   a. Greatest stability comes from the medial side due to the medial collateral ligament, especially its anterior oblique fibers; it stabilizes the elbow to both valgus and distractional forces with the forearm flexion to about 90°
   b. In extension, the joint capsule is the primary restraint to distraction forces
   c. Laterally, the joint stability is essentially due to the lateral collateral ligament, the anconeus muscle, and the joint capsule
3. The elbow joint is the weight-bearing joint in patients with crutches
4. The elbow joint is the "fulcrum" (support around which a lever turns) for forearm lever; thus, in throwing something, it functions primarily as a means of transferring energy from the shoulder and trunk to the forearm and hand
5. Major muscle forces in the elbow joint biomechanics:
   a. Flexion: primarily the brachialis and biceps brachii (also brachioradialis and pronator teres)
   b. Extension: primarily the triceps (also the anconeus)
   c. Pronation: the pronators teres and quadratus
   d. Supination: the biceps brachii and the supinator (Note: because the biceps brachii inserts close to the joint, it is relatively inefficient and must support 3 times the weight of the arm and any objects held in the hand)

IV. Clinical Considerations

A. Because the ulna cannot be anteriorly dislocated without a concomitant fracture, most dislocations at the elbow are posterior; the ulnar nerve is frequently injured
B. Dislocation of the head of the radius alone is usually anterior and is common in children ("pulled elbow")
C. Carrying angle: long axis of the extended forearm lies at an angle of about 170° (male) and 167° (female) to long axis of arm; disappears when the elbow joint is fully flexed

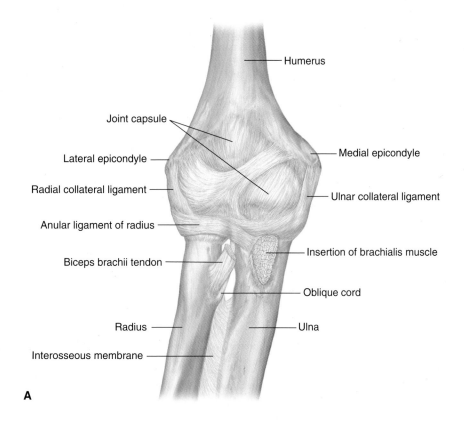

Humerus

Joint capsule

Lateral epicondyle

Radial collateral ligament

Anular ligament of radius

Biceps brachii tendon

Radius

Interosseous membrane

Medial epicondyle

Ulnar collateral ligament

Insertion of brachialis muscle

Oblique cord

Ulna

A

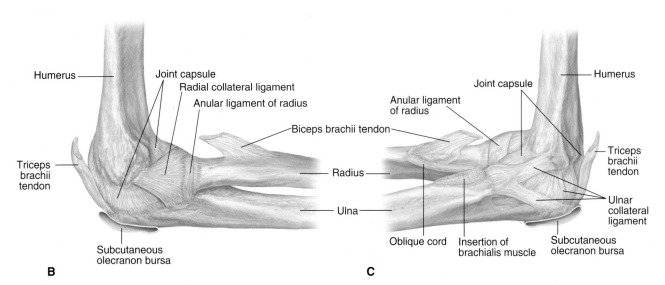

Humerus

Joint capsule

Radial collateral ligament

Anular ligament of radius

Biceps brachii tendon

Radius

Ulna

Triceps
brachii
tendon

Subcutaneous
olecranon bursa

B

Anular ligament
of radius

Joint capsule

Humerus

Triceps
brachii
tendon

Ulnar
collateral
ligament

Oblique cord

Insertion of
brachialis muscle

Subcutaneous
olecranon bursa

C

Figure 2.25A–C. Elbow Joint. **A.** Anterior View. **B.** Lateral View. **C.** Medial View.

Joints of the Wrist and Hand

I. Joints (Fig. 2.26A–E)

A. Radioulnar joint
1. Proximal: considered with the elbow joint
2. Middle: considered a syndesmosis; the shafts of the radius and ulna joined by the oblique cord and interosseous membrane
3. Distal:
   a. Type: trochoid (pivot)
   b. Bones: head of the ulna and the ulnar notch of radius
   c. Movements: rotation (pronation, supination)
   d. Ligaments
      i. Articular capsule with palmar and dorsal radioulnar ligaments
      ii. Articular disc
B. Wrist joint (radiocarpal articulation)
1. Type: condyloid
2. Bones: distal radius and articular disc with proximal row of carpals
3. Movements: flexion, extension, abduction, and adduction
4. Ligaments
   a. Palmar radiocarpal
   b. Dorsal radiocarpal
   c. Ulnar carpal collateral
   d. Radial carpal collateral
5. Muscles acting on the wrist joint

Flexion	Extension	Abduction	Adduction
Flexor carpi ulnaris	Extensor carpi radialis longus	Flexor carpi radialis	Flexor carpi ulnaris
Flexor carpi radialis	Extensor carpi radialis brevis	Extensor carpi radialis longus	Extensor carpi ulnaris
Palmaris longus	Extensor carpi ulnaris	Extensor carpi radialis brevis	Extensor indicis
Flexor digitorum superficialis	Extensor digitorum	Extensor pollicis longus	
Flexor digitorum profundus		Extensor pollicis brevis	

C. Intercarpal articulation
1. Articulations of carpals with each other: arthrodial joints with dorsal, palmar, and interosseous ligaments
2. Articulations between the 2 rows of carpals (the midcarpal joint): a hinge joint, acting with wrist; has dorsal, palmar, and collateral ligaments
D. Carpometacarpal joint
1. Between the 1st metacarpal and trapezium: a saddle joint, permitting flexion, extension, abduction, adduction, and opposition
2. All others between the distal row of carpals and bases of metacarpals: arthrodial, with dorsal, palmar, and interosseous ligaments
E. Intermetacarpal joints
1. Among bases of metacarpals: dorsal, palmar, and interosseous ligaments
2. Deep transverse metacarpal ligaments join heads of metacarpals
F. Metacarpophalangeal joints
1. Type: condyloid
2. Joined by 1 palmar and 2 collateral ligaments
G. Interphalangeal joints
1. Type: hinge
2. Joined by 1 palmar and 2 collateral ligaments

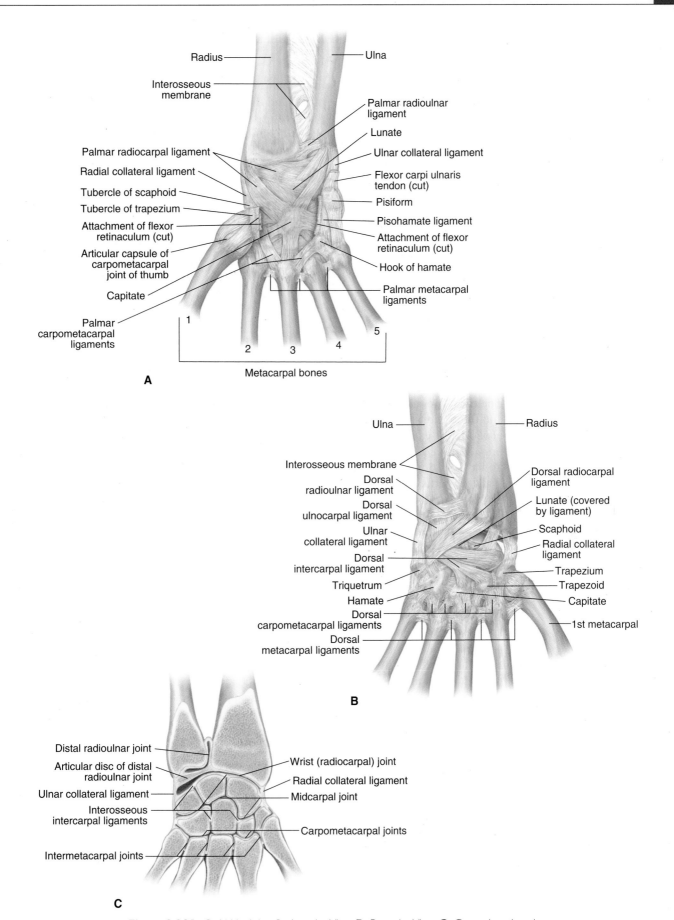

Radius

Ulna

Interosseous membrane

Palmar radioulnar ligament

Lunate

Palmar radiocarpal ligament

Ulnar collateral ligament

Radial collateral ligament

Flexor carpi ulnaris tendon (cut)

Tubercle of scaphoid

Tubercle of trapezium

Pisiform

Attachment of flexor retinaculum (cut)

Pisohamate ligament

Attachment of flexor retinaculum (cut)

Articular capsule of carpometacarpal joint of thumb

Hook of hamate

Capitate

Palmar metacarpal ligaments

Palmar carpometacarpal ligaments

1

5

2   3   4

Metacarpal bones

A

Ulna

Radius

Interosseous membrane

Dorsal radioulnar ligament

Dorsal radiocarpal ligament

Dorsal ulnocarpal ligament

Lunate (covered by ligament)

Ulnar collateral ligament

Scaphoid

Radial collateral ligament

Dorsal intercarpal ligament

Triquetrum

Trapezium

Hamate

Trapezoid

Dorsal carpometacarpal ligaments

Capitate

1st metacarpal

Dorsal metacarpal ligaments

B

Distal radioulnar joint

Articular disc of distal radioulnar joint

Wrist (radiocarpal) joint

Ulnar collateral ligament

Radial collateral ligament

Midcarpal joint

Interosseous intercarpal ligaments

Carpometacarpal joints

Intermetacarpal joints

C

Figure 2.26A–C. Wrist Joint. **A.** Anterior View. **B.** Posterior View. **C.** Coronal section view.

II. Essentials of ROM

A. Inferior radioulnar joint
1. Pronation:
   a. Head of the radius rotates within the anular ligament (superior radioulnar joint), whereas the distal end of the radius and the hand moves forward, the ulnar notch of the radius moving around the circumference of the head of the ulna
   b. Distal end of the ulna moves laterally, so the hand remains in line with the upper limb and is not medially displaced
2. Supination reverses the process, and the hand returns to its anatomical position (palm facing anteriorly)

B. Wrist (radiocarpal) joint

Flexion	Extension	Radial Deviation (Abduction)	Ulnar Deviation (Adduction)
65°–80°	55°–70°	15°–20°	30°–35°
Functional: 10°	Functional: 35°	Functional: 10°	Functional: 15°

The ulna is excluded from the wrist joint; thus, the radius carries the carpus and hand in pronation and supination.

Note: Movements take place in the radioulnar, radiocarpal, and intercarpal joints together. Major movements are flexion, extension, abduction, and adduction. The neck of the capitate is usually considered to be the axis around which the movements take place.

1. Head of the ulna is separated from the carpal bones by a fibrocartilaginous articular disc, which unites the radius and ulna
2. The carpal bones of the wrist joint, from lateral to medial, are the scaphoid, the lunate, and the triquetral
3. Flexion and extension are primarily radiocarpal (2/3), but intercarpal movement is important (1/3)
4. Radial deviation is primarily due to intercarpal movement
5. Ulnar deviation relies on radiocarpal and intercarpal motion
6. The instant center for wrist motion is the head of the capitate bone (but this is variable).
7. Distal radius normally bears about 80% of the distal radioulnar joint load and the distal ulna 20%

C. Joints of the hand
1. Metacarpophalangeal joints

Flexion	Extension	Abduction–Adduction
100°	0° (hyperextension: 0°–30°–40°)	20°–60°

   a. Stability of MP: provided by the volar plate and collateral ligaments
   b. Abduction: from the axial line through the middle finger
   c. Adduction: fingers come together and touch after abduction
2. Fingers (digits 2 to 5): Proximal interphalangeal joints

Flexion	Extension
100°–110°	0° (hyperextension: 20°)

3. Fingers (digits 2 to 5): Distal interphalangeal joints

Flexion	Extension
80°–90°	0°

4. Thumb

Joint	Flexion	Extension	Abduction–Adduction
Carpometacarpal	50°	50°	70°
Metacarpophalangeal	90°	0° Hyperextension: 30°	—
Interphalangeal	90°	0°	—

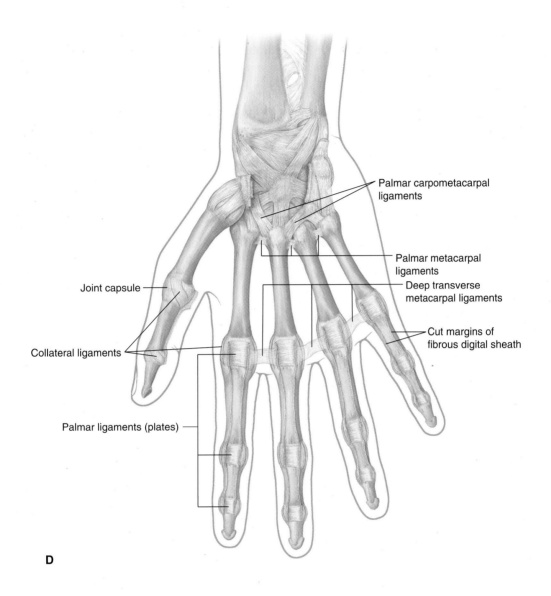

Palmar carpometacarpal
ligaments

Palmar metacarpal
ligaments

Deep transverse
metacarpal ligaments

Cut margins of
fibrous digital sheath

Joint capsule

Collateral ligaments

Palmar ligaments (plates)

D

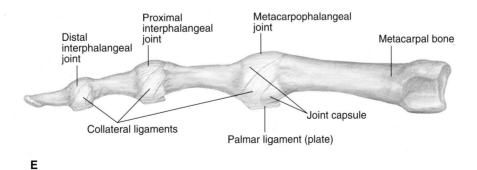

Distal
interphalangeal
joint

Proximal
interphalangeal
joint

Metacarpophalangeal
joint

Metacarpal bone

Collateral ligaments

Joint capsule

Palmar ligament (plate)

E

Figure 2.26. D. Hand and Digital Joints. Anterior View. **E.** Digital Joints. Lateral View.

5. The pulleys (the flexor sheath covering the flexor tendons forms 5 pulleys with 3 intervening cruciate attachments) in the hand prevent bowstringing and decrease tendon excursion
6. The hand "grasps" with the fingers flexing tightly around an object, and the thumb, by opposing, reinforces the grip outside of the flexed fingers
    a. Normal grasp of the hand for men is 50 kg and for women is 25 kg (Note: only about 4 kg is necessary for normal, everyday function)
    b. Normal pinch for men is 8 kg and for women is 4 kg (daily usage usually only requires about 1 kg)
    c. Compression at the thumb due to pinching includes 3 kg at the interphalangeal joint, 5 kg at the metacarpophalangeal joint, and 12 kg at the thumb carpometacarpal joint, which is an unstable joint susceptible to degeneration from these pressures
7. The hand is an important sense organ able to differentiate shapes, sizes, and textures as well as temperature changes
8. The hand is capable of precise movement, being capable of picking up small objects between its thumb and fingers (and between fingers) and can also make rapid as well as finely graded movements
9. The hand can bear the body weight (as in doing a handstand or pushup or pulling the body upward when grasping a bar); in addition, it can exert the full body weight by "pushing" light or heavy objects

III. Clinical Considerations: Wrist Arthrodesis

A. Surgical fixation of a joint to accomplish fusion of the joint surfaces
B. Unilateral fusion should position the joint in 10% to 20% dorsiflexion
C. Avoid bilateral fusion, but if necessary, the other wrist should be fused in a 0° to 10° position of palmar flexion

Specific Nerve Injury: Median Nerve (C5-T1)

I. Injury above the Elbow (Fig. 2.27A–C)

A. Muscles in arm are not involved; muscles in forearm and hand are involved because nerve supplies them only after it has entered the forearm

B. All flexors of wrist are out of action except the flexor carpi ulnaris and medial 2 tendons of the flexor digitorum profundus

    1. Flexion and abduction of wrist are considerably weakened but not abolished

    2. Thumb condition similar to nerve injury at the wrist, but the long flexor now is also paralyzed, and the thumb cannot flex at all (therefore, is practically useless); it can be used like a lobster claw to nip objects between its medial surface and index finger (intact adductor and 1st dorsal interosseus muscles)

    3. Long flexor tendons to index and middle fingers are paralyzed

        a. These fingers cannot be flexed at the interphalangeal joints, though flexion at the metacarpophalangeal joints is still possible due to the intact interossei (ulnar nerve)

        b. However, movement is greatly weakened due to loss of lumbricals 1 and 2

    4. Superficialis tendons to ring and little fingers are inoperable, but profundus tendons are intact, permitting flexion at all joints of these fingers

    5. Pronation in the forearm is impossible (pronators inoperable)

    6. Sensory loss is the same as that seen when the nerve is interrupted at the wrist

    7. The grip of such a hand is greatly deficient, though small objects can be held between the medial 2 fingers and the palm

        a. Nothing heavy can be carried

        b. Without the thumb, no precision grip is possible

        c. Hand is unable to do manual labor or be used in dressing

        d. Writing is possible with pen between the thumb and the index finger or between 2 fingers and using the shoulder muscles

II. Injury at the Wrist

A. Nerve is most vulnerable as it crosses the wrist just proximal to the flexor retinaculum (suicide attempts, putting the hand through a window, etc.); loss of function of the palmaris longus is not significant

B. Short muscles of the thumb will usually be put out of action with the exception of the adductor pollicis muscle (ulnar nerve)

C. The thumb, deprived of tone of short abductor, cannot abduct at right angles to the palm, and, due to loss of opponens pollicis, it cannot be opposed to fingers; it tends to be pulled into plane of the palm by the intact adductor and 1st dorsal interosseus

D. Thenar eminence is grossly wasted (atrophies with a flattened eminence, termed **ape hand**)

E. Long flexor of thumb is working (supplied by the median nerve in the forearm)

F. Lateral (radial) 2 lumbrical muscles are usually paralyzed, affecting the ability of the index and middle fingers to make independent movements, but their power is not much affected because the long flexors and interossei are still intact

G. Sensory loss

    1. Areas generally include the lateral side of the palm, the palmar surface of the thumb, index, middle, and 1/2 of ring finger, including the nail beds over the middle and terminal phalanges of these fingers

    2. Sense of joint movement is abolished in the interphalangeal joints of the thumb, index, and middle fingers but is partly compensated for by the activity of the stretch receptors in the flexor and extensor muscles

III. Carpal Tunnel Syndrome

A. Compression of the median nerve (due to inflammation of the flexor retinaculum, arthritis, or tenosynovitis) as it passes through the osseofibrous carpal tunnel along with the tendons of the long digital flexor muscles

B. Results in paresthesia (tingling), anesthesia (loss of tactile sensation), or hypesthesia (diminished sensation) in skin areas related to the thumb, index, middle, and lateral 1/2 of ring fingers

C. Palm may be saved due to the palmar cutaneous branch arising superficial to the flexor retinaculum

D. Progressive loss of strength and coordination in the thumb with diminished use of the thumb, index, and middle fingers as nerve is compressed

E. Relieved by partial or complete division of the flexor retinaculum

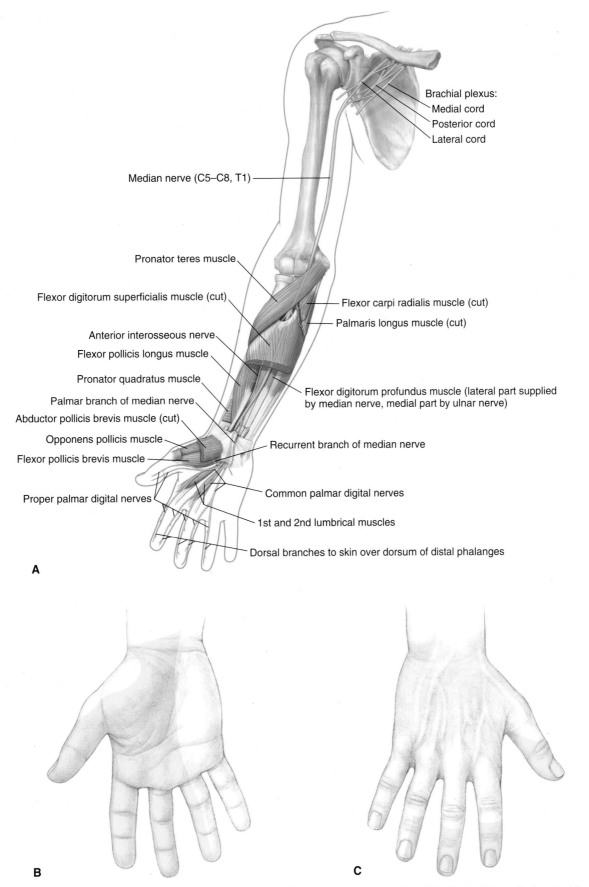

Brachial plexus:
Medial cord
Posterior cord
Lateral cord

Median nerve (C5–C8, T1)

Pronator teres muscle

Flexor digitorum superficialis muscle (cut)

Flexor carpi radialis muscle (cut)

Palmaris longus muscle (cut)

Anterior interosseous nerve

Flexor pollicis longus muscle

Pronator quadratus muscle

Flexor digitorum profundus muscle (lateral part supplied by median nerve, medial part by ulnar nerve)

Palmar branch of median nerve

Abductor pollicis brevis muscle (cut)

Opponens pollicis muscle

Recurrent branch of median nerve

Flexor pollicis brevis muscle

Common palmar digital nerves

Proper palmar digital nerves

1st and 2nd lumbrical muscles

Dorsal branches to skin over dorsum of distal phalanges

A

B

C

Figure 2.27A. Distribution of the Median Nerve. **A.** Anterior View. Cutaneous Distribution of the Median Nerve. **B.** Anterior View. **C.** Posterior View

Specific Nerve Injury: Ulnar Nerve (C8, T1)

I. Injury at the Wrist (Fig. 2.28A–C)

A. Hand takes up a striking and characteristic posture called a "**claw hand**"

B. Fingers are hyperextended at the metacarpophalangeal joints and flexed at the interphalangeal joints because of paralysis of the interossei and medial 2 lumbrical muscles

   1. This upsets the balance of strength (power) on these joints

   2. The 2 radial fingers are less flexed at the interphalangeal joints than the 2 medial ones because the 2 lateral lumbricals are usually intact, being innervated by the median nerve

C. Tendons of the flexor digitorum profundus to the 2 medial fingers are paralyzed, so no flexion is possible at the distal interphalangeal joints of the ring and little fingers, but the superficialis tendons are operable (median nerve), so the proximal interphalangeal joints can be flexed

D. Small muscles of the little finger are all paralyzed and wasted, but the small muscles of the thumb are intact except for the adductor pollicis (in 10% of the population, they are all paralyzed because the ulnar nerve also supplies the thenar muscles)

E. Adduction and abduction of the fingers is impaired due to paralysis of the interossei, muscles

   1. Adduction of the thumb is lost, but other movements are normal

   2. Interosseous spaces are empty of their muscles due to atrophy, and metacarpal bones protrude under the skin

F. Produces a sensory change in the medial part of the hand and in the ring and little fingers

G. Tests for ulnar weakness

   1. Have patient abduct the little finger against resistance (abductor digiti minimi)

   2. Grip a card between the finger and the thumb without bending the tip of the finger (tests adductor pollicis and 1st dorsal interosseus muscles)

II. Injury at or near the Elbow

A. The shoulder and elbow are unaffected because the ulnar innervates no muscles in the arm

B. Injuries here paralyze the flexor carpi ulnaris and the medial portion (ulnar 1/2) of the flexor digitorum profundus

   1. Ulnar deviation of the wrist is weakened, and the hand is slightly extended and abducted in position

   2. Motor loss is predominantly one of fine movements of the fingers, as described above, with injury at the wrist

   3. Impaired flexion and adduction of the wrist with impaired movement of the thumb, ring, and little fingers

   4. Inability to abduct and adduct the medial 4 digits due to loss of strength of the interossei muscles

   5. The fingers can still be flexed, and the grip is strong except for the 2 medial fingers

   6. Heavy tools can be carried and used, but sewing or knitting, piano playing, writing, etc., are difficult, even though it is possible to oppose the thumb to the fingers

C. Sensory loss in ulnar nerve paralysis is not of great importance and involves the 2 least important fingers and the medial side of the palm

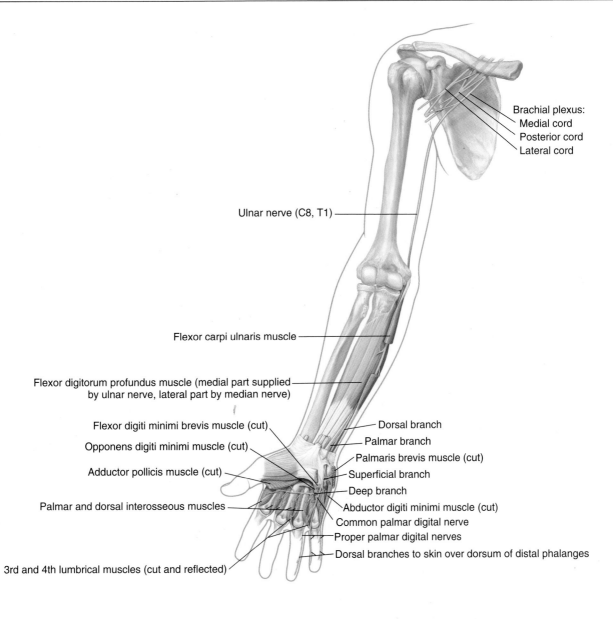

Brachial plexus:
Medial cord
Posterior cord
Lateral cord

Ulnar nerve (C8, T1)

Flexor carpi ulnaris muscle

Flexor digitorum profundus muscle (medial part supplied by ulnar nerve, lateral part by median nerve)

Flexor digiti minimi brevis muscle (cut)

Opponens digiti minimi muscle (cut)

Adductor pollicis muscle (cut)

Palmar and dorsal interosseous muscles

3rd and 4th lumbrical muscles (cut and reflected)

Dorsal branch

Palmar branch

Palmaris brevis muscle (cut)

Superficial branch

Deep branch

Abductor digiti minimi muscle (cut)

Common palmar digital nerve

Proper palmar digital nerves

Dorsal branches to skin over dorsum of distal phalanges

A

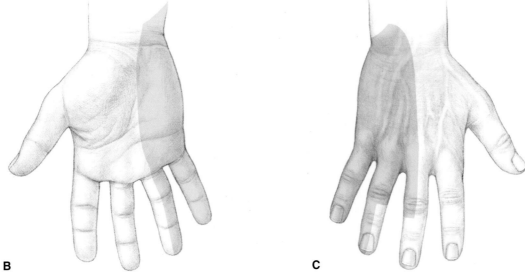

B   **C**

Figure 2.28A–C. Distribution of the Ulnar Nerve. **A.** Anterior View. Cutaneous Distribution of the Ulnar Nerve. **B.** Anterior View. **C.** Posterior View.

Specific Nerve Injury: Radial Nerve (C5-T1)

I. Injury Proximal to Origin of the Triceps Muscle (Fig. 2.29A,B)

A. Paralysis of the triceps muscle (the elbow is flexed and cannot be extended against resistance, but extremity hangs down straight at side due to gravity overcoming the tone of the flexors); absence of the triceps reflex; and paralysis of the brachioradialis, supinator (supination, however, is only weakened, not abolished, because the biceps is still functional), and extensors of the wrist, thumb, and fingers (the wrist is flexed, the forearm is pronated, the thumb is flexed and adducted, and there is a tendency for the fingers to be flexed, but not severely, due to loss of the extensor digitorum)

B. Characteristic clinical sign is **wrist drop,** in which the hand is flexed at the wrist and lies flaccid with an inability to extend the hand at the wrist and digits at the metacarpophalangeal joints, and lateral movements of the hand are difficult because the ulnar and radial extensors are paralyzed

C. Adducted position of the thumb and position of the already-flexed hand make flexion of the fingers difficult; the thumb cannot be extended or abducted because of paralysis of the abductor pollicis longus and extensor pollicis longus and brevis

D. Interphalangeal joints can be weakly extended via action of the intact lumbrical and interossei muscles (median and ulnar nerves)

E. While the hand is in its "dropped" position, the metacarpophalangeal joints are not flexed, as might be expected, but extended, due to passive stretching of the extensor tendons by the flexion of the wrist
   1. Grip is poor as a result
   2. When the wrist is passively dorsiflexed, the metacarpophalangeal joints flex under the pull of the flexor muscles, and the hand curls up with the thumb coming across the palm
      a. In this, position, the flexor muscles can take firm hold of anything put in their grasp, and the hand becomes useful
      b. Thus, by wearing a "cork-up" splint, dorsiflexion can be obtained, but the hand is not fully functional because the fingers cannot open properly to get hold of their objective, which must be placed into the hand between the half-closed fingers

F. The bulge of the dorsal forearm group of muscles (extensor-supinator group) is flattened or hollowed

G. Absence of the periosteal reflex on tapping of the radius

H. Results in anesthesia of the dorsolateral aspects of the distal end of the arm, the posterior surface of the forearm, the dorsum of the hand, and proximal phalanges on the radial side
   1. The radial nerve has only a small region of exclusive cutaneous supply on the hand, and the extent of anesthesia is minimal even in serious nerve injury (confined to a small area on the lateral aspect of the dorsum of the hand)
   2. Note: the radial nerve supplies no muscles in the hand itself

II. Injury in the Radial Groove

A. Most likely site of injury, where the nerve is affected by a fracture of the humerus; does not normally affect branches to the triceps because these come off very early in the course of the nerve

B. Total paralysis of extensor muscles of the forearm and hand results
   1. Inability to extend the hand at the wrist indicates damage of the nerve proximal to the elbow
   2. Extension of wrist is impossible (see I.B), and the hand assumes a flexed position (see discussion above)

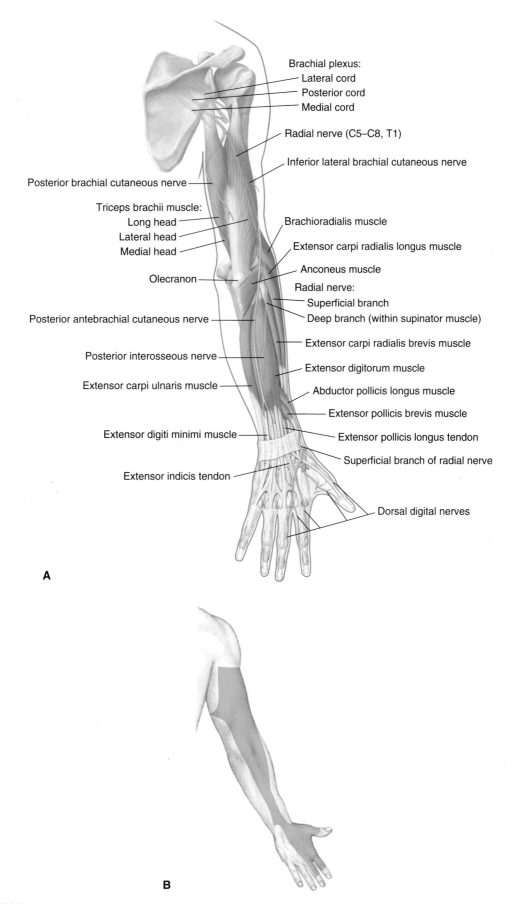

Figure 2.29A,B. A. Distribution of the Radial Nerve. Posterior View. **B.** Cutaneous Distribution of the Radial Nerve. Posterior View.

   3. Sensory loss
      a. May be minimal because the area of exclusive radial supply is small due to overlapping innervation
      b. Sensory loss on the back of the arm and the forearm is not vital

III. Injury in the Forearm

   A. Deep wounds may injure the deep radial nerve as it passes through the supinator muscle
   B. Results in inability to extend the thumb as well as the metacarpophalangeal joints of the fingers
   C. No loss of sensation occurs because the deep radial nerve is entirely a muscular and articular nerve
   D. Nerve supply to the extensor carpi radialis longus is intact (arises from the radial before its superficial and deep branches), as is that of the supinator and extensors

Lower Limbs

3.1	Introduction to the Lower Limb	150
3.2	Cutaneous Innervation of the Lower Limb	152
3.3	Superficial Veins and Deep Fascia of the Lower Limb	155
3.4	Lymphatic Drainage of the Lower Limb	158
3.5	The Pelvic Girdle	160
3.6	Articulations of the Pelvic Girdle	164
	Bones of the Thigh	166
3.8	Bones of the Leg	169
9	Bones of the Ankle and Foot	172
3.10	Compartments of the Thigh	176
3.11	Muscles of the Anterior Thigh	178
3.12	Femoral Triangle and Femoral Sheath	180
3.13	Muscles of the Medial Thigh	182
3.14	Femoral and Obturator Vessels and Nerves	184
3.15	Muscles of the Gluteal Region	188
3.16	Vessels and Nerves of the Gluteal Region	190
3.17	Muscles of the Posterior Thigh	194
3.18	Popliteal Region and Anastomosis Around the Knee	196
3.19	Compartments of the Leg	198
3.20	Muscles of the Posterior Leg	200
3.21	Muscles of the Lateral and Anterior Leg	204
3.22	Vessels and Nerves of the Leg	207
3.23	Dorsum of the Foot	211
3.24	Plantar Aponeurosis and Cutaneous Nerves of the Sole of the Foot	214
3.25	Muscles of the Sole of the Foot	216
3.26	Vessels and Nerves of the Sole of the Foot	220
3.27	The Hip Joint	222
3.28	The Knee Joint	226
3.29	Bursae of the Knee Joint and the Tibiofibular Joints	233
3.30	Joints of the Ankle and Foot	236
3.31	Arches of the Foot	242
3.32	Disorders of the Feet	244
3.33	Walking (Bipedal Locomotion), Part 1	246
3.34	Walking (Bipedal Locomotion), Part 2	248
3.35	Walking (Bipedal Locomotion), Part 3	250
3.36	Nerve Injuries in the Lower Limb	254

Introduction to the Lower Limb

I. Organ of Locomotion

A. Joints, especially hip, emphasize stability rather than mobility

II. General Organization (Fig. 3.1A–D)

A. Pelvic girdle (hip girdle)
  1. Paired bones (os coxae) that articulate with sacrum behind and with each other anteriorly at pubic symphysis
  2. Each coxal (hip) bone is formed by fusion of 3 bones: ilium, ischium, and pubis
B. Hip
  1. Extends from the iliac crest to the greater trochanter
  2. Contains powerful muscles for hip movements
C. Thigh
  1. Extends from hip to knee
  2. 1 bone: femur
  3. 3 compartments
    a. Anterior: flexors
    b. Posterior: extensors
    c. Medial: adductors
  4. Femoral triangle
    a. Bounded by sartorius, inguinal ligament, and adductor longus
    b. Contains the femoral nerve, artery, and vein
D. Knee
  1. Primarily the joint between femoral and tibial condyles
  2. Patella and fibula also involved
E. Leg
  1. Extends from knee to ankle
  2. 2 bones: fibula (lateral) and tibia (medial)
  3. 4 compartments
    a. Anterior: dorsiflexors
    b. Lateral: evertors
    c. Posterior (subdivided into superficial and deep compartments): plantarflexors
  4. Popliteal fossa: space posterior to knee
F. Ankle
  1. Medial and lateral malleoli form the mortise joint with talus
G. Foot
  1. Skeleton of the foot consists of 7 tarsal bones, 5 metatarsal bones, 14 phalanges
  2. Arches protect neurovascular structures on plantar surface (sole)

III. General Relations

A. In erect position, the coccyx, pubic crest, middle of acetabulum, head of the femur, and tip of the greater trochanter are all in the same horizontal plane
B. Femoral artery can be compressed by pressing directly backward at the midinguinal point
C. Lowest level of the knee joint is at a level at the margins of the tibial condyles (about 1 cm below the apex of the patella).
D. Highest level of the ankle joint is about 1 cm above the tip of the medial malleolus
E. Medial edge of the sustentaculum tali is about 2 to 3 cm below the tip of the medial malleolus
F. Transverse tarsal joint is indicated by a line from the back of the tuberosity of the navicular to a point halfway between the lateral malleolus and tuberosity of the 5th metatarsal bone
G. Nélaton line joins the anterior superior iliac spine to the most prominent part of the ischial tuberosity
  1. Tip of the greater trochanter should lie on this line or just below
  2. If the tip lies above, it indicates an upward displacement of the trochanter, due to either dislocation of the hip joint or neck fracture of the femur (common in elderly people)

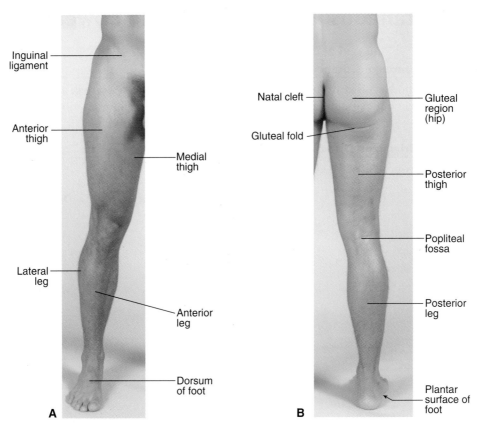

Figure 3.1A,B. Surface Anatomy of the Lower Limb. **A.** Anterior View. **B.** Posterior View.

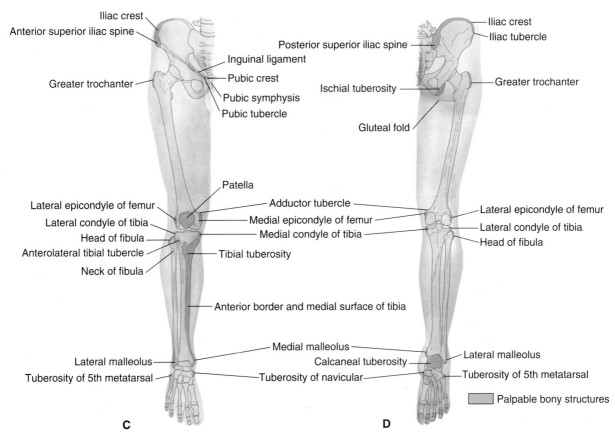

Figure 3.1C,D. Palpable Features of the Lower Limb. **C.** Anterior View. **D.** Posterior View.

Cutaneous Innervation of the Lower Limb

I. Source of Cutaneous Nerves

A. Lumbar plexus: anterior and medial thigh, upper anterior leg, and medial leg

B. Sacral plexus: lower buttocks, posterior thigh and leg, lower anterior leg, and foot

C. Posterior rami of lumbar and sacral nerves: upper buttocks

II. Origin and Distribution (Fig. 3.2A,B)

A. From lumbar plexus (L1-4)

Nerve	Spinal Component	Distribution to Lower Limb
Iliohypogastric	LI	
Lateral cutaneous branch		Lateral gluteal region
Ilioinguinal	LI	Upper medial thigh
Genitofemoral	LI, L2	
Genital branch		Upper medial thigh
Femoral branch		Upper anterior thigh
Lateral femoral cutaneous[a]	L2, L3	Lateral and anterolateral thigh
Obturator	L2-4	Medial thigh, just above knee
Femoral		
Anterior cutaneous branches	L2, L3	Anterior and anteromedial thigh
Saphenous	L3, L4	Medial side of knee, leg, ankle

[a]Meralgia paresthetica common disorder due to compression of the lateral femoral cutaneous nerve as it passes deep to the inguinal ligament. Due to obesity, weight loss, constrictive clothing, heavy tool belt, or object carried on a belt. Symptoms: burning, tingling, or anesthesia on the proximal lateral thigh.

B. From sacral plexus (L4-S3)

Nerve	Spinal Component	Distribution to Lower Limb
Posterior femoral cutaneous	SI-3	Lower buttock, posterior thigh
Inferior cluneal branches		Lower buttock
Perineal branch		Upper medial thigh
Sural	S1, S2	Posterior leg, lateral side and the dorsum of the foot
Lateral sural cutaneous	S1, S2	Lateral side of the leg
Medial calcaneal	S1, S2	Heel
Medial plantar	L4, L5	Sole of the foot, adjacent sides first 4 toes
Lateral plantar	S1, S2	Lateral sole of the foot, sides of toes 4 and 5
Deep fibular	L4, L5	Adjacent sides of the dorsum, toes 1 and 2
Superficial fibular	L4, L5, SI	Anterior lower leg and ankle, the dorsum of the foot, adjacent sides toes 1–4

C. From posterior rami of lumbar and sacral nerves

Nerve	Spinal Component	Distribution to Lower Limb
Superior cluneal	LI-3	Upper buttock
Middle cluneal	SI-3	Medial aspect of buttock

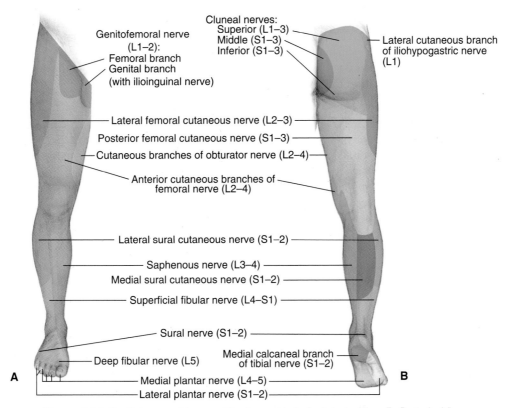

Genitofemoral nerve
(L1–2):
Femoral branch
Genital branch
(with ilioinguinal nerve)

Cluneal nerves:
Superior (L1–3)
Middle (S1–3)
Inferior (S1–3)

Lateral cutaneous branch
of iliohypogastric nerve
(L1)

Lateral femoral cutaneous nerve (L2–3)

Posterior femoral cutaneous nerve (S1–3)

Cutaneous branches of obturator nerve (L2–4)

Anterior cutaneous branches of
femoral nerve (L2–4)

Lateral sural cutaneous nerve (S1–2)

Saphenous nerve (L3–4)

Medial sural cutaneous nerve (S1–2)

Superficial fibular nerve (L4–S1)

Sural nerve (S1–2)

Deep fibular nerve (L5)

Medial calcaneal branch
of tibial nerve (S1–2)

Medial plantar nerve (L4–5)

Lateral plantar nerve (S1–2)

A   **B**

Figure 3.2A,B. Cutaneous Nerves of the Lower Limb. **A.** Anterior View. **B.** Posterior View.

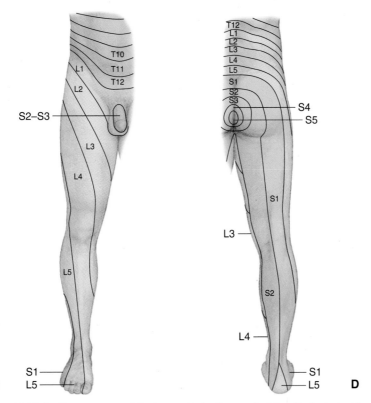

C   **D**

Figure 3.2C,D. Dermatomes of the Lower Limb. **C.** Anterior View. **D.** Posterior View.

III. Dermatomes (Fig. 3.2C,D)

A. Definition: specific skin areas supplied by specific spinal nerves, regardless of the named cutaneous nerves that are distributed to the same general territory

B. Arrangement: dermatomes of the lower extremity are related to the development of the limb; their spiral course in the lower extremity is an expression of the rotation of the limb as an adaptation to the erect position

IV. Clinical Considerations

A. Dermatomes: numbness in certain dermatomes can be related to definite spinal cord levels; thus, a lesion in the central nervous system (CNS) can be located readily

B. Spinal-vertebral segments: patient with numbness between the hallux and second toe and anterolateral leg may have a lesion in the 5th lumbar spinal nerve or dorsal root ganglion

    1. Most frequently the herniated intervertebral disc is at L4/L5, which often affects the L5 spinal nerve

    2. Recall that the L5 spinal cord segment lies at the level of the 11th thoracic vertebra

Superficial Veins and Deep Fascia of the Lower Limb

I. General Features

A. Superficial veins lie between the layers of the superficial fascia; valves are more numerous in the veins of the lower extremity than they are in the upper

B. Dorsal digital veins run along the two dorsal margins of each toe and unite at the webs of the toes to form **dorsal metatarsal veins**, which empty into the **dorsal venous arch** (overlies metatarsal bones and lies in the subcutaneous tissue)

   1. Arch receives communications from the plantar venous arch
   2. Proximally, it is connected with the irregular dorsal venous network of the foot

II. Specific Veins (Fig. 3.3A,B)

A. Great saphenous vein: longest vein in body

   1. Origin: medial side of the dorsal venous arch of the foot (accompanied by the saphenous nerve inferior to the knee)
   2. Course: ascends in front of the medial malleolus, along the medial side of the leg, behind the medial condyles of tibia and the femur, along the medial side of the thigh to the saphenous hiatus, where it pierces the cribriform fascia, and the femoral sheath
   3. Termination: in femoral vein about 3.75 cm before the inguinal ligament
   4. Tributaries
       a. Superficial external pudendal from the genital area
       b. Superficial circumflex iliac from the upper lateral thigh
       c. Superficial epigastric from abdomen, has communication with lateral thoracic vein by way of thoracoepigastric vein
       d. Variable number of other unnamed tributaries from the foot, leg, and thigh

B. Small saphenous vein

   1. Origin: lateral side of the dorsal venous arch of the foot
   2. Course: from behind the lateral malleolus along the lateral side of tendo calcaneus (Achilles), crosses the latter to middle of back of the leg, runs straight upward to pierce the deep fascia in the lower popliteal space
   3. Termination: in popliteal vein between heads of gastrocnemius muscle
   4. Tributaries: especially from the lateral foot and leg, send communication upward to join great saphenous vein

III. Clinical Considerations

A. Varicose veins: abnormal dilation and loss of valvular competence in superficial veins of lower extremity, especially the great saphenous system

1. Prevalent in the lower limb because of the great weight of the long column of blood (heart to foot)
   a. Because venous blood flow depends on muscular movement, longstanding or increased pressure on the more caudal part of the system (as in pregnancy) causes venous stasis
   b. This, in turn, causes walls to dilate in regions of the numerous valves
2. To relieve this condition, superficial veins can be ligated, stripped, etc., without interference with venous return because of the numerous communications with the deep veins

B. Venipuncture: great saphenous vein, especially its lower end, is often used for emergency access to a large vein

1. "Saphenous vein cutdown" is made about 1.25 cm anterior to the medial malleolus (when necessary, the cephalic portion may be used, although here it may be embedded in fat)
2. Proximal site is often described as 2 fingerbreadths medial and 1 fingerbreadth below the pubic tubercle
3. Another method of finding the vein is given as 1 fingerbreadth below the inguinal ligament just medial to the point where the pulsating femoral artery can be palpated

C. Vein grafts: great saphenous vein is often used for coronary bypass procedures

D. Saphenous nerve accompanies the great saphenous vein anterior to the medial malleolus; if trapped by a ligature in a saphenous vein cutdown, the patient may complain of pain along the medial side of the foot

E. Thrombophlebitis: marked inflammation of a vein with secondary thrombus or clot formation

1. May destroy valves of the deep veins, resulting in varicosities
2. May lead to a traveling thrombus and eventual pulmonary embolus

F. Phlebothrombosis: inflammatory element is mild, and the thrombosis takes the form of a loosely attached clot, originating peripherally and propagating centrally

IV. Fascia of the Lower Limb

A. Superficial fascia

1. Continuous with that of the abdomen; the deeper, membranous layer of the superficial fascia of the abdomen attaches to the fascia lata just below the inguinal ligament
2. Cribriform fascia: deep layer of the superficial fascia located over the saphenous hiatus (fossa ovalis)

B. Fascia lata: tubular deep fascial investment of the thigh; attached above to the os coxae and inguinal ligament and below is continuous with the crural fascia of the leg

1. Iliotibial tract: thickened part of the fascia lata overlying vastus lateralis
   a. Forms an envelope for the tensor fasciae latae muscle
   b. Attachment of most of gluteus maximus fibers
   c. Inserts onto lateral tibial condyle
2. Saphenous hiatus (fossa ovalis): passageway through the fascia lata in the upper medial thigh for great saphenous vein and superficial lymphatic channels, which penetrate the cribriform fascia covering the saphenous hiatus

C. Crural fascia: deep fascia of the leg, forming a tubular investment

1. Popliteal fascia: continuous with the fascia lata above and the crural fascia below; covers popliteal fossa
2. Patellar retinacula: crural fascia blends with vastus aponeurotic fibers to form medial and lateral patellar retinacula
3. Extensor, flexor, and fibular retinacula: thickenings of the crural fascia at the ankle that prevent bowstringing of tendons

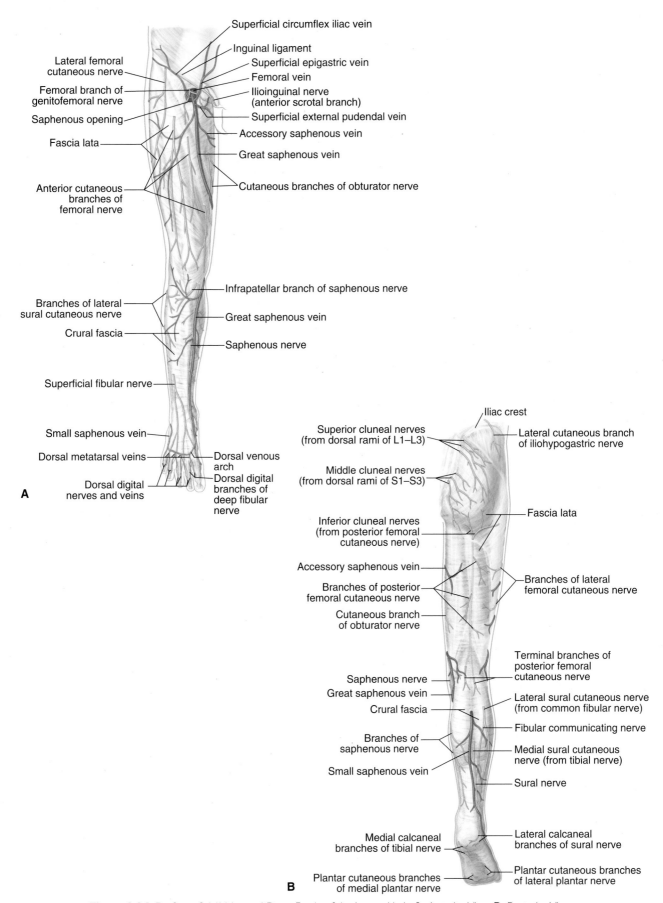

Superficial circumflex iliac vein

Inguinal ligament

Lateral femoral cutaneous nerve

Superficial epigastric vein

Femoral vein

Femoral branch of genitofemoral nerve

Ilioinguinal nerve (anterior scrotal branch)

Saphenous opening

Superficial external pudendal vein

Accessory saphenous vein

Fascia lata

Great saphenous vein

Cutaneous branches of obturator nerve

Anterior cutaneous branches of femoral nerve

Infrapatellar branch of saphenous nerve

Branches of lateral sural cutaneous nerve

Great saphenous vein

Crural fascia

Saphenous nerve

Superficial fibular nerve

Small saphenous vein

Dorsal metatarsal veins

Dorsal venous arch

Dorsal digital nerves and veins

Dorsal digital branches of deep fibular nerve

A

Iliac crest

Superior cluneal nerves (from dorsal rami of L1–L3)

Lateral cutaneous branch of iliohypogastric nerve

Middle cluneal nerves (from dorsal rami of S1–S3)

Fascia lata

Inferior cluneal nerves (from posterior femoral cutaneous nerve)

Accessory saphenous vein

Branches of lateral femoral cutaneous nerve

Branches of posterior femoral cutaneous nerve

Cutaneous branch of obturator nerve

Terminal branches of posterior femoral cutaneous nerve

Saphenous nerve

Great saphenous vein

Lateral sural cutaneous nerve (from common fibular nerve)

Crural fascia

Fibular communicating nerve

Branches of saphenous nerve

Medial sural cutaneous nerve (from tibial nerve)

Small saphenous vein

Sural nerve

Medial calcaneal branches of tibial nerve

Lateral calcaneal branches of sural nerve

Plantar cutaneous branches of medial plantar nerve

Plantar cutaneous branches of lateral plantar nerve

B

Figure 3.3A,B. Superficial Veins and Deep Fascia of the Lower Limb. **A.** Anterior View. **B.** Posterior View.

Lymphatic Drainage
of the Lower Limb

I. Superficial Vessels Lie in the Superficial Fascia (Fig. 3.4A,B)

A. Medial group follow great saphenous vein (3 to 7 trunks)
  1. Origin and course: the medial side of the dorsum of the foot, pass on both sides of the medial malleolus, run behind medial femoral condyle
  2. Termination: superficial inguinal nodes
B. Lateral group (1 to 2 main trunks)
  1. Origin and course: lateral side of the foot, ascend the leg on both posterior and anterior sides; those on the anterior side join the medial group (see above)
  2. Termination: for anterior vessels, see A.2. above; the posterior group end in the popliteal nodes

II. Deep Vessels Accompany Deep Blood Vessels

A. Anterior and posterior tibial, fibular (peroneal), and femoral sets, 2 or 3 lymphatics with each artery
B. Terminate in popliteal and deep inguinal nodes
C. Deep lymphatics of the gluteal region follow gluteal vessels to internal iliac nodes

III. Lymph Nodes: 2 Sets

A. Popliteal nodes: usually 6 or 7 scattered in fat of popliteal fossa (Fig. 3.4B)
  1. Afferents: vessels running with lesser (small) saphenous vein, vessels from the knee joint running with genicular arteries, and vessels running with anterior and posterior tibial arteries
  2. Efferents: some follow great saphenous vein to superficial inguinal nodes; most follow femoral vessels to deep inguinal nodes
B. Inguinal nodes: vary from 12 to over 20, located in proximal part of femoral triangle (Fig. 3.4A)
  1. Superficial inguinal: numerous large nodes arranged as slanted "T" parallel and distal to the inguinal ligament and inferiorly along the proximal portion of great saphenous vein
     a. Afferents: follow superficial vessels of the lower limb, especially those with great saphenous vein; also from penis, scrotum, perineum, buttock, and abdominal wall
     b. Efferents: to external iliac nodes and deep inguinal nodes
  2. Deep inguinal: under deep fascia on the medial side of femoral vein; 1 to 3 in number; one of these may lie in the femoral canal (node of Cloquet)
     a. Afferents: deep lymphatics of the lower extremity; from superficial inguinal nodes
     b. Efferents: to external iliac nodes

IV. Clinical Considerations

A. External genitalia, perineum, buttock, and lower anal canal drain into the inguinal nodes
B. Uterus adjoining the attachment of the round ligament sends its lymphatics along the ligament to drain into the superficial inguinal nodes
C. As they course upward in the thigh, the superficial lymphatics from the lateral side run anteriorly and then medially, and those from the medial side run anteriorly and then laterally, to converge toward the path of the great saphenous vein, thus creating a sort of "lymphatic divide" on the back of the thigh
D. Injection of radiopaque material into the lymphatics of the lower limb can demonstrate the lymphatics as well as lymph nodes
E. Enlargement of superficial inguinal lymph nodes is extremely common and in most cases is due to minor superficial infections; if the size and texture of nodes suggest malignant disease, a careful search for the primary lesion is necessary

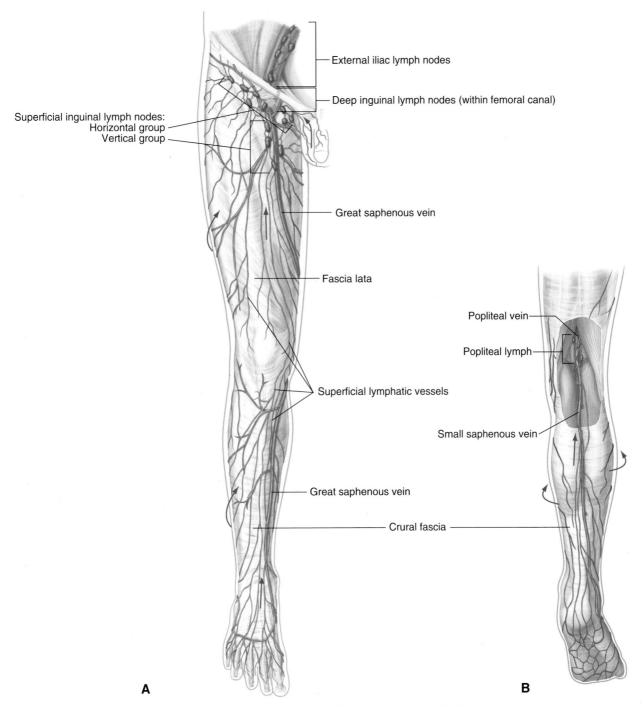

External iliac lymph nodes

Deep inguinal lymph nodes (within femoral canal)

Superficial inguinal lymph nodes:
Horizontal group
Vertical group

Great saphenous vein

Fascia lata

Superficial lymphatic vessels

Great saphenous vein

Crural fascia

Popliteal vein

Popliteal lymph

Small saphenous vein

A

B

Figure 3.4A,B. Lymphatics of the Lower Limb. **A.** Anterior View. **B.** Posterior View.

The Pelvic Girdle

I. Definition

A. Bones through which the lower extremity is attached to the trunk
B. Sacrum and paired os coxae

II. Os Coxae or Hip Bone (Fig. 3.5A–D)

A. Parts: ilium, ischium, and pubis
1. Ilium: ala showing an arched iliac crest with an iliac tubercle; anterior, posterior, and inferior gluteal lines on the lateral surface; anterior superior and anterior inferior iliac spines projecting ventrally; posterior superior and posterior inferior iliac spines projecting dorsally; iliac fossa, arcuate line, auricular surface, and iliac tuberosity on the medial side
2. Ischium: shows an ischial spine, ischial tuberosity, and ischial ramus; the ischial ramus unites with the inferior pubic ramus to form the ischiopubic ramus
3. Pubis: shows superior and inferior rami, pubic crest, pubic tubercle, pubic pectin, and iliopubic eminence; the paired pubic bones are united by the pubic symphysis
B. Special features
1. Acetabulum: formed by the union of ilium, ischium, and pubis
2. Obturator foramen and groove
3. Greater and lesser sciatic notches

III. Ossification: From 8 Centers

Location	Appears	Fuses
Lower ilium	8th–9th fetal week	18th year
Ischial ramus	3rd fetal month	18th year
Superior pubic ramus	4th–5th fetal month	18th year
Acetabulum (1 or more)	12th year	18th year
Iliac crest	Puberty	20th–25th year
Ischial tuberosity	Puberty	20th–25th year
Body of pubis	Puberty	20th–25th year

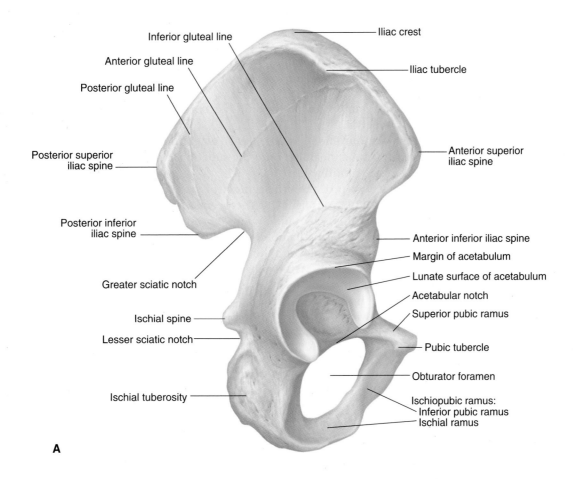

Inferior gluteal line
Anterior gluteal line
Posterior gluteal line
Iliac crest
Iliac tubercle
Posterior superior iliac spine
Anterior superior iliac spine
Posterior inferior iliac spine
Anterior inferior iliac spine
Margin of acetabulum
Lunate surface of acetabulum
Acetabular notch
Greater sciatic notch
Superior pubic ramus
Ischial spine
Lesser sciatic notch
Pubic tubercle
Obturator foramen
Ischial tuberosity
Ischiopubic ramus:
Inferior pubic ramus
Ischial ramus

A

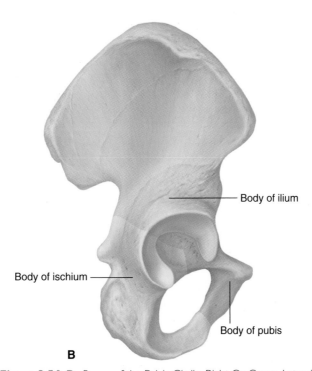

Body of ilium
Body of ischium
Body of pubis

B

Figure 3.5A,B. Bones of the Pelvic Girdle, Right Os Coxae. Lateral View.

IV. Special Features

A. Pelvis serves 2 purposes:
   1. Transmits the weight of the body to the lower limbs
   2. Forms the lower part of the abdominopelvic cavity and houses part of the abdominopelvic viscera

B. Pelvic inlet
   1. Divides pelvis into an "open" anterosuperior region and a confined posteroinferior tunnel, the **true pelvis**
   2. Extends from sacral promontory across each ala of the sacrum and the sacroiliac joint and along each iliopectineal line onto the superior aspect of each pubic bone beside the centrally located symphysis

C. Pelvic outlet: from the tip of the 5th segment of sacrum (not the tip of coccyx), then on each side the sacrotuberous ligament (between sacrum and ischial tuberosity), to the ischial tuberosity, then the ischiopubic ramus, and finally, anteriorly, the anteroinferior aspect of the symphysis pubis (a diamond-shaped area)

D. Pelvic cavity lies between the inlet and the outlet

E. False pelvis (greater pelvis): above the pelvic inlet
   1. Formed by ala of sacrum, iliac fossa, L5 and S1 vertebrae, and abdominal wall
   2. Its cavity is part of the abdominal cavity and contains abdominal viscera

F. True pelvis (lesser pelvis)
   1. Between the pelvic inlet (above) and the pelvic outlet (below); sacrum and coccyx, posterior; symphysis pubis, body of pubis, and pubic rami, anterior; pelvic aspects of ilium and ischium, lateral
   2. Contains pelvic viscera (bladder, rectum, and parts of urogenital organs), blood vessels, nerves, and lymphatics

V. Clinical Considerations

A. Fractures: most commonly due to crushing forces occurring at thinnest places, either ala of ilium or ischiopubic rami; usually little displacement

B. Bursitis: inflammation, especially of bursa, over the ischial tuberosity caused by sitting for long hours on hard seat; also called "tailor's" or "weaver's bottom"

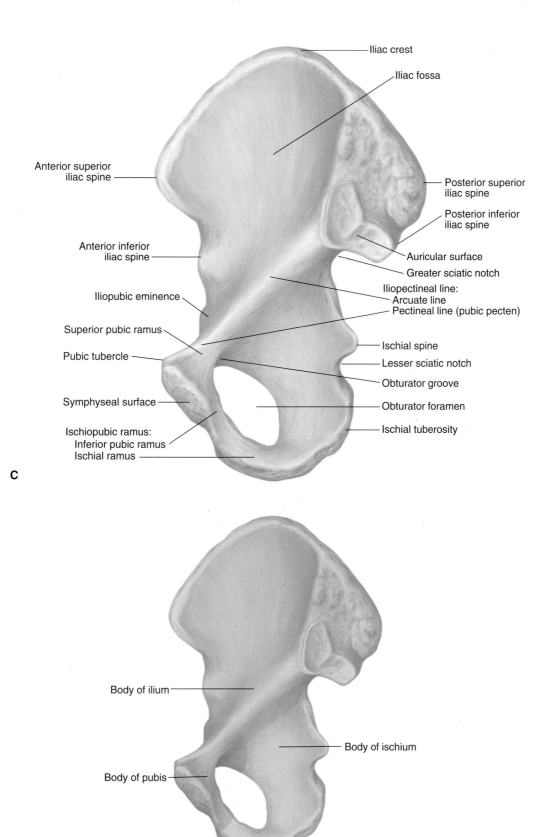

Iliac crest

Iliac fossa

Anterior superior
iliac spine

Posterior superior
iliac spine

Posterior inferior
iliac spine

Anterior inferior
iliac spine

Auricular surface

Greater sciatic notch

Iliopubic eminence

Iliopectineal line:
Arcuate line
Pectineal line (pubic pecten)

Superior pubic ramus

Ischial spine

Pubic tubercle

Lesser sciatic notch

Obturator groove

Symphyseal surface

Obturator foramen

Ischiopubic ramus:
Inferior pubic ramus
Ischial ramus

Ischial tuberosity

C

Body of ilium

Body of ischium

Body of pubis

D

Figure 3.5C,D. Bones of the Pelvic Girdle, Right Os Coxae. Medial View.

Articulations of the Pelvic Girdle

I. Joints (Fig. 3.6A,B)

A. Iliolumbar: between the 5th lumbar vertebra and the iliac crest
   1. Type: amphiarthrodial (syndesmosis)
   2. Iliolumbar ligament: from transverse process of the 5th lumbar vertebra to iliac crest

B. Sacroiliac: between auricular surfaces of sacrum and ilium
   1. Type: amphiarthrodial (syndesmosis)
   2. Ligaments
      a. Anterior: from anterolateral sacrum to auricular and preauricular sulcus of ilium
      b. Posterior: from first 3 transverse tubercles of sacrum to the iliac tuberosity and the posterior superior iliac spine
      c. Interosseous: short fibers between tuberosities of sacrum and ilium

C. Ligaments between sacrum and ischium
   1. Sacrotuberous from the posterior inferior iliac spine, 4th and 5th transverse tubercles and sides of sacrum, and side of coccyx to the ischial tuberosity
   2. Sacrospinous from the side of sacrum and coccyx to the ischial spine

D. Interpubic: between the pubic bones of opposite sides
   1. Type: amphiarthrodial (symphysis)
   2. Pubic symphysis: fibrocartilaginous disc
   3. Ligaments
      a. Superior pubic: connects bones superiorly
      b. Arcuate pubic: connects bones inferiorly

E. Sacrococcygeal: between the apex of sacrum and the base of coccyx
   1. Type: amphiarthrodial (symphysis)
   2. Intervertebral disc: fibrocartilaginous disc
   3. Ligaments: anterior, posterior, lateral, and intercornual

II. Special Features

A. Obturator membrane: attached to bony margins of foramen, which the membrane nearly fills, leaving the obturator canal superiorly for passage of obturator neurovascular bundle. Obturator internus and externus muscles arise from inner and outer surfaces

B. Greater sciatic foramen
   1. Boundaries: greater sciatic notch of ilium; sacrotuberous ligament; sacrospinous ligament
   2. Structures passing through or lying in it: piriformis muscle, superior gluteal vessels and nerve, inferior gluteal vessels and nerve, internal pudendal vessels and pudendal nerve, sciatic nerve, posterior femoral cutaneous nerve, and nerves to obturator internus and quadratus femoris

C. Lesser sciatic foramen
   1. Boundaries: ischial tuberosity, ischial spine and sacrospinous ligament, sacrotuberous ligament
   2. Structures passing through: tendon of obturator internus muscle, nerve to obturator internus, internal pudendal vessels and pudendal nerve

III. Clinical Considerations

A. Sacroiliac strain is quite rare, although formerly often misdiagnosed, due to great strength of supporting ligaments

B. During pregnancy:
   1. Ligaments of pelvic girdle progressively relax and movements between the vertebral column and pelvis become freer
   2. Symphysis pubis relaxes (due to hormone relaxin) and the distance between pubic bones increases considerably
   3. This facilitates passage of fetus through the birth canal during parturition

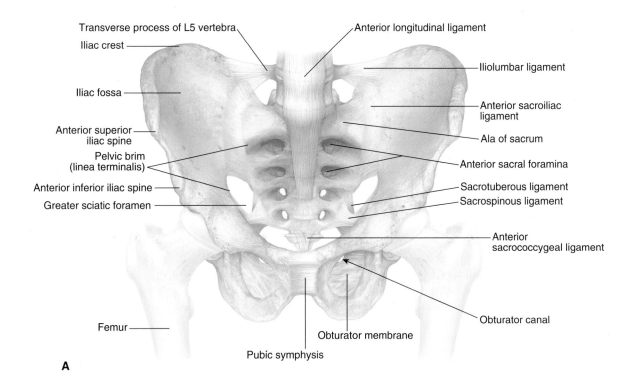

Transverse process of L5 vertebra
Iliac crest
Iliac fossa
Anterior superior iliac spine
Pelvic brim (linea terminalis)
Anterior inferior iliac spine
Greater sciatic foramen
Femur
Pubic symphysis
Obturator membrane

Anterior longitudinal ligament
Iliolumbar ligament
Anterior sacroiliac ligament
Ala of sacrum
Anterior sacral foramina
Sacrotuberous ligament
Sacrospinous ligament
Anterior sacrococcygeal ligament
Obturator canal

A

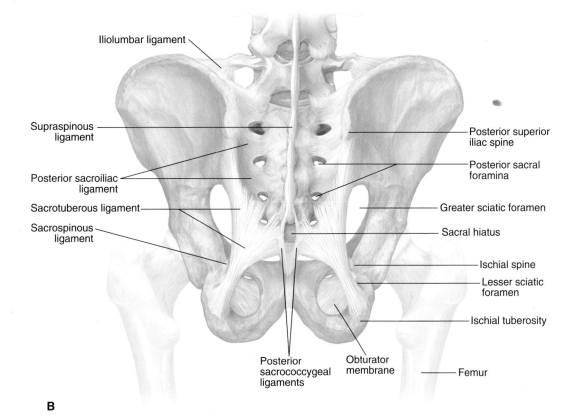

Iliolumbar ligament
Supraspinous ligament
Posterior sacroiliac ligament
Sacrotuberous ligament
Sacrospinous ligament
Posterior sacrococcygeal ligaments
Obturator membrane

Posterior superior iliac spine
Posterior sacral foramina
Greater sciatic foramen
Sacral hiatus
Ischial spine
Lesser sciatic foramen
Ischial tuberosity
Femur

B

Figure 3.6A,B. Articulations of the Pelvic Girdle. **A.** Anterior View. **B.** Posterior View.

Bones of the Thigh

I. Femur (Fig. 3.7A–C)

A. Parts: proximal extremity, shaft, distal extremity
1. Proximal: head with fovea, neck (constricted portion between the head and the intertrochanteric crest and line); lesser trochanter, intertrochanteric crest with the quadrate tubercle, intertrochanteric line, gluteal tuberosity, and greater trochanter
2. Shaft: linea aspera with a medial and lateral lip; pectineal line (an upward continuation of the medial lip); continuation of the lateral lip to gluteal tuberosity; inferior continuation of lips of linea aspera as supracondylar lines; nutrient foramen
3. Distal: popliteal surface (flat space between supracondylar lines); medial and lateral condyles and epicondyles; intercondylar fossa; adductor tubercle

B. Special features
1. Longest, largest, heaviest bone of body
2. Angle between the shaft and the neck: 120°–125°; smaller in female, greater in children
3. In erect posture, shaft runs obliquely; medial distal ends of femora in contact
4. Anatomical neck: epiphyseal line between the head and the neck
5. Surgical neck: junction of shaft and proximal extremity just below the lesser trochanter
6. In standing position, the femur transmits weight from the hip bone to tibia
7. Because the femur is covered with muscles, only its upper and lower ends are palpable

C. Ossification, from 5 centers

Location	Appears	Fuses
Body	7th fetal week	
Distal end	9th fetal week	20th year
Head	1st year	After puberty, last to close
Greater trochanter	4th year	After puberty, 2nd to close
Lesser trochanter	13th–14th year	After puberty, 1st to close

II. Clinical Considerations

A. Fracture
1. **Subtrochanteric:** a break just below the lesser trochanter
   a. Due to the power of iliopsoas, the proximal fragment of the bone is flexed, adducted, and laterally rotated
   b. Distal part will be shortened by the pull of hamstrings, rectus femoris, adductors, and sartorius muscles; abducted by gluteal muscles
2. Fractures in the lower 3rd
   a. Proximal part is fairly stable, but the distal part will override (shorten) by the pull of the hamstrings, rectus femoris, sartorius, and adductor magnus muscles and will be pulled backward by attachments of the gastrocnemius and plantaris muscles
   b. Could lead to damage of the popliteal artery, which lies close to the bone in that position
3. Fractures of the neck, intertrochanteric (between trochanters) or pertrochanteric (through the trochanters), are common over 60 years of age and are more common in older women than men, because women's bones are weakened due to senile and postmenopausal osteoporosis
4. The usual "broken hip" is most often a fracture of the femoral neck

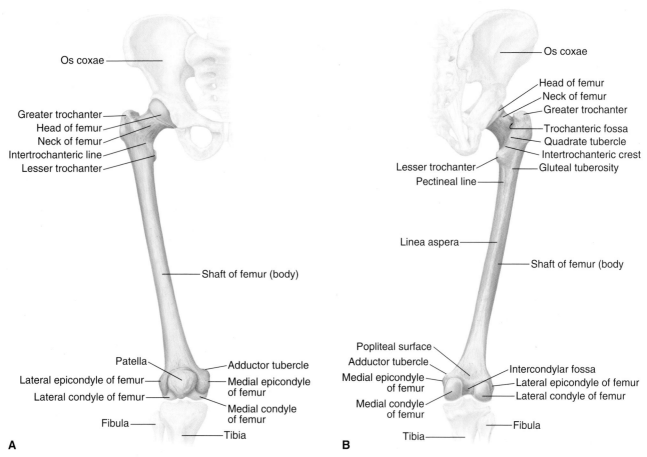

Os coxae

Greater trochanter
Head of femur
Neck of femur
Intertrochanteric line
Lesser trochanter

Shaft of femur (body)

Patella
Lateral epicondyle of femur
Lateral condyle of femur
Fibula
Adductor tubercle
Medial epicondyle of femur
Medial condyle of femur
Tibia

A

Os coxae

Head of femur
Neck of femur
Greater trochanter
Trochanteric fossa
Quadrate tubercle
Intertrochanteric crest
Gluteal tuberosity
Lesser trochanter
Pectineal line

Linea aspera

Shaft of femur (body)

Popliteal surface
Adductor tubercle
Medial epicondyle of femur
Medial condyle of femur
Intercondylar fossa
Lateral epicondyle of femur
Lateral condyle of femur
Fibula
Tibia

B

Figure 3.7A,B. Femur. **A.** Anterior View. **B.** Posterior View.

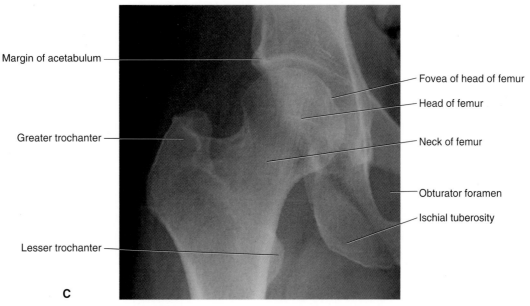

Margin of acetabulum

Greater trochanter

Lesser trochanter

Fovea of head of femur
Head of femur
Neck of femur
Obturator foramen
Ischial tuberosity

C

Figure 3.7C. Hip Joint, Radiograph. PA View.

VI. Clinical Considerations

B. Decrease or increase in the **angle of inclination** between the neck and the body of the femur

1. **Coxa vara** (bent hip): a marked decrease in the angle of inclination (a more transverse direction of the neck)

    a. Results from weight bearing on a bone not capable of supporting it

    b. Usually due to rickets but also can result from bone disease or an improperly set fracture of the neck

2. **Coxa valga:** an increase in the angle of inclination

C. Blood supply of femur consists of multiple arteries entering at each end and one or two nutrient arteries entering the body

1. **Nutrient arteries** are derived from upper perforating branches of the profunda femoris (deep femoral)

2. Principle blood supply to the femoral head in the adult is the medial circumflex femoral artery, which may be disrupted in **femoral neck fracture**, leading to **avascular necrosis of the femoral head**

Bones of the Leg

I. Patella (Knee Cap)

A. Sesamoid bone in tendon of quadriceps femoris muscle
B. Flat and triangular
  1. Superior border convex upward, apex downward
  2. Anterior surface convex and rough
  3. Posterior or articular surface is smooth and divided by a ridge into a larger lateral and smaller medial facet

II. Tibia (Shin Bone) (Fig. 3.8A–C)

A. 2d longest bone of body
B. Parts: proximal extremity, shaft (body), and distal extremity
  1. Proximal extremity shows medial and lateral condyles, anterior and posterior intercondylar areas, intercondylar eminence, tibial tuberosity, and an articular facet for head of fibula
  2. Shaft shows an anterior border; a broad, convex, smooth medial (subcutaneous) surface; and a lateral (interosseous) border
  3. Distal extremity shows a medial malleolus; a smooth, concave inferior articular surface for talus; a fibular notch; a posterior groove for flexor hallucis longus muscle; and a medial malleolar sulcus for tibialis posterior and flexor digitorum longus muscles

III. Fibula (Calf Bone)

A. Most slender of long bones
B. Parts: body and 2 extremities
  1. Proximal extremity shows a head, with superior articular surfaces, and an apex
  2. Shaft is described as having 3 borders and 3 surfaces
  3. Distal extremity shows a lateral malleolus, with a smooth articular and inferior extremity for the talus and a roughened medial area for the tibia

IV. Ossification

A. Tibia, from 3 centers

Location	Appears	Fuses
Body	7th fetal week	—
Proximal end	At time of birth	20th year
Distal end	2nd year	18th year

B. Fibula, from 3 centers

Location	Appears	Fuses
Body	8th fetal week	—
Proximal end	4th year	25th year
Distal end	2nd year	20th year

C. Patella

Location	Appears	Fuses
Patella, from 1 center	2nd or 3rd year	At puberty

V. Clinical Considerations

A. **Fracture of patella** can be due to the muscle pull; fragments are usually drawn apart by the muscle pull, making closed reduction difficult due to tendons being caught in the break

B. **Fractures of fibular neck** may damage the common fibular nerve

C. In case of fracture of either fibula or tibia individually, the unbroken bone helps to splint the other with little displacement
1. If tibia is broken, look for break in fibula at another level
2. Fracture of both bones is referred to as **Pott fracture**

D. Lateral malleolus is often snapped off in **overinversion of the foot** (ankle turn); overeversion may break the medial malleolus, and, if force is strong enough, the lateral may also break

E. Body of tibia is narrowest at junction of middle and lower 3rds; this is the most frequent site of fracture and the region where rickets affects bone during childhood

F. **Spiral fracture** of tibia is caused by severe torsion at junction of middle and lower 3rds (usually see fractures of fibular neck, in addition)

G. Patellar (knee) reflex is blocked by damage to the femoral nerve supplying the quadriceps muscle; damage to spinal cord reflex centers (L2-4) also affects the reflex

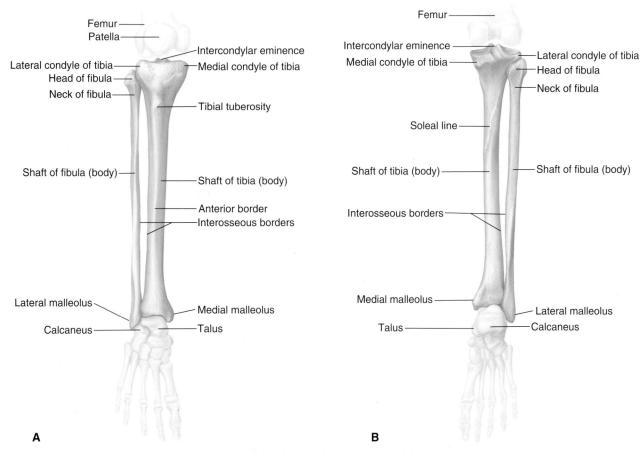

Figure 3.8A,B. Bones of the Leg and Foot. **A.** Anterior View. **B.** Posterior View.

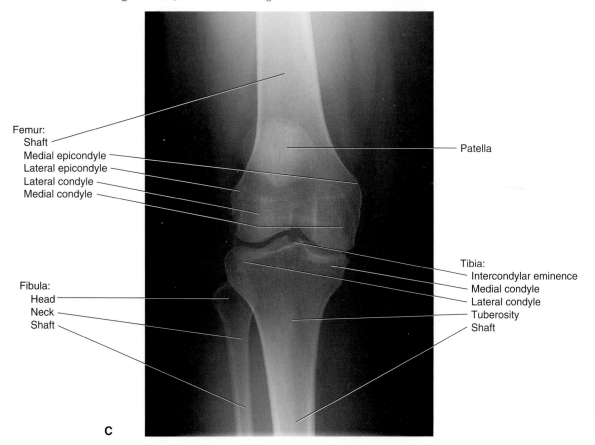

Figure 3.8C. Knee Joint, Radiograph. PA View.

Bones of the Ankle and Foot

I. Tarsals: Talus, Calcaneus, Navicular, Cuboid, and 3 Cuneiforms (Fig. 3.9A–F)

A. Talus (ankle bone): 3 parts
   1. Body: behind, rests on the anterior part of calcaneus; above, lies under the tibia and is gripped by both malleoli; posteriorly has a medial and lateral tubercle with intervening groove for flexor hallucis longus muscle tendon; inferiorly has deep groove—*sulcus tali*
   2. Head: in front, articulates with navicular and calcaneus
   3. Neck: constriction between 1 and 2, above
B. Calcaneus (heel bone) has the following features:
   1. Sustentaculum tali: medial shelf to hold the head of talus
   2. Groove for flexor hallucis longus muscle tendon runs below sustentaculum
   3. Posterior 3rd ("heel") projects behind the ankle joint
   4. Tuberosity: in contact with ground; plantar surface has medial and lateral tubercles (processes)
   5. Fibular (peroneal) trochlea on the lateral aspect
   6. Groove corresponding to sulcus tali with which it forms **sinus tarsi**
C. Navicular (boat-shaped): tuberosity on the medial side
D. Cuboid: groove on plantar surface for fibularis (peroneus) longus muscle tendon
E. 3 cuneiforms (wedge-shaped):
   1. Medial
   2. Intermediate
   3. Lateral

II. Metatarsals (5)

A. Numbered from medial to lateral
B. Each consists of:
   1. Head (distal end): articulates with the proximal phalanx
   2. Body (midportion)
   3. Base (proximal end): articulates with tarsals and bases of other metatarsals
C. 1st: shortest, stoutest; 2 sesamoid bones at the plantar surface of the distal end
D. 5th has a tuberosity projecting posteriorly

III. Phalanges (14)

A. 3 for toes 2 to 5: proximal, middle, and distal
B. 2 for large toe (hallux)
C. Each phalanx consists of the base (proximal end), body, and head (distal end)

IV. Ossification

A. Tarsals: all from 1 center except calcaneus, which has a 2nd center for heel

Location	Appears	Fuses
Calcaneus	6th fetal month	—
Talus	7th fetal month	—
Cuboid	9th fetal month	—
3rd cuneiform	1st year	—
2nd cuneiform	4th year	—
1st cuneiform	3rd year	—
Navicular	4th year	—
Heel	10th year	Puberty

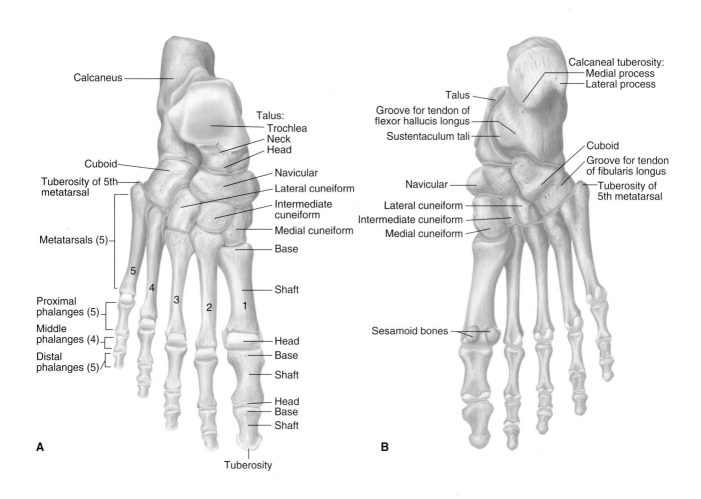

Calcaneus

Talus:
— Trochlea
— Neck
— Head

Cuboid

— Navicular
— Lateral cuneiform

Tuberosity of 5th metatarsal

— Intermediate cuneiform

— Medial cuneiform

Metatarsals (5)

— Base

Proximal phalanges (5)

— Shaft

Middle phalanges (4)

— Head
— Base
— Shaft

Distal phalanges (5)

— Head
— Base
— Shaft

A

Tuberosity

Calcaneal tuberosity:
— Medial process
— Lateral process

Talus

Groove for tendon of flexor hallucis longus

Sustentaculum tali

Cuboid

Groove for tendon of fibularis longus

Navicular

Tuberosity of 5th metatarsal

Lateral cuneiform
Intermediate cuneiform
Medial cuneiform

Sesamoid bones

B

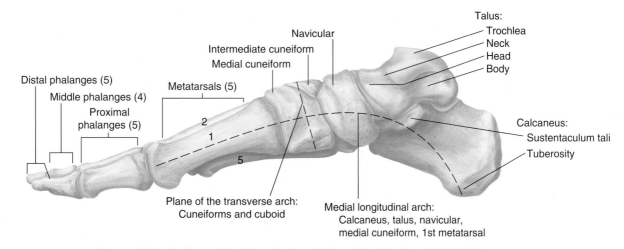

Navicular

Intermediate cuneiform
Medial cuneiform

Talus:
— Trochlea
— Neck
— Head
— Body

Distal phalanges (5)

Metatarsals (5)

Middle phalanges (4)

Proximal phalanges (5)

Calcaneus:
— Sustentaculum tali
— Tuberosity

Plane of the transverse arch:
Cuneiforms and cuboid

Medial longitudinal arch:
Calcaneus, talus, navicular, medial cuneiform, 1st metatarsal

C

Figure 3.9A–C. Bones of the Foot. **A.** Superior View. **B.** Inferior View. **C.** Medial View.

B. Metatarsals: from 2 centers—the body and the head for 2 to 5; the body and the base for 1st

Location	Appears	Fuses
Body	9th fetal week	18th–20th year
Base of 1st	3rd year	18th–20th year
Heads of 2nd–5th	5th–8th year	18th–20th year

C. Phalanges: from 2 centers—the body and the base

Location	Appears	Fuses
Body	10th fetal week	18th year
Base	4th–10th years	18th year

V. Clinical Considerations

A. Fractures of the bones of the foot are common: jumping from a height, landing on the heels, fractures the calcanei (very disabling due to disruption of the subtalar joint)

B. Fractures of the neck of talus occur during severe dorsiflexion of the ankle

C. Fractures of metatarsals and phalanges
  1. Usually occur when a heavy object falls on the foot
  2. Phalangeal fracture may occur when stubbing the bare toes
  3. Fracture of the 5th metatarsal is common in forced eversion

D. Talus has no muscular attachments

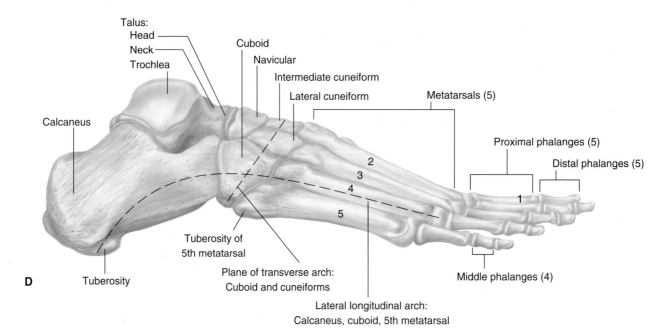

Figure 3.9D. Bones of the Foot. Lateral View.

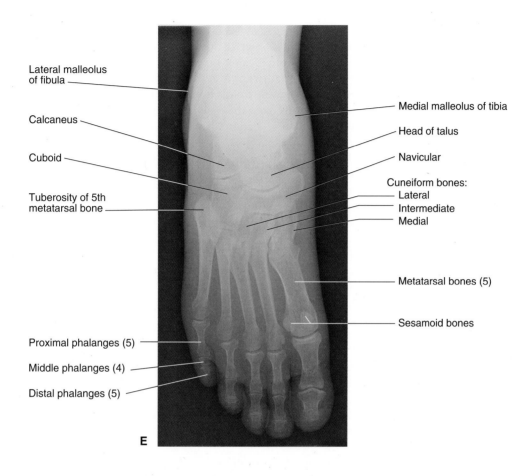

Lateral malleolus of fibula

Calcaneus

Cuboid

Tuberosity of 5th metatarsal bone

Medial malleolus of tibia

Head of talus

Navicular

Cuneiform bones:
Lateral
Intermediate
Medial

Metatarsal bones (5)

Sesamoid bones

Proximal phalanges (5)

Middle phalanges (4)

Distal phalanges (5)

E

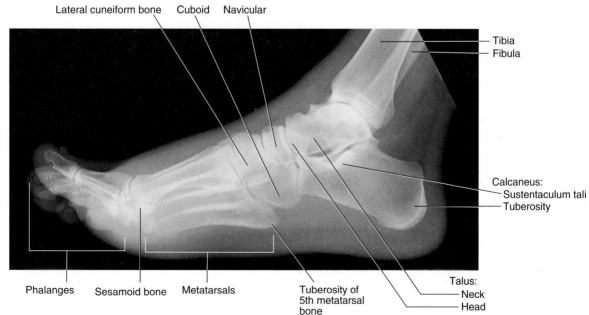

Lateral cuneiform bone   Cuboid   Navicular

Tibia
Fibula

Calcaneus:
Sustentaculum tali
Tuberosity

Phalanges   Sesamoid bone   Metatarsals   Tuberosity of 5th metatarsal bone

Talus:
Neck
Head

Figure 3.9E,F. Radiograph of the Foot. **E.** Anterior View. **F.** Lateral View.

Compartments of the Thigh

I. Definition and Number (Fig. 3.10A–C)

A. Defined by the fascia lata and the medial and lateral intermuscular septa

1. Medial intermuscular septum: divides the extensors from the adductors; extends inward to the bone between the quadriceps femoris and adductor muscles

2. Lateral intermuscular septum: extends inward from the fascia lata to the linea aspera; separates the vastus lateralis from the biceps femoris muscle

B. 3 compartments in the thigh and 1 compartment in the hip/gluteal region

1. Anterior compartment
   a. Primary action: flexion of the thigh; sartorius, quadriceps femoris, iliopsoas
   b. Nerve: femoral
   c. Artery: femoral

2. Medial compartment
   a. Primary action: adduction of the thigh; pectineus, adductor longus, adductor brevis, adductor magnus, gracilis, obturator externus
   b. Nerve: obturator
   c. Artery: deep femoral, medial circumflex femoral

3. Posterior compartment
   a. Primary action: extension of the thigh; semitendinosus, semimembranosus, biceps femoris
   b. Nerve: sciatic
   c. Artery: deep femoral

4. Hip/gluteal region
   a. Primary actions: extension, abduction, and lateral rotation of the thigh; gluteus maximus, gluteus medius, gluteus minimus, tensor fasciae latae, piriformis, obturator internus, superior and inferior gemellus, quadratus femoris
   b. Nerves: superior and inferior gluteal, nerves to obturator internus and quadratus femoris
   c. Arteries: superior and inferior gluteal

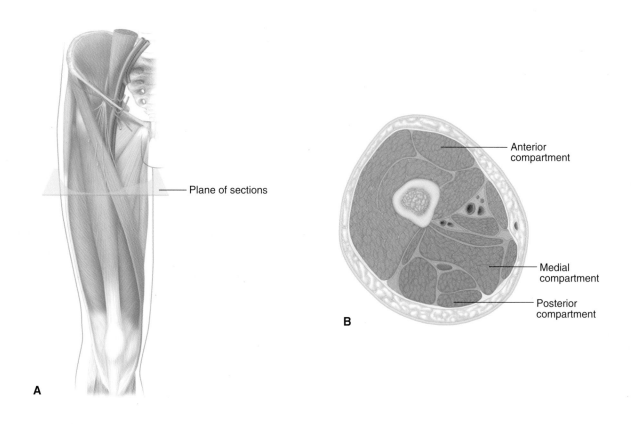

Plane of sections

Anterior compartment

Medial compartment

Posterior compartment

B

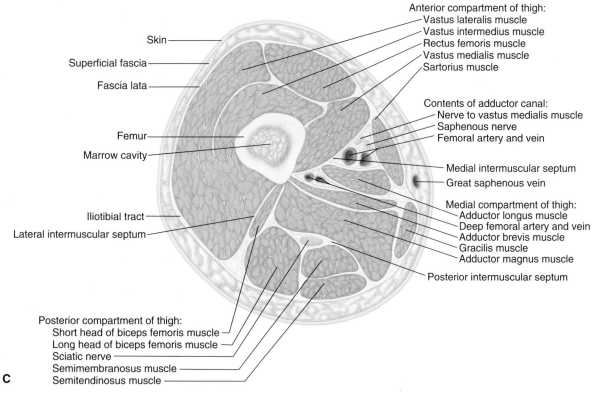

Skin

Superficial fascia

Fascia lata

Femur

Marrow cavity

Iliotibial tract

Lateral intermuscular septum

Anterior compartment of thigh:
Vastus lateralis muscle
Vastus intermedius muscle
Rectus femoris muscle
Vastus medialis muscle
Sartorius muscle

Contents of adductor canal:
Nerve to vastus medialis muscle
Saphenous nerve
Femoral artery and vein

Medial intermuscular septum

Great saphenous vein

Medial compartment of thigh:
Adductor longus muscle
Deep femoral artery and vein
Adductor brevis muscle
Gracilis muscle
Adductor magnus muscle

Posterior intermuscular septum

Posterior compartment of thigh:
Short head of biceps femoris muscle
Long head of biceps femoris muscle
Sciatic nerve
Semimembranosus muscle
Semitendinosus muscle

C

Figure 3.10A–C. Compartments of the Thigh. **A.** Orientation. **B.** Cross-section View. **C.** Cross-section View.

Muscles of the Anterior Thigh

I. Muscles of the Anterior Thigh (Fig. 3.11A,B)

Muscle	Origin	Insertion	Action	Nerve
Iliopsoas	Combination of iliacus (from iliac fossa) and psoas major (from lumbar vertebrae)	Lesser trochanter	Flexes the thigh at the hip joint; laterally rotates the thigh	Branches from L2-4
Sartorius	Anterior superior iliac spine	Upper medial tibia via pes anserinus	Flexes, abducts, and rotates the thigh laterally, flexes the leg and medially rotates when the knee is flexed	Femoral (L2, L3)
Quadriceps femoris Rectus femoris	Anterior inferior iliac spine, rim of acetabulum	Tibial tuberosity via patellar ligament from patella (sesamoid bone within tendon of quadriceps)	Flexes the thigh and extends the leg; steadies the hip joint	Femoral (L2-4)
Vastus lateralis	Intertrochanteric line, the greater trochanter, the lateral lip of linea aspera	Patella and lateral patellar retinaculum	Extends the leg	Femoral (L2-4)
Vastus medialis	Intertrochanteric line, the medial lip of linea aspera	Patella and medial patellar retinaculum	Extends the leg	Femoral (L2-4)
Vastus intermedius	Anterior and lateral shaft of the femur	Patella (and tibial tuberosity via patellar ligament)	Extends the leg	Femoral (L2-4)

II. Clinical Considerations

A. In general, the iliopsoas and pectineus (a flexor in the medial thigh) act only at the hip joint; the sartorius and rectus femoris act both at the hip and knee joints (but with opposite actions at the knee joint); and the vastus muscles act only at the knee joint

B. **Paralysis of the quadriceps femoris muscle:** knee cannot be extended, but patient can stand erect since the body weight tends to overextend the knee; patient also may be able to walk with short steps if the pelvis is rotated to prevent overextension of the hip, which would flex the knee

C. **Hip pointer:** a bruise or contusion over a bony prominence, particularly the anterior superior iliac spine from which the sartorius muscle and inguinal ligament arise

D. **"Charley horse":** a contusion and tearing of muscle fibers sufficient enough to cause a thigh hematoma (local blood collection from damaged vessels)
  1. Most common site: quadriceps muscle
  2. Associated with localized pain and/or muscle stiffness, usually the result of trauma

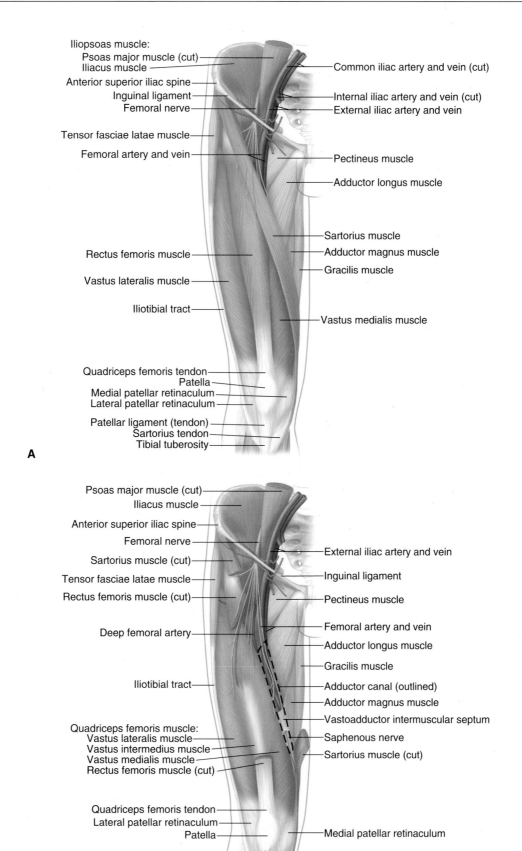

Iliopsoas muscle:
Psoas major muscle (cut)
Iliacus muscle
Anterior superior iliac spine
Inguinal ligament
Femoral nerve

Tensor fasciae latae muscle

Femoral artery and vein

Rectus femoris muscle

Vastus lateralis muscle

Iliotibial tract

Quadriceps femoris tendon
Patella
Medial patellar retinaculum
Lateral patellar retinaculum
Patellar ligament (tendon)
Sartorius tendon
Tibial tuberosity

Common iliac artery and vein (cut)

Internal iliac artery and vein (cut)
External iliac artery and vein

Pectineus muscle

Adductor longus muscle

Sartorius muscle
Adductor magnus muscle
Gracilis muscle

Vastus medialis muscle

A

Psoas major muscle (cut)
Iliacus muscle
Anterior superior iliac spine
Femoral nerve
Sartorius muscle (cut)
Tensor fasciae latae muscle
Rectus femoris muscle (cut)

Deep femoral artery

Iliotibial tract

Quadriceps femoris muscle:
Vastus lateralis muscle
Vastus intermedius muscle
Vastus medialis muscle
Rectus femoris muscle (cut)

Quadriceps femoris tendon
Lateral patellar retinaculum
Patella

Patellar ligament (tendon)

Tibial tuberosity

External iliac artery and vein

Inguinal ligament

Pectineus muscle

Femoral artery and vein
Adductor longus muscle
Gracilis muscle

Adductor canal (outlined)
Adductor magnus muscle
Vastoadductor intermuscular septum
Saphenous nerve
Sartorius muscle (cut)

Medial patellar retinaculum

Sartorius tendon

B

Figure 3.11A,B. Muscles of the Anterior Thigh. **A.** Superficial Dissection, Anterior View. **B.** Deep Dissection, Anterior View.

Femoral Triangle and Femoral Sheath

I. Femoral Triangle (Fig. 3.12A)

A. Bounded: above, inguinal ligament; laterally, sartorius muscle; medially, medial border of adductor longus muscle

B. Floor, from lateral to medial: iliopsoas, pectineus, and adductor longus muscles

C. Roof: formed by skin and fascia of the thigh

D. Contents: terminal part of the femoral nerve and its branches, femoral sheath, femoral artery and its branches, femoral vein and its tributaries, and the deep inguinal lymph nodes

II. Adductor (Hunter) Canal

A. Musculofibrous canal in the middle of the thigh, beginning at the apex of the femoral triangle and ending in tendinous adductor hiatus in the adductor magnus muscle

B. Bounded: laterally, vastus medialis; posteriorly, adductor longus and magnus muscles; covered (roofed) anteromedially by sartorius muscle (and vastoadductor membrane distally)

III. Interval Behind Inguinal Ligament (Fig. 3.12B)

A. Iliopectineal arch: a septum of iliopectineal fascia extends between the iliopubic eminence to the inguinal ligament, dividing the area into 2 compartments

    1. Muscular: contains iliacus and psoas major muscles, the femoral nerve, and the lateral femoral cutaneous nerve

    2. Vascular: contains the femoral sheath and its contents (see below)

IV. Femoral Sheath

A. Prolongation of transversalis fascia from abdomen, fusing to iliac fascia dorsally

B. Funnel-shaped: narrow end fuses with the intrinsic fascia of vessels contained about 5 cm below the inguinal ligament

C. 2 vertical septa divide the sheath into 3 compartments:

    1. Lateral, for the artery and femoral branch of genitofemoral nerve

    2. Intermediate, for vein

    3. Medial, for the femoral canal, containing a few small lymphatics and a deep inguinal lymph node (node of Cloquet)

D. Femoral ring: the cephalic opening of the femoral canal

    1. Bounded: medially, aponeurosis and fascia of transversus abdominis muscle; laterally, fascia over femoral veins; anteriorly, inguinal ligament; posteriorly, superior ramus of pubic bone and pectineal ligament

V. Clinical Considerations

A. Femoral canal is the most common site for femoral herniations

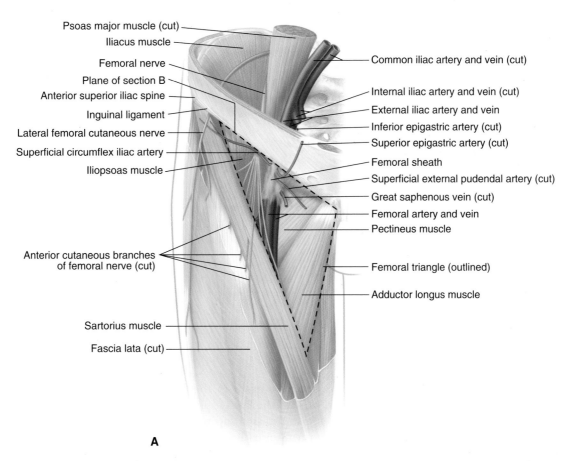

Psoas major muscle (cut)
Iliacus muscle
Femoral nerve
Plane of section B
Anterior superior iliac spine
Inguinal ligament
Lateral femoral cutaneous nerve
Superficial circumflex iliac artery
Iliopsoas muscle

Common iliac artery and vein (cut)
Internal iliac artery and vein (cut)
External iliac artery and vein
Inferior epigastric artery (cut)
Superior epigastric artery (cut)
Femoral sheath
Superficial external pudendal artery (cut)
Great saphenous vein (cut)
Femoral artery and vein
Pectineus muscle

Anterior cutaneous branches
of femoral nerve (cut)

Femoral triangle (outlined)

Adductor longus muscle

Sartorius muscle

Fascia lata (cut)

A

Figure 3.12. A. Femoral Triangle. Anterior View.

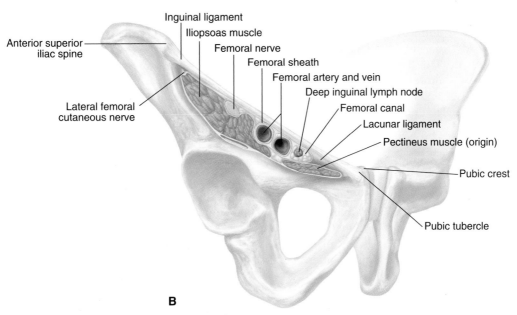

Inguinal ligament
Iliopsoas muscle
Femoral nerve
Femoral sheath
Femoral artery and vein
Deep inguinal lymph node
Femoral canal
Lacunar ligament
Pectineus muscle (origin)

Anterior superior
iliac spine

Lateral femoral
cutaneous nerve

Pubic crest

Pubic tubercle

B

Figure 3.12. B. Femoral Sheath. Anterior View.

Muscles of the Medial Thigh

I. Muscles of the Medial Thigh (Fig. 3.13A–C)

Muscle	Origin	Insertion	Action	Nerve
Pectineus	Pecten (superior ramus) of pubis	Pectineal line of the femur	Flexes, adducts, and medially rotates the thigh	Femoral (L2, L3) (obturator may also innervate)
Adductor longus	Body of pubis below pubic crest	Medial lip of linea aspera of the femur	Adducts, flexes, and medially rotates the thigh	Obturator (L2-4)
Gracilis	Body and the inferior pubic ramus	Upper medial tibia, below condyle	Adducts and medially rotates the thigh, flexes the leg	Obturator (L2, L3)
Adductor brevis	Body and the inferior pubic ramus	Pectineal line and the upper medial lip of linea aspera of the femur	Adducts, flexes, and assists in medial rotation of the thigh	Obturator (L2, L3)
Adductor magnus				
Adductor part	Inferior pubic ramus, the ischial ramus	Medial lip of linea aspera, the medial supracondylar line	Adducts, flexes, and medially rotates the thigh	Obturator (L2-4)
Hamstring (ischiocondylar) part	Ischial tuberosity	Adductor tubercle of the femur	Extends the thigh	Tibial part of sciatic (L4)

II. Special Features

A. A series of small tendinous arches attach to the bone at the insertion of the adductor magnus muscle along and close to the linea aspera

  I. Upper 4 are small apertures transmitting perforating branches of the deep femoral artery, which supply hamstring muscles at the back of the thigh as well as a nutrient vessel to the femur

  2. 5th and lowest is the largest: **adductor hiatus**, which represents the caudal end of the adductor canal through which the femoral vessels enter the popliteal space

B. Most of these muscles are supplied by the obturator nerve except for the pectineus, which is usually supplied by the femoral (or both); the ischiocondylar (extensor) part of the adductor magnus muscle is considered part of the hamstrings and is supplied by the tibial part of the sciatic nerve

C. The 3 adductors (helped by the pectineus) are powerful muscles and are used in all movements where the thighs are approximated

  I. They are stabilizers during flexion and extension

  2. Longus and magnus are active during medial rotation

  3. Ischiocondylar portion of the magnus helps the hamstrings in extending the thigh

D. Gracilis acts at both the hip and the knee but is chiefly an adductor, flexor, and medial rotator, especially during the swing phase of walking; it has no postural function

III. Clinical Considerations: Groin Strain

A. Straining, stretching, and some tearing away of attachments of the anterior and medial thigh muscles

B. Usually involves the iliopsoas and/or the adductor group

C. Injury often occurs in sports requiring "quick starts," that is, racing, basketball, etc.

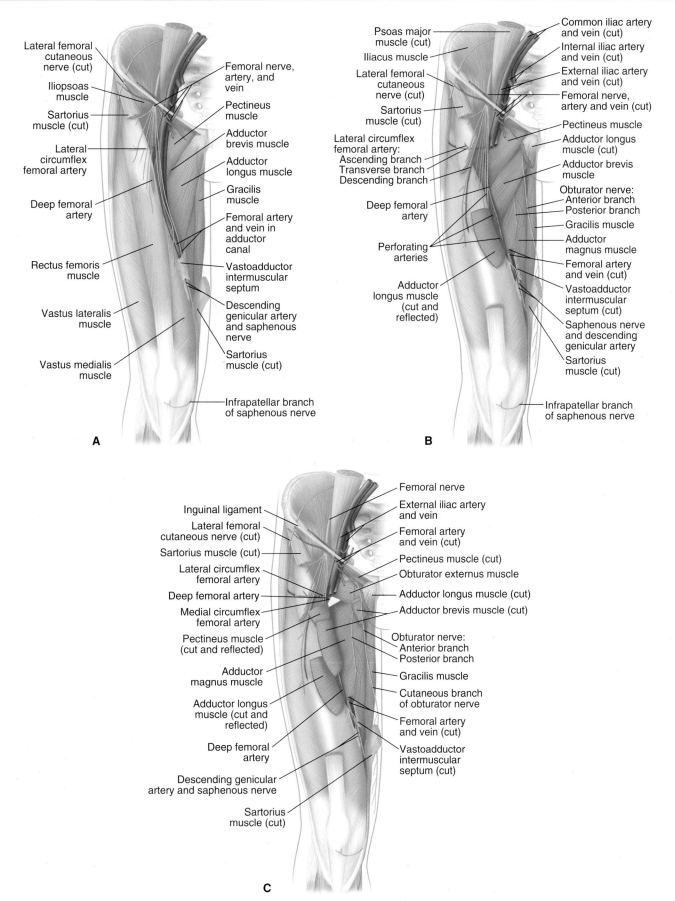

Lateral femoral cutaneous nerve (cut)
Iliopsoas muscle
Sartorius muscle (cut)
Lateral circumflex femoral artery
Deep femoral artery
Rectus femoris muscle
Vastus lateralis muscle
Vastus medialis muscle

Femoral nerve, artery, and vein
Pectineus muscle
Adductor brevis muscle
Adductor longus muscle
Gracilis muscle
Femoral artery and vein in adductor canal
Vastoadductor intermuscular septum
Descending genicular artery and saphenous nerve
Sartorius muscle (cut)
Infrapatellar branch of saphenous nerve

A

Psoas major muscle (cut)
Iliacus muscle
Lateral femoral cutaneous nerve (cut)
Sartorius muscle (cut)
Lateral circumflex femoral artery:
  Ascending branch
  Transverse branch
  Descending branch
Deep femoral artery
Perforating arteries
Adductor longus muscle (cut and reflected)

Common iliac artery and vein (cut)
Internal iliac artery and vein (cut)
External iliac artery and vein (cut)
Femoral nerve, artery and vein (cut)
Pectineus muscle
Adductor longus muscle
Adductor brevis muscle
Obturator nerve:
  Anterior branch
  Posterior branch
Gracilis muscle
Adductor magnus muscle
Femoral artery and vein (cut)
Vastoadductor intermuscular septum (cut)
Saphenous nerve and descending genicular artery
Sartorius muscle (cut)
Infrapatellar branch of saphenous nerve

B

Inguinal ligament
Lateral femoral cutaneous nerve (cut)
Sartorius muscle (cut)
Lateral circumflex femoral artery
Deep femoral artery
Medial circumflex femoral artery
Pectineus muscle (cut and reflected)
Adductor magnus muscle
Adductor longus muscle (cut and reflected)
Deep femoral artery
Descending genicular artery and saphenous nerve
Sartorius muscle (cut)

Femoral nerve
External iliac artery and vein
Femoral artery and vein (cut)
Pectineus muscle (cut)
Obturator externus muscle
Adductor longus muscle (cut)
Adductor brevis muscle (cut)
Obturator nerve:
  Anterior branch
  Posterior branch
Gracilis muscle
Cutaneous branch of obturator nerve
Femoral artery and vein (cut)
Vastoadductor intermuscular septum (cut)

C

Figure 3.13A–C. Muscles of the Medial Thigh. **A.** Superficial Dissection, Anterior View. **B.** Intermediate Dissection, Anterior View. **C.** Deep Dissection, Anterior View.

Femoral and Obturator Vessels and Nerves

I. Femoral Artery (Fig. 3.14A,B)

A. Relations

	Anterior	
	Fascia lata, nerve to vastus medialis, saphenous nerve, sartorius muscle, vastoadductor membrane	
Lateral	**Femoral Artery**	**Medial**
Vastus intermedius muscle		Adductor longus and sartorius (distally) muscles, femoral vein
	Posterior	
	Iliopsoas, pectineus, adductor longus, and adductor magnus muscles, deep femoral and femoral veins	

B. Branches: superficial epigastric, superficial circumflex iliac, superficial and deep external pudendal, deep femoral and descending genicular arteries

II. Deep Femoral Artery

A. Arises from the back of the femoral artery
   1. Initially lies lateral to, then behind, the femoral artery as far as the medial side of the femur; it then runs behind the adductor longus muscle to end as the 4th perforating artery
B. Branches:
   1. Medial circumflex femoral winds around the medial side of the femur between the pectineus and iliopsoas muscles and then between the obturator externus and adductor brevis muscles to the back of the thigh, where it anastomoses with the inferior gluteal, lateral circumflex femoral, and 1st perforating artery of the profunda femoris to form the cruciate (arterial) anastomosis.
   2. Lateral circumflex femoral arises from the lateral side, behind the sartorius and rectus femoris muscles; runs beneath the rectus femoris to anastomose with the superior gluteal, deep circumflex iliac, and superior lateral genicular arteries
   3. 4 perforating arteries pierce adductor brevis and magnus muscles to reach the back of the thigh, forming anastomotic loops
C. Termination: 4th perforating artery

III. Femoral Vein

A. Begins at adductor hiatus in adductor magnus muscle as the continuation of popliteal vein
B. Receives muscular tributaries, deep femoral vein, and great saphenous vein

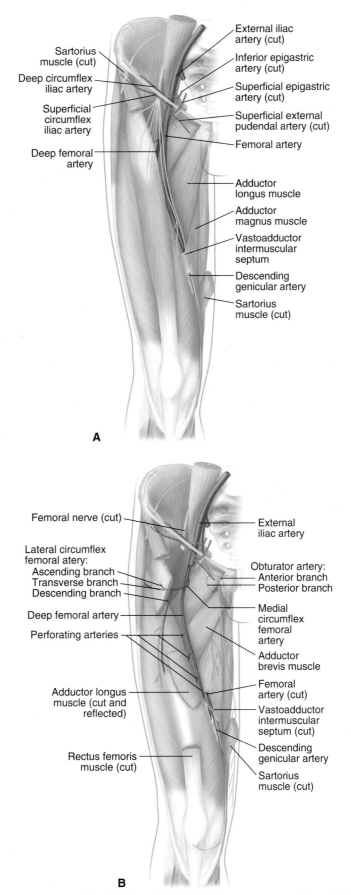

Sartorius muscle (cut)

Deep circumflex iliac artery

Superficial circumflex iliac artery

Deep femoral artery

External iliac artery (cut)

Inferior epigastric artery (cut)

Superficial epigastric artery (cut)

Superficial external pudendal artery (cut)

Femoral artery

Adductor longus muscle

Adductor magnus muscle

Vastoadductor intermuscular septum

Descending genicular artery

Sartorius muscle (cut)

A

Femoral nerve (cut)

Lateral circumflex femoral atery:
Ascending branch
Transverse branch
Descending branch

Deep femoral artery

Perforating arteries

Adductor longus muscle (cut and reflected)

Rectus femoris muscle (cut)

External iliac artery

Obturator artery:
Anterior branch
Posterior branch

Medial circumflex femoral artery

Adductor brevis muscle

Femoral artery (cut)

Vastoadductor intermuscular septum (cut)

Descending genicular artery

Sartorius muscle (cut)

B

Figure 3.14A,B. Arteries of the Anterior and Medial Thigh. **A.** Superficial Dissection, Anterior View. **B.** Deep Dissection, Anterior View.

IV. Femoral Nerve (Fig. 3.14C–E)

A. Muscular to pectineus, sartorius, and quadriceps femoris muscles

B. Cutaneous

   1. Anterior branches to the anterior and medial thigh

   2. Saphenous runs with the femoral artery, crossing it from the lateral to medial, in the adductor canal; it becomes superficial at the medial side of the knee to supply skin over the patella and on the medial side of the leg and ankle

C. Sensory nerves to the hip joint and knee joint (Hilton's law: a nerve that supplies a muscle that moves a joint must also send sensory [proprioceptive] branches to the joint)

V. Obturator Vessels and Nerve

A. Artery

   1. Distributed to the origins of obturator externus, pectineus, gracilis, and adductor muscles and hip joint

   2. Anastomoses with the inferior gluteal and medial circumflex femoral arteries

B. Nerve:

   1. Anterior branch

      a. Passes inferiorly deep to pectineus and adductor longus muscles and superficially to adductor brevis muscle

      b. Supplies adductor longus, brevis, and gracilis muscles; skin of the medial thigh; the hip joint

   2. Posterior branch

      a. As it enters the thigh, passes through and innervates obturator externus

      b. Passes inferiorly posterior to adductor brevis muscle but superficial to adductor magnus muscle

      c. In addition to obturator externus, supplies adductor magnus, sometimes adductor brevis, and also the knee joint

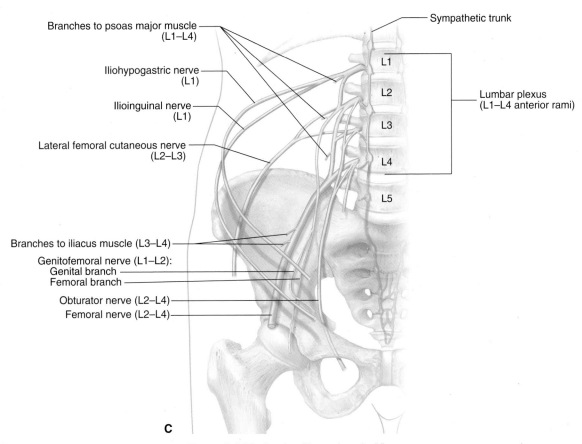

Branches to psoas major muscle
(L1–L4)

Iliohypogastric nerve
(L1)

Ilioinguinal nerve
(L1)

Lateral femoral cutaneous nerve
(L2–L3)

Sympathetic trunk

L1

L2

L3

L4

L5

Lumbar plexus
(L1–L4 anterior rami)

Branches to iliacus muscle (L3–L4)

Genitofemoral nerve (L1–L2):
Genital branch
Femoral branch

Obturator nerve (L2–L4)
Femoral nerve (L2–L4)

C

Figure 3.14C. Lumbar Plexus. Anterior View.

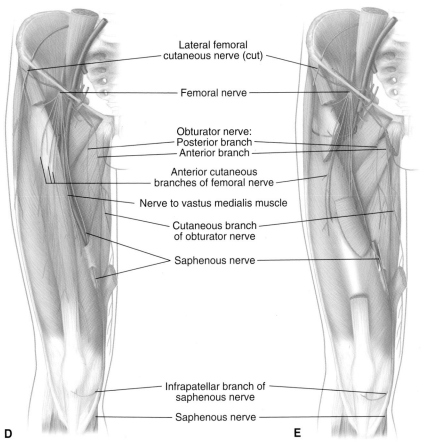

Lateral femoral
cutaneous nerve (cut)

Femoral nerve

Obturator nerve:
Posterior branch
Anterior branch

Anterior cutaneous
branches of femoral nerve

Nerve to vastus medialis muscle

Cutaneous branch
of obturator nerve

Saphenous nerve

Infrapatellar branch of
saphenous nerve

Saphenous nerve

D

E

Figure 3.14D,E. Nerves of the Anterior and Medial Thigh. **D.** Superficial Dissection, Anterior View.
E. Deep Dissection, Anterior View.

Muscles of the Gluteal Region

I. Muscles of the Gluteal Region (Fig. 3.15A,B)

Muscle	Origin	Insertion	Action	Nerve
Gluteus maximus	Ilium behind the posterior gluteal line, sacrotuberous ligament	Iliotibial band gluteal tuberosity of the femur	Extends and laterally rotates the thigh, braces the knee	Inferior gluteal (L5, S1, S2)
Gluteus medius	Outer ilium and crest between anterior and posterior gluteal lines	Lateral surface of the greater trochanter	Abducts the thigh, the anterior part rotates the thigh medially, the posterior part rotates the thigh laterally	Superior gluteal (L4, L5, S1)
Gluteus minimus	Outer ilium, between anterior and inferior gluteal lines, sciatic notch	Anterior surface of the greater trochanter of the femur	Abducts and medially rotates the thigh	Superior gluteal (L4, L5, S1)
Tensor fasciae latae	Anterior iliac crest, the anterior superior iliac spine	Iliotibial band	Flexes, abducts, and medially rotates the thigh	Superior gluteal (L4, L5, S1)
Piriformis	Anterior sacrum, the greater sciatic notch	Upper medial border of the greater trochanter	Abducts and laterally rotates the thigh	Nerve to piriformis (anterior rami of S1, S2)
Obturator internus	Margins of obturator foramen and the inner surface of obturator membrane	Medial surface of the greater trochanter	Laterally rotates and abducts the thigh	Nerve to obturator internus (L5, S1, S2)
Gemellus superior	Outer surface of the ischial spine	Tendon of obturator internus muscle	See obturator internus	Nerve to obturator internus (L5, S1, S2)
Gemellus inferior	Ischial tuberosity	Tendon of obturator internus muscle	See obturator internus	Nerve to quadratus femoris (L4, L5, S1)
Obturator externus	Margins of obturator foramen and the outer surface of obturator membrane	Trochanteric fossa	Rotates the thigh laterally	Obturator (L2-4)
Quadratus femoris	Ischial tuberosity	Quadrate line	Rotates the thigh laterally	Nerve to quadratus femoris (L4, L5, S1)

II. Special Features

A. Piriformis arises inside pelvis and divides the greater sciatic foramen into superior and inferior portions

B. Obturator internus muscle arises inside pelvis and passes through the lesser sciatic foramen

C. Gemelli insert into tendon of obturator internus muscle

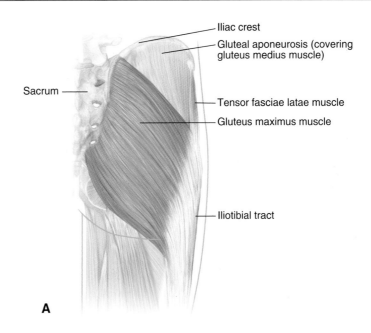

Iliac crest

Gluteal aponeurosis (covering gluteus medius muscle)

Sacrum

Tensor fasciae latae muscle

Gluteus maximus muscle

Iliotibial tract

A

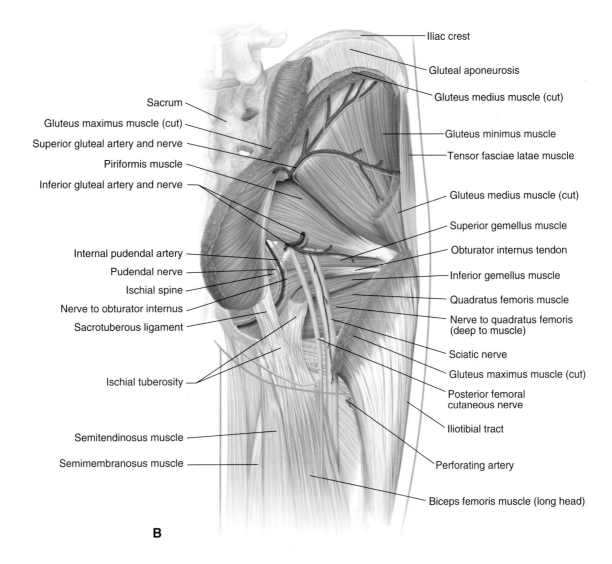

Iliac crest

Gluteal aponeurosis

Gluteus medius muscle (cut)

Sacrum

Gluteus maximus muscle (cut)

Gluteus minimus muscle

Superior gluteal artery and nerve

Tensor fasciae latae muscle

Piriformis muscle

Inferior gluteal artery and nerve

Gluteus medius muscle (cut)

Superior gemellus muscle

Internal pudendal artery

Obturator internus tendon

Pudendal nerve

Inferior gemellus muscle

Ischial spine

Quadratus femoris muscle

Nerve to obturator internus

Nerve to quadratus femoris (deep to muscle)

Sacrotuberous ligament

Sciatic nerve

Gluteus maximus muscle (cut)

Ischial tuberosity

Posterior femoral cutaneous nerve

Iliotibial tract

Semitendinosus muscle

Perforating artery

Semimembranosus muscle

Biceps femoris muscle (long head)

B

Figure 3.15A,B. Muscles of the Gluteal Region. **A.** Superficial Dissection, Posterior View. **B.** Deep Dissection, Posterior View.

Vessels and Nerves of the Gluteal Region

I. Arteries (Fig. 3.16A,B)

A. Superior gluteal: largest branch of the internal iliac artery
   1. Leaves pelvis through the greater sciatic foramen, above piriformis muscle
   2. Branches
      a. Superficial branch enters gluteus maximus muscle and anastomoses with the inferior gluteal artery
      b. Deep branch runs forward under gluteus medius muscle
         i. Superior division continues along the upper border of gluteus minimus muscle to the anterior superior iliac spine to anastomose with deep circumflex iliac and lateral circumflex femoral arteries
         ii. Inferior division passes downward over the surface of gluteus minimus muscle to the greater trochanter and anastomoses with the lateral circumflex femoral artery

B. Inferior gluteal
   1. From the internal iliac artery, leaves pelvis through the greater sciatic foramen below the piriformis muscle
   2. Branches:
      a. Sciatic: runs with the sciatic nerve
      b. Anastomotic: forms the cruciate anastomosis by uniting with the lateral and medial circumflex femoral and the 1st perforating artery from the deep femoral

C. Internal pudendal: from the internal iliac artery, leaves pelvis through the greater sciatic foramen, below piriformis muscle, crosses the spine of ischium, and enters ischioanal fossa through the lesser sciatic foramen

II. Cutaneous Nerves

See Section 3.2, pages 153-154.

III. Sacral Plexus and Derivatives (Fig. 3.16C–E)

A. Components: lumbosacral trunk (L4 and L5) plus anterior rami of sacral nerves S1-4 inclusive
B. Location: posterolateral pelvis, between internal iliac vessels and piriformis muscle
C. Branches
   1. Superior gluteal (L4, L5, S1): follows the superior gluteal artery; supplies gluteus medius, gluteus minimus, and tensor fasciae latae muscles
   2. Nerve to quadratus femoris (L4, L5, S1): leaves pelvis through the greater sciatic foramen below piriformis muscle; supplies quadratus femoris and inferior gemellus muscles
   3. Inferior gluteal (L5, S1, S2): follows inferior gluteal vessels; supplies gluteus maximus muscle
   4. Nerve to obturator internus (L5, S1, S2): leaves pelvis through the greater sciatic foramen below piriformis muscle and enters ischioanal fossa through the lesser sciatic foramen
   5. Sciatic: the largest nerve of body
      a. Actually 2 nerves, tibial and common fibular (peroneal) within the same sheath
         i. Tibial (L4, L5, Sl-3): supplies all hamstrings except the short head of biceps, and then enters the leg to supply the posterior leg and the plantar foot
         ii. Common fibular (peroneal) (L4, L5, S1, S2): supplies short head of biceps and enters the leg to supply the lateral and anterior leg and the dorsal foot (Note: occasionally [slightly more than 10%], common fibular passes through or even above piriformis muscle and may travel distally separate from the tibial nerve)
      b. Leaves pelvis through the greater sciatic foramen below the piriformis muscle, passes inferiorly on obturator internus, gemelli, and quadratus femoris muscles; deep to the gluteus maximus muscle
      c. Distally it runs on the adductor magnus muscle and is crossed by the long head of the biceps muscle; splits above popliteal space into its 2 parts

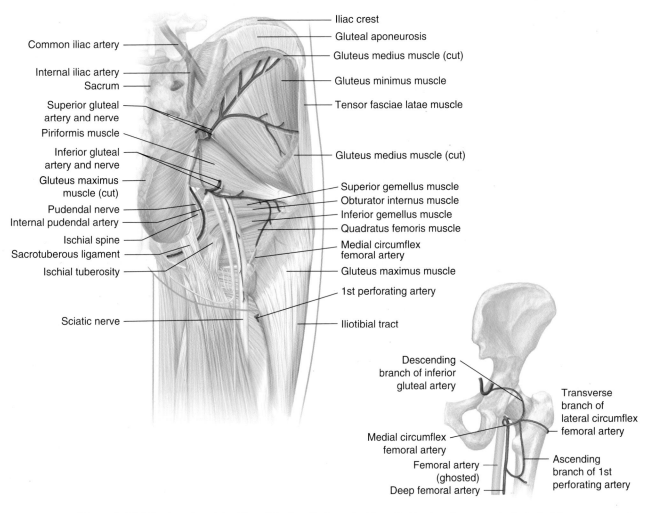

Iliac crest
Gluteal aponeurosis
Gluteus medius muscle (cut)
Common iliac artery
Gluteus minimus muscle
Internal iliac artery
Sacrum
Tensor fasciae latae muscle
Superior gluteal artery and nerve
Piriformis muscle
Inferior gluteal artery and nerve
Gluteus medius muscle (cut)
Gluteus maximus muscle (cut)
Superior gemellus muscle
Obturator internus muscle
Pudendal nerve
Inferior gemellus muscle
Internal pudendal artery
Quadratus femoris muscle
Ischial spine
Medial circumflex femoral artery
Sacrotuberous ligament
Ischial tuberosity
Gluteus maximus muscle
1st perforating artery
Sciatic nerve
Iliotibial tract

Descending branch of inferior gluteal artery
Transverse branch of lateral circumflex femoral artery
Medial circumflex femoral artery
Femoral artery (ghosted)
Ascending branch of 1st perforating artery
Deep femoral artery

Figure 3.16A,B. Arteries of the Gluteal Region. **A.** Posterior View. **B.** Cruciate Anastomosis, Posterior View.

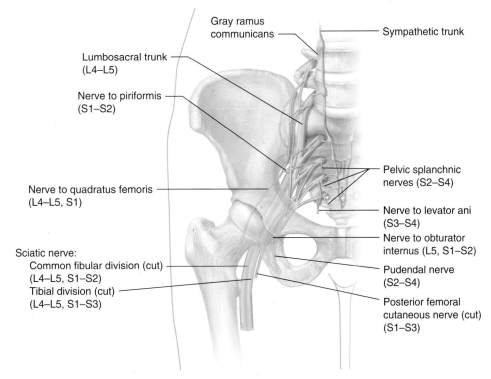

Gray ramus communicans
Sympathetic trunk
Lumbosacral trunk (L4–L5)
Nerve to piriformis (S1–S2)
Pelvic splanchnic nerves (S2–S4)
Nerve to quadratus femoris (L4–L5, S1)
Nerve to levator ani (S3–S4)
Nerve to obturator internus (L5, S1–S2)
Sciatic nerve:
 Common fibular division (cut) (L4–L5, S1–S2)
 Tibial division (cut) (L4–L5, S1–S3)
Pudendal nerve (S2–S4)
Posterior femoral cutaneous nerve (cut) (S1–S3)

Figure 3.16C. Sacral Plexus. Anterior view.

6. Nerve to piriformis muscle (S1, S2): muscle does not leave pelvis
7. Posterior femoral cutaneous (S1-3): leaves pelvis through the greater sciatic foramen to reach the skin over the lower part of gluteus maximus muscle with inferior cluneal branches and then distribute to the posterior thigh skin
8. Perforating cutaneous (S2, S3): pierces sacrotuberous ligament; supplies the lower and medial buttock
9. Pudendal (S2-4): leaves pelvis through the greater sciatic foramen, crosses the ischial spine, and enters ischioanal fossa through the lesser sciatic foramen

IV. Clinical Considerations

A. **Sciatica** is characterized by intense pain at the back of the thigh, most often caused by prolapse of intervertebral disc L4-5
B. Lesions of the sciatic nerve lead to paralysis of all of the muscles below the knee; sensation on the lateral side of the leg and both surfaces of the foot is also lost
C. The sciatic nerve leaves the buttock by passing just lateral to the ischial tuberosity, and thereafter runs downward in the posterior midline, behind the adductor magnus but deep to the other muscles arising from the tuberosity
D. Gluteal region is a common site of intramuscular injection of drugs
   1. Injection can only be made safely into the superolateral quadrant just inferior to the iliac crest where it penetrates the belly of the gluteus medius and possibly the gluteus minimus
   2. Injections into either 2 inferior quadrants will endanger and possibly injure the sciatic or other nerves and vessels that emerge inferior to the piriformis muscle
   3. Injection into superomedial quadrant may injure the superior gluteal nerve and/or vessels
E. "Driver's thigh" is a neuralgia caused by pressure on gluteal nerves
F. Lesions of the superior gluteal nerve cause a drastic sag of the pelvis toward the side of the "swing phase" in walking, called Trendelenburg sign or gluteal gait
G. Injuries to sacral plexus are uncommon, but nerves arising from it can be compressed by pelvic tumors resulting in lower limb pain, which can be severe

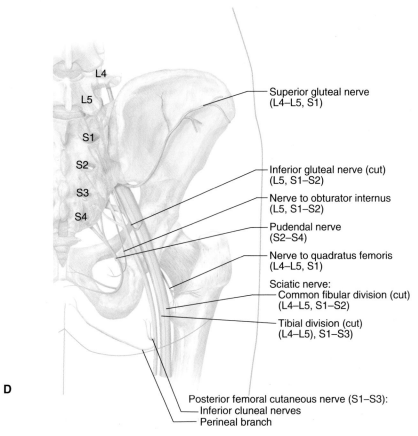

Superior gluteal nerve
(L4–L5, S1)

Inferior gluteal nerve (cut)
(L5, S1–S2)

Nerve to obturator internus
(L5, S1–S2)

Pudendal nerve
(S2–S4)

Nerve to quadratus femoris
(L4–L5, S1)

Sciatic nerve:
Common fibular division (cut)
(L4–L5, S1–S2)

Tibial division (cut)
(L4–L5), S1–S3)

L4

L5

S1

S2

S3

S4

D

Posterior femoral cutaneous nerve (S1–S3):
Inferior cluneal nerves
Perineal branch

Figure 3.16D. Sacral Plexus. Posterior View.

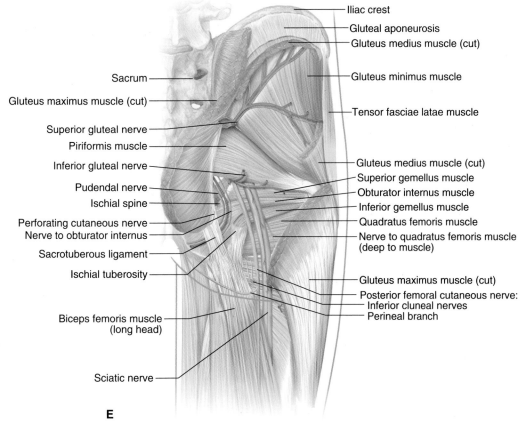

Iliac crest

Gluteal aponeurosis

Gluteus medius muscle (cut)

Gluteus minimus muscle

Tensor fasciae latae muscle

Gluteus medius muscle (cut)

Superior gemellus muscle

Obturator internus muscle

Inferior gemellus muscle

Quadratus femoris muscle

Nerve to quadratus femoris muscle
(deep to muscle)

Gluteus maximus muscle (cut)

Posterior femoral cutaneous nerve:
Inferior cluneal nerves
Perineal branch

Sacrum

Gluteus maximus muscle (cut)

Superior gluteal nerve

Piriformis muscle

Inferior gluteal nerve

Pudendal nerve

Ischial spine

Perforating cutaneous nerve

Nerve to obturator internus

Sacrotuberous ligament

Ischial tuberosity

Biceps femoris muscle
(long head)

Sciatic nerve

E

Figure 3.16E. Nerves of the Gluteal Region. Posterior View.

Muscles of the Posterior Thigh

I. Muscles of the Posterior Thigh (Fig. 3.17A,B)

Muscle	Origin	Insertion	Action	Nerve
Biceps femoris:				
Long head	Ischial tuberosity	Head of fibula	Extends the thigh, flexes the leg	Tibial (L5, S1, S2)
Short head	Lateral lip of linea aspera, lateral intermuscular septum		Flexes the leg	Common fibular (peroneal) (L5, S1, S2)
Semitendinosus	Lower medial surface of ischial tuberosity	Medial surface of proximal tibia via pes anserinus	Extends the thigh, flexes the leg	Tibial (L5, S1, S2)
Semimembranosus	Upper lateral surface of the ischial tuberosity	Posterior aspect of medial tibial condyle	Extends the thigh, flexes the leg	Tibial (L5, S1, S2)

II. Clinical Considerations

A. Charley horse: expressed as pain or muscle stiffness after a bruise or excessive athletic activity; frequently occurs in the hamstring muscles

B. In their actions, all muscles arising from the ischial tuberosity assist the gluteus maximus to extend the hip joint and, because they normally maintain more tone than the gluteus maximus, patients with paralyzed hamstrings tend to fall forward

C. Short head of biceps can act only at the knee; it is a more efficient flexor at the knee than the long head because the long head apparently relaxes during the last half of flexion, while the short head continues to contract

D. Pulled hamstrings are common sports injuries in people who run hard
   1. There may be a tearing off or avulsion of part of the tendinous origin of the hamstrings from the ischial tuberosity
   2. Contusion (bruising) and tearing of some muscle fibers, resulting in blood vessel rupture that creates a hematoma held in the dense fascia lata, is usually seen

E. Pain from an abscess or tumor in the popliteal region is usually severe due to the tenseness of popliteal fascia not allowing for expansion

F. Injury to the common fibular (peroneal) nerve results in loss of eversion and dorsiflexion of the foot (footdrop) and sensory loss to the lateral leg and the dorsum of the foot

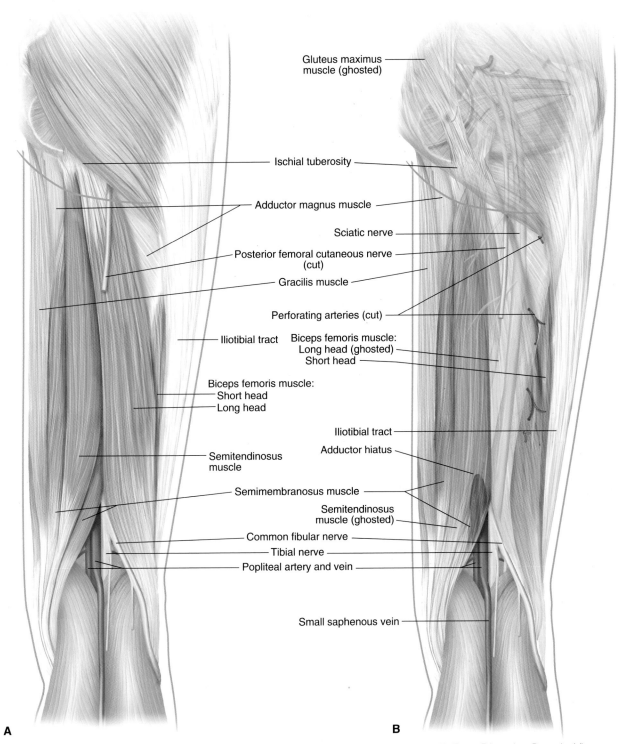

Gluteus maximus
muscle (ghosted)

Ischial tuberosity

Adductor magnus muscle

Sciatic nerve

Posterior femoral cutaneous nerve
(cut)

Gracilis muscle

Perforating arteries (cut)

Iliotibial tract

Biceps femoris muscle:
Long head (ghosted)
Short head

Biceps femoris muscle:
Short head
Long head

Iliotibial tract

Adductor hiatus

Semitendinosus
muscle

Semimembranosus muscle

Semitendinosus
muscle (ghosted)

Common fibular nerve

Tibial nerve

Popliteal artery and vein

Small saphenous vein

A

B

Figure 3.17A,B. Muscles of the Posterior Thigh. **A.** Superficial Dissection, Posterior View. **B.** Deep Dissection, Posterior View.

Popliteal Region and Anastomosis Around the Knee

I. Popliteal Fossa (Fig. 3.18A)

A. Definition: diamond-shaped space behind the knee

B. Bounded: laterally and above, biceps femoris muscle; medially and above, semimembranosus and semitendinosus muscles; laterally and below, lateral head of the gastrocnemius and plantaris muscle; medially and below, medial head of the gastrocnemius muscle

C. Floor: from above downward, is formed by popliteal surface of the femur, oblique popliteal ligament, and popliteus muscle

D. Roof: covered by popliteal fascia (a distal extension of the fascia lata), superficial fascia, and skin

E. Contents (superficial to deep): termination of lesser saphenous vein, tibial and common fibular (peroneal) nerves, popliteal vein, popliteal artery, articular branch of the obturator nerve, and a few small lymph nodes and fat

II. Tibial Nerve

A. Relations: enters fossa from beneath biceps femoris muscle, lateral to popliteal vessels, and crosses superficial to vessels to reach the medial side

B. Proprioceptive sensory branches follow the superior, inferior medial, and middle genicular arteries to the joint

III. Common Fibular (Peroneal) Nerve

A. Relations: along the lateral side of fossa at the medial border of biceps femoris muscle

B. Proprioceptive sensory branches follow the superior and inferior lateral genicular arteries to the joint

C. Nerve leaves popliteal fossa by crossing the lateral head of the gastrocnemius; becomes subcutaneous just behind the head of fibula and divides into 2 branches:

1. Deep fibular (peroneal): runs around fibula deep to fibularis longus and enters the anterior compartment; gives off a branch to fibularis longus muscle and supplies muscles of the anterior compartment

2. Superficial fibular (peroneal): descends in the lateral compartment, supplies fibularis longus and brevis, and emerges to supply skin (sensory) of the lower 3rd of the leg and the dorsum of the foot and digits (L5 dermatome)

IV. Popliteal Vein

A. Formed by anterior and posterior tibial veins at the lower border of popliteus muscle

B. At first medial and then crosses superficial to the popliteal artery to the lateral side; becomes femoral vein as it passes through adductor hiatus

C. Receives lesser saphenous vein

V. Popliteal Artery (Fig. 3.18B)

A. Continuation of the femoral artery as it passes through adductor hiatus in adductor magnus muscle

B. Relations

	Anterior	
	Femur, oblique popliteal ligament, popliteus muscle	
Lateral	*Popliteal Artery*	*Medial*
Biceps and lateral head gastrocnemius muscles; plantaris muscle; lateral condyle of femur		Semimembranosus, medial head of gastrocnemius muscles, medial condyle femur
	Posterior	
	Popliteal vein, tibial nerve, gastrocnemius, plantaris	

C. Branches: medial and lateral superior genicular, middle genicular, medial and lateral inferior genicular; terminates as anterior and posterior tibial arteries

VI. Genicular Anastomosis: Collateral Circulation around the Knee

A. Lateral arteries
  1. Descending branch of the lateral circumflex femoral
  2. Superior and inferior lateral genicular arteries from popliteal
B. Medial arteries
  1. Descending genicular branch of femoral
  2. Superior and inferior medial genicular from popliteal
C. Other anastomosing arteries
  1. Middle genicular from popliteal
  2. Anterior and posterior tibial recurrent from the anterior tibial

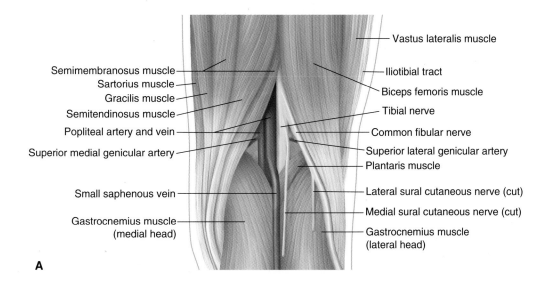

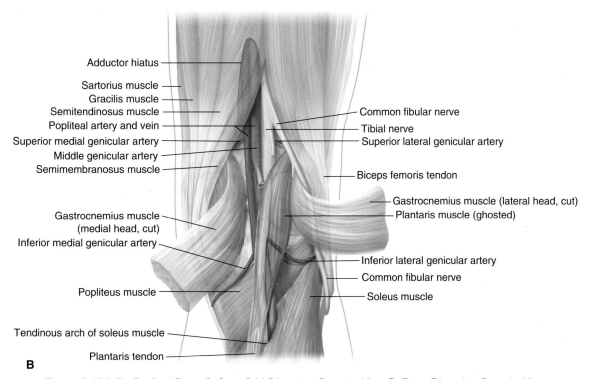

Figure 3.18A,B. Popliteal Fossa. **A.** Superficial Dissection, Posterior View. **B.** Deep Dissection, Posterior View.

Compartments of the Leg

I. Intermuscular Septa: Inward Extensions of the Crural Fascia to Anterior and Lateral Crests of Fibula (Fig. 3.19A–C)

A. Anterior intermuscular septum: attached to anterior border of fibula; separates extensor muscles of the anterior compartment from fibular (peroneal) muscles of the lateral compartment

B. Posterior intermuscular septum: attached to the posterior border of fibula; separates fibular (peroneal) muscles from flexors of the back of the leg

C. Transverse intermuscular septum: extends medially from posterior intermuscular septum; separates superficial and deep groups of the posterior leg, or calf, muscles; ends medially on tibia and in the crural fascia covering flexor digitorum longus muscle

D. These septa, plus tibia, fibula, and interosseous membrane, divide the leg into anterior, lateral, and superficial and deep posterior compartments

II. Compartments

A. Anterior compartment
   1. Primary action: dorsiflexion of the foot; tibialis anterior, extensor hallucis longus, extensor digitorum longus, fibularis tertius
   2. Nerve: deep fibular
   3. Artery: anterior tibial

B. Lateral compartment
   1. Primary action: eversion of the foot
   2. Nerve: superficial fibular
   3. Artery: branches of fibular (which travels within the posterior compartment)

C. Posterior compartment
   1. Primary action: plantarflexion and inversion of the foot
   2. Nerve: tibial
   3. Artery: posterior tibial

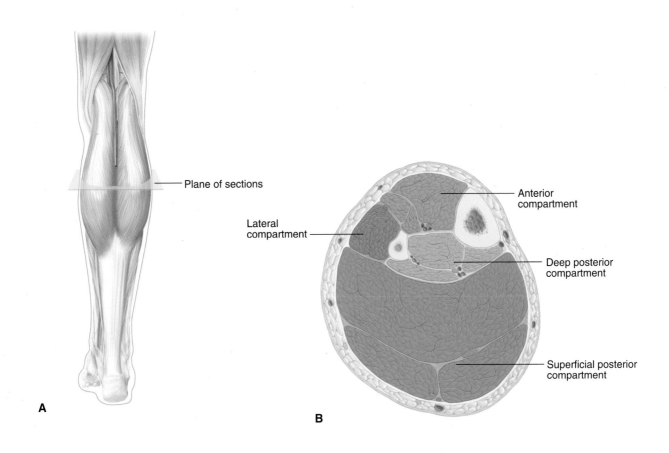

Plane of sections

Anterior compartment

Lateral compartment

Deep posterior compartment

Superficial posterior compartment

A

B

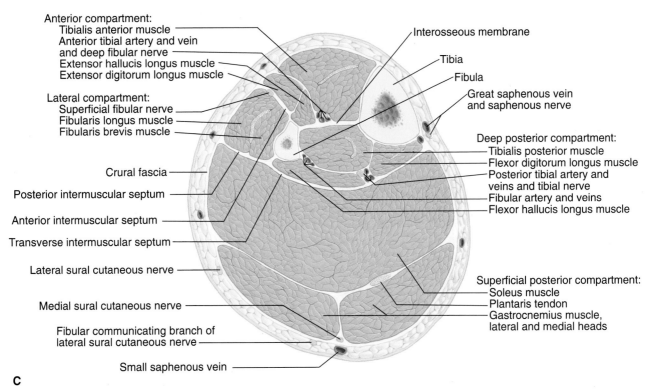

Anterior compartment:
Tibialis anterior muscle
Anterior tibial artery and vein and deep fibular nerve
Extensor hallucis longus muscle
Extensor digitorum longus muscle

Lateral compartment:
Superficial fibular nerve
Fibularis longus muscle
Fibularis brevis muscle

Crural fascia

Posterior intermuscular septum

Anterior intermuscular septum

Transverse intermuscular septum

Lateral sural cutaneous nerve

Medial sural cutaneous nerve

Fibular communicating branch of lateral sural cutaneous nerve

Small saphenous vein

Interosseous membrane

Tibia

Fibula

Great saphenous vein and saphenous nerve

Deep posterior compartment:
Tibialis posterior muscle
Flexor digitorum longus muscle
Posterior tibial artery and veins and tibial nerve
Fibular artery and veins
Flexor hallucis longus muscle

Superficial posterior compartment:
Soleus muscle
Plantaris tendon
Gastrocnemius muscle, lateral and medial heads

C

Figure 3.19A–C. Compartments of the Leg. **A.** Orientation, Posterior View. **B.** Cross-Section View. **C.** Cross-Section View.

Muscles of the Posterior Leg

I. Muscles of the Posterior Leg

A. Superficial compartment (Fig. 3.20A,B)

Muscle	Origin	Insertion	Action	Nerve
Gastrocnemius:				
Medial head	Upper posterior surface of medial condyle of the femur	Dorsum of calcaneus through calcaneal tendon	Flexes the leg, plantar flexes the foot	Tibial (S1, S2)
Lateral head	Upper posterior surface of lateral condyle of the femur	Same	Same	Same
Soleus	Head and upper fibula, soleal line, upper medial tibia	Dorsum of calcaneus through calcaneal tendon	Plantar flexes the foot	Tibial (S1, S2)
Plantaris	Lower lateral supracondylar line	Posterior calcaneus	Flexes the leg, plantar flexes the foot	Tibial (S1, S2)

B. Deep compartment (Fig. 3.20C)

Muscle	Origin	Insertion	Action	Nerve
Popliteus	Lateral surface of lateral condyle of the femur	Posterior tibia above soleal line	Flexes leg, rotates leg medially	Tibial (L4-5, S1)
Flexor hallucis longus	Distal 2/3 of the posterior tibia	Base of the distal phalanx of hallux	Flexes the distal phalanx of hallux, plantar flexes and inverts the foot	Tibial (S2, S3)
Flexor digitorum longus	Posterior tibia distal to soleal line	Base of the distal phalanx of lateral 4 toes	Flexes toes, plantar flexes and inverts the foot	Tibial (L4, L5)
Tibialis posterior	Posterior surface of tibia, fibula, and interosseous membrane	Tuberosity of navicular, cuboid cuneiforms, sustentaculum tali of calcaneus, and bases of metatarsals 2–4	Plantar flexes, adducts, and inverts the foot (supports the medial longitudinal arch)	Tibial (L4, L5)

II. Special Features

A. Long, slender plantaris tendon running on the medial border of calcaneal tendon may rupture

B. Flexor hallucis longus tendon runs in a groove on the posterior inferior tibia, posterior talus, and under sustentaculum tali

C. Flexor digitorum longus tendon runs in a groove behind the medial malleolus with tibialis posterior muscle, obliquely forward and lateralward superficial to the deltoid ligament into the sole of the foot, where it crosses inferior to flexor hallucis longus

D. Tibialis posterior tendon runs in front of flexor digitorum longus in a groove with this muscle as they lie behind the medial malleolus, under flexor retinaculum, but superficial to the deltoid ligament; it passes under the calcaneonavicular ligament

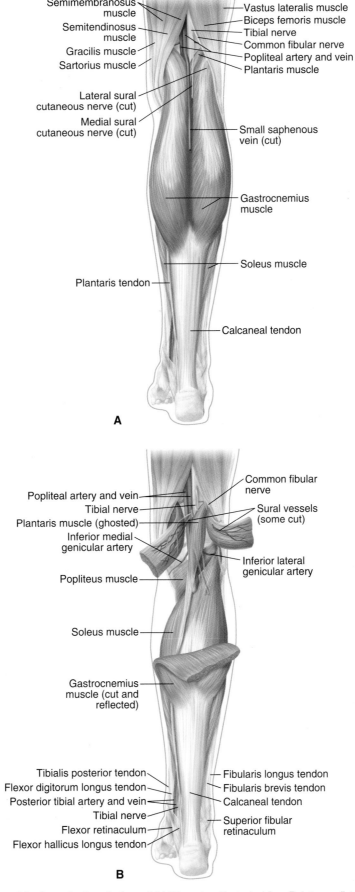

Semimembranosus muscle

Semitendinosus muscle

Gracilis muscle

Sartorius muscle

Lateral sural cutaneous nerve (cut)

Medial sural cutaneous nerve (cut)

Plantaris tendon

Vastus lateralis muscle

Biceps femoris muscle

Tibial nerve

Common fibular nerve

Popliteal artery and vein

Plantaris muscle

Small saphenous vein (cut)

Gastrocnemius muscle

Soleus muscle

Calcaneal tendon

A

Popliteal artery and vein

Tibial nerve

Plantaris muscle (ghosted)

Inferior medial genicular artery

Popliteus muscle

Soleus muscle

Gastrocnemius muscle (cut and reflected)

Tibialis posterior tendon

Flexor digitorum longus tendon

Posterior tibial artery and vein

Tibial nerve

Flexor retinaculum

Flexor hallucis longus tendon

Common fibular nerve

Sural vessels (some cut)

Inferior lateral genicular artery

Fibularis longus tendon

Fibularis brevis tendon

Calcaneal tendon

Superior fibular retinaculum

B

Figure 3.20A,B. Muscles of the Posterior Leg. **A.** Superficial Dissection, Posterior View. **B.** Intermediate Dissection, Posterior View.

    E. Flexor retinaculum holds long flexor tendons at the medial side of the ankle

      I. Extends from margins of the medial malleolus to calcaneus, passes over tendon of tibialis posterior muscle, attaches to bone behind this, and then forms superficial and deep layers

        a. Superficial extends to tuberosity of calcaneus

        b. Deep passes over flexor digitorum longus and flexor hallucis longus muscles and is attached to bone on either side of these, forming separate osseofibrous canals

      2. Converts bony grooves into 4 osseofibrous canals for the following structures (from medial to lateral):

        a. Tendon of tibialis posterior muscle

        b. Tendon of flexor digitorum longus muscle

        c. Posterior tibial artery and vein and the tibial nerve

        d. Tendon of the flexor hallucis longus muscle

    F. Tendon sheaths: Behind the medial malleolus, the tendon of tibialis posterior muscle lies in front of but in the same groove with flexor digitorum longus muscle

      I. Both have separate sheaths

        a. Sheath for tibialis posterior starts 5 cm above the malleolus and extends to tuberosity of navicular

        b. Sheath for flexor digitorum longus begins just above the tip of the malleolus and ends opposite the first cuneiform

      2. Tendon of flexor hallucis longus muscle lies dorsal to that of flexor digitorum longus muscle and crosses it from the lateral to medial; its sheath starts at the tip of the malleolus and extends to the base of the 1st metatarsal

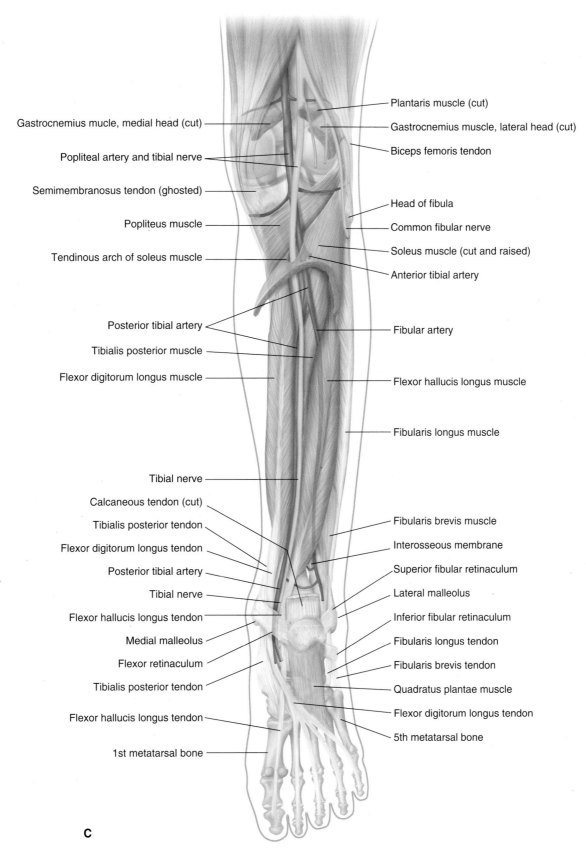

Gastrocnemius mucle, medial head (cut)

Popliteal artery and tibial nerve

Semimembranosus tendon (ghosted)

Popliteus muscle

Tendinous arch of soleus muscle

Posterior tibial artery

Tibialis posterior muscle

Flexor digitorum longus muscle

Tibial nerve

Calcaneous tendon (cut)

Tibialis posterior tendon

Flexor digitorum longus tendon

Posterior tibial artery

Tibial nerve

Flexor hallucis longus tendon

Medial malleolus

Flexor retinaculum

Tibialis posterior tendon

Flexor hallucis longus tendon

1st metatarsal bone

Plantaris muscle (cut)

Gastrocnemius muscle, lateral head (cut)

Biceps femoris tendon

Head of fibula

Common fibular nerve

Soleus muscle (cut and raised)

Anterior tibial artery

Fibular artery

Flexor hallucis longus muscle

Fibularis longus muscle

Fibularis brevis muscle

Interosseous membrane

Superior fibular retinaculum

Lateral malleolus

Inferior fibular retinaculum

Fibularis longus tendon

Fibularis brevis tendon

Quadratus plantae muscle

Flexor digitorum longus tendon

5th metatarsal bone

C

Figure 3.20C. Muscles of the Posterior Leg. Deep Dissection, Posterior View.

Muscles of the Lateral and Anterior Leg

I. Muscles of the Lateral and Anterior Leg

A. Lateral (Fig. 3.21A)

Muscle	Origin	Insertion	Action	Nerve
Fibularis (peroneus) longus	Head and upper 2/3 of the lateral surface of fibula	Inferior surface of the first cuneiform and the base of the first metatarsal	Everts and plantar flexes the foot (supports lateral longitudinal and transverse arches of the foot)	Superficial fibular (peroneal) (L5, S1, S2)
Fibularis (peroneus) brevis	Lower 2/3 of the lateral surface of fibula	Tuberosity of the 5th metatarsal	Everts and plantar flexes the foot	Superficial fibular (peroneal) (L5, S1, S2)

B. Anterior (Fig. 3.21B)

Muscle	Origin	Insertion	Action	Nerve
Tibialis anterior	Lateral tibial condyle and the upper lateral surface of tibia	Inferomedial surface of 1st cuneiform and the base of the 1st metatarsal	Dorsiflexes and inverts the foot	Deep fibular (peroneal) (L4, L5)
Extensor digitorum longus	Lateral tibial condyle, the anterior surface of fibula, and lthe ateral anterior surface of interosseous membrane	Dorsum of lateral 4 toes via extensor expansions (central slip inserts on the base of the middle phalanx, lateral slips on the base of distal phalanx)	Extends toes, dorsiflexes the foot	Deep fibular (peroneal) (L5, S1)
Fibularis (peroneus) tertius	Distal anterior surface of fibula	Dorsum of shaft of the 5th metatarsal	Dorsiflexes and everts the foot	Deep fibular (peroneal) (L5, S1)
Extensor hallucis longus	Middle half of the anterior surface of fibula and interosseous membrane	Base of the distal phalanx of hallux	Extends hallux, dorsiflexes the ankle	Deep fibular (peroneal) (L5, S1)

II. Special Features

A. Superior and inferior fibular retinacula: prevent lateral compartment tendons from bowstringing
   1. Superior: from the lateral malleolus to fascia of the back of the leg and the lateral side of calcaneus
   2. Inferior: overlies tendons on the lateral calcaneus and is attached to bone on either side of the tendons; joins superficial part of the inferior extensor retinaculum
B. Synovial sheaths: both fibularis muscles lie in a common sheath extending 4 cm above and below the tip of the malleolus
C. Course of tendon of fibularis (peroneus) longus
   1. Passes behind the lateral malleolus with tendon of fibularis (peroneus) brevis muscle but lies posteriorly, under fibular (peroneal) retinacula
   2. Along the lateral side of calcaneus, passes over the lateral side of cuboid bone and then in a groove on the plantar surface of this bone; held in groove by the **long plantar ligament**
   3. Then crosses the foot obliquely to first cuneiform and metatarsal bones
D. The 4 anterior muscles of the leg lie in a fascial compartment between the anterior intermuscular septum and the tibia
   1. All 4 are innervated by the deep fibular (peroneal) nerve
   2. All dorsiflex the foot, although with varying strength

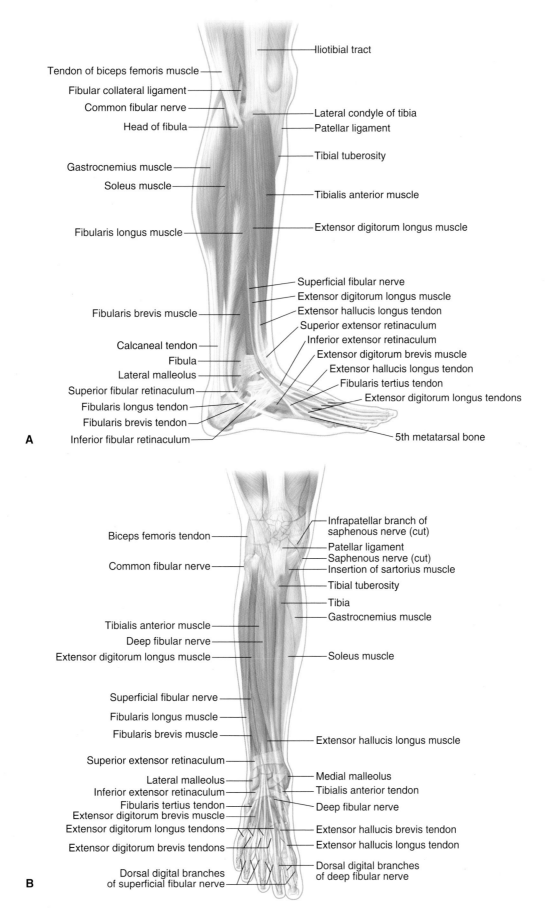

Iliotibial tract

Tendon of biceps femoris muscle

Fibular collateral ligament

Common fibular nerve

Head of fibula

Lateral condyle of tibia

Patellar ligament

Tibial tuberosity

Gastrocnemius muscle

Soleus muscle

Tibialis anterior muscle

Fibularis longus muscle

Extensor digitorum longus muscle

Superficial fibular nerve

Extensor digitorum longus muscle

Extensor hallucis longus tendon

Superior extensor retinaculum

Fibularis brevis muscle

Inferior extensor retinaculum

Extensor digitorum brevis muscle

Calcaneal tendon

Extensor hallucis longus tendon

Fibula

Fibularis tertius tendon

Lateral malleolus

Superior fibular retinaculum

Extensor digitorum longus tendons

Fibularis longus tendon

Fibularis brevis tendon

5th metatarsal bone

Inferior fibular retinaculum

A

Infrapatellar branch of
saphenous nerve (cut)

Biceps femoris tendon

Patellar ligament

Saphenous nerve (cut)

Common fibular nerve

Insertion of sartorius muscle

Tibial tuberosity

Tibia

Gastrocnemius muscle

Tibialis anterior muscle

Deep fibular nerve

Extensor digitorum longus muscle

Soleus muscle

Superficial fibular nerve

Fibularis longus muscle

Fibularis brevis muscle

Extensor hallucis longus muscle

Superior extensor retinaculum

Medial malleolus

Lateral malleolus

Tibialis anterior tendon

Inferior extensor retinaculum

Deep fibular nerve

Fibularis tertius tendon

Extensor digitorum brevis muscle

Extensor digitorum longus tendons

Extensor hallucis brevis tendon

Extensor digitorum brevis tendons

Extensor hallucis longus tendon

Dorsal digital branches
of superficial fibular nerve

Dorsal digital branches
of deep fibular nerve

B

Figure 3.21A,B. Muscles of the Lateral and Anterior Leg. **A.** Lateral View. **B.** Anterior View.

E. Extensor retinacula: hold extensor tendons in place

  1. Thickenings of crural fascia

  2. Superior (transverse) and inferior (cruciate crural) extensor retinacula: prevent bowstringing of the anterior compartment muscles

    a. Inferior retinaculum: divided into a superficial Y-shape with a stem attached to the lateral side of the calcaneus

      i. Splits into an upper limb that attaches to the medial malleolus and a lower limb that inserts on the 1st cuneiform and the sole of the foot, after passing over the extensor digitorum longus muscle

      ii. There is also a deep limb beneath the Y-split, which passes deep to the fibularis tertius and extensor longus muscles

F. Synovial tendon sheaths of anterior muscles

  1. Tibialis anterior: from above superior extensor retinaculum, under inferior extensor retinaculum to the level of the talonavicular joint

  2. Extensor hallucis longus: from just above the superior limb of the inferior extensor retinaculum, beneath both limbs of retinaculum to the level of the 1st tarsometatarsal joint

  3. Extensor digitorum longus: envelops this and fibularis (peroneus) tertius muscle from above the inferior extensor retinaculum to the middle of the cuboid bone

III. Clinical Considerations

A. Shin splints: painful condition of the anterior compartment of the leg after vigorous and/or lengthy exercise. The muscles in the anterior compartment swell from overuse, reducing blood flow to muscles, and cramps develop; this is a mild form of compartment syndrome

B. Foot drop: results if tibialis anterior is paralyzed due to injury of the common fibular nerve or its deep branch

Vessels and Nerves of the Leg

I. Posterior Tibial Artery (Fig. 3.22A,B)

A. Direct continuation of the popliteal artery after the branching of the anterior tibial artery

B. Relations

	Anterior	
	Tibialis posterior and flexor digitorum longus muscles, tibia, ankle joint	
Lateral	**Posterior Tibial Artery**	**Medial**
Vena comitans		Vena comitans
	Posterior	
	Skin and fascia, gastrocnemius and soleus muscles, tibial nerve, and transverse intermuscular septum	

C. Branches: fibular (peroneal), posterior medial malleolar, communicating, medial calcaneal, muscular, and nutrient (tibial)

II. Fibular (Peroneal) Artery

A. Arises from the posterior tibial artery, approaches fibula, and passes in a fibrous canal between tibialis posterior and flexor hallucis longus muscles to come to lie beneath flexor hallucis longus

B. Relations

	Anterior	
	Tibialis posterior muscle, interosseous membrane	
Lateral	**Fibular (Peroneal) Artery**	**Medial**
Flexor hallucis longus, fibula		Flexor hallucis longus muscle
	Posterior	
	Soleus, flexor hallucis longus muscle, transverse intermuscular septum	

C. Branches: perforating, communicating, lateral calcaneal, muscular, and nutrient

III. Anterior Tibial Artery

A. Branches from the popliteal artery at the lower border of popliteus muscle; it passes between 2 heads of tibialis posterior muscle and above interosseous membrane to the anterior compartment of the leg, where it is joined by the deep fibular (peroneal) nerve

B. Relations

	Anterior	
	Tibialis anterior, extensor digitorum longus, and extensor hallucis longus muscles; deep fibular (peroneal) nerve	
Lateral	**Anterior Tibial Artery**	**Medial**
Extensor digitorum longus and extensor hallucis longus muscles; deep fibular (peroneal) nerve		Deep fibular (peroneal) nerve and extensor hallucis longus muscle
	Posterior	
	Interosseous membrane, tibia, ankle joint	

C. Branches: anterior and posterior tibial recurrent; fibular; anterior medial and anterior lateral malleolar; and muscular

IV. Anastomoses About the Ankle

Medial Malleolar Network	**Lateral Malleolar Network**
Anterior medial malleolar from the anterior tibial artery	Anterior lateral malleolar from the anterior tibial artery
Medial tarsal from the dorsalis pedis artery	Lateral tarsal from the dorsalis pedis artery
Posterior medial malleolar from the posterior tibial artery	Perforating branch from the fibular (peroneal) artery
Medial calcaneal from the posterior tibial artery	Lateral calcaneal from the fibular (peroneal) artery
	Arcuate from the dorsalis pedis artery

V. Relations of Vessels

A. Dorsalis pedis artery is a continuation of the anterior tibial artery in front of the ankle; has a deep fibular (peroneal) nerve on its lateral side and tendon of flexor hallucis longus muscle on its medial side as they pass under the extensor retinacula

B. Tibial nerve lies lateral to the posterior tibial artery as they pass in the 3rd compartment beneath the flexor retinaculum

C. Fibular (peroneal) vessels lie behind the inferior tibiofibular articulation

VI. Tibial Nerve (L4, L5, SI-3) (Fig. 3.22C,D)

A. Branches from sciatic superior to popliteal fossa

B. Provides branches within popliteal fossa
   1. Innervates both heads of gastrocnemius, plantaris, popliteus, and soleus
   2. Cutaneous branch: medial sural cutaneous nerve, which combines with a communicating branch of lateral sural cutaneous nerve to form sural nerve
   3. Proprioceptive branches to knee joint

C. Passes beneath soleus muscle to pass through and innervate deep posterior compartment of the leg: flexor digitorum longus, tibialis posterior, and flexor hallucis longus

D. Passes deep to flexor retinaculum behind tendon of flexor digitorum longus with posterior tibial vessels

E. Ends by dividing at ankle into medial and lateral plantar nerves

VII. Common Fibular (Peroneal) Nerve (L4, L5, SI-2)

A. Branches from sciatic superior to popliteal fossa

B. Provides branches within popliteal fossa
   1. Cutaneous branch: lateral sural cutaneous nerve, whose communicating branch unites with medial sural cutaneous nerve to form sural nerve
   2. Proprioceptive branches to knee joint

C. Passes along posterior edge of biceps femoris muscle to enter lateral leg compartment

D. Divides at neck of fibula deep to fibularis longus into superficial and deep fibular nerves

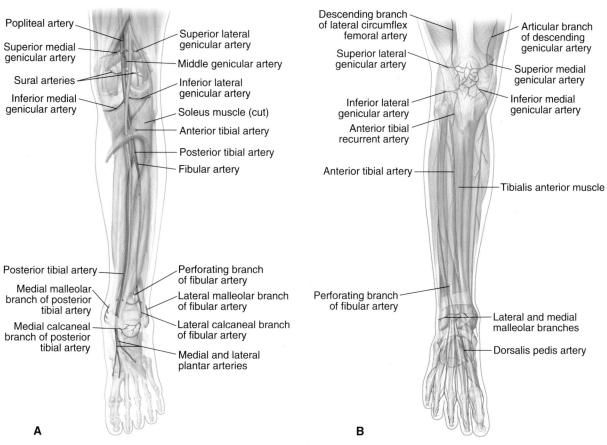

Popliteal artery

Superior medial genicular artery

Sural arteries

Inferior medial genicular artery

Superior lateral genicular artery

Middle genicular artery

Inferior lateral genicular artery

Soleus muscle (cut)

Anterior tibial artery

Posterior tibial artery

Fibular artery

Posterior tibial artery

Medial malleolar branch of posterior tibial artery

Medial calcaneal branch of posterior tibial artery

Perforating branch of fibular artery

Lateral malleolar branch of fibular artery

Lateral calcaneal branch of fibular artery

Medial and lateral plantar arteries

Descending branch of lateral circumflex femoral artery

Superior lateral genicular artery

Inferior lateral genicular artery

Anterior tibial recurrent artery

Anterior tibial artery

Perforating branch of fibular artery

Articular branch of descending genicular artery

Superior medial genicular artery

Inferior medial genicular artery

Tibialis anterior muscle

Lateral and medial malleolar branches

Dorsalis pedis artery

A

B

Figure 3.22A,B. Arteries of the Leg. **A.** Posterior View. **B.** Anterior View.

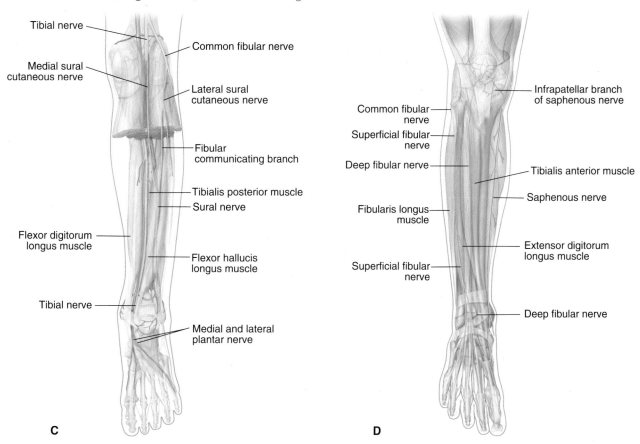

Tibial nerve

Medial sural cutaneous nerve

Flexor digitorum longus muscle

Tibial nerve

Common fibular nerve

Lateral sural cutaneous nerve

Fibular communicating branch

Tibialis posterior muscle

Sural nerve

Flexor hallucis longus muscle

Medial and lateral plantar nerve

Common fibular nerve

Superficial fibular nerve

Deep fibular nerve

Fibularis longus muscle

Superficial fibular nerve

Infrapatellar branch of saphenous nerve

Tibialis anterior muscle

Saphenous nerve

Extensor digitorum longus muscle

Deep fibular nerve

C

D

Figure 3.22C,D. Nerves of the Leg. **C.** Posterior View. **D.** Anterior View.

VIII. Superficial Fibular (Peroneal) Nerve (L4, L5, Sl-2)

A. Branches from common fibular at neck of fibula

B. Passes through and innervates lateral leg compartment: fibularis longus and brevis

C. Leaves lateral compartment near mid-leg to penetrate crural fascia and become cutaneous

    1. Innervates skin of anterolateral leg from mid-leg distally

    2. Divides into 2 or more branches as it descends distally on extensor digitorum longus

    3. Innervates skin of dorsum of foot except first web space between hallux and 2nd toe

IX. Deep Fibular (Peroneal) Nerve (L4, L5, Sl-2)

A. Branches from common fibular at neck of fibula

B. Passes into and innervates anterior leg compartment: extensor digitorum longus, extensor hallucis longus, tibialis anterior, and fibularis tertius

C. Passes deep to extensor retinacula to enter foot and innervate extensor digitorum brevis and extensor hallucis brevis

D. Ends as cutaneous branches to skin of first web space between hallux and second toe

X. Clinical Considerations

A. Pulse of the posterior tibial artery is usually palpated about halfway between the posterior surface of the medial malleolus and the medial border of the calcaneal tendon

B. Dorsalis pedis pulse can be felt where it passes over the navicular and cuneiform bones lateral to the extensor hallucis longus tendon or distal to this at the proximal end of the 1st interosseous space (10% to 20% may be too small to palpate or are found in unusual positions)

C. Tibial nerve is deep and not commonly injured

    1. If damaged proximally, there is paralysis of all muscles in the posterior compartment of the leg and intrinsic muscles in the sole of the foot

    2. There is also loss of sensation in the sole of the foot (vulnerable to development of pressure sores)

D. Compartment syndromes of the leg

    1. Anterior compartment: severe pain, loss of dorsiflexion of the ankle and extension of toes; severe pain on passive plantar flexion of the ankle, eversion of the foot, and passive flexion of toes

    2. Lateral compartment: severe pain, anesthesia over the dorsum of the foot and toes; severe pain on passive dorsiflexion and inversion of the foot; inability to plantar flex and evert the foot (weakness in the dorsiflexion and inversion is seen due to involvement of the deep fibular [peroneal] nerve before it leaves the lateral compartment to enter the anterior compartment)

    3. Posterior compartment: pain, inability to plantar flex the ankle, anesthesia over the distribution of the sural nerve and pain on passive dorsiflexion

    4. Deep compartment: severe pain, weakness of plantar flexion and toe flexion, anesthesia of most of the sole and plantar surface of the toes and severe pain on passive extension of the toes or passive dorsiflexion of the ankle

Dorsum of the Foot

I. Cutaneous Nerves and Superficial Veins (Fig. 3.23A,B)

A. Superficial fibular nerve: the dorsum of the foot except medial and lateral sides and the skin between hallux and the 2nd toe

B. Deep fibular nerve: skin between hallux and the 2nd toe

C. Saphenous nerve: medial surface of the foot as far distally as hallux

D. Sural nerve: variably along the lateral side of the foot, especially near the ankle

E. Dorsal venous arch: drains dorsal metatarsal veins and is drained by great and small saphenous vein

II. Muscles (Fig. 3.23C,D)

Muscle	Origin	Insertion	Action	Nerve
Extensor hallucis brevis	Superolateral surface of calcaneus	Dorsum of the base of the proximal phalanx of hallux	Extends hallux	Deep fibular (peroneal) (L5, S1)
Extensor digitorum brevis	Superolateral surface of calcaneus	Extensor expansion of toes 2–4	Extends toes	Deep fibular (peroneal) (L5, S1)
Dorsal interossei (4)	Adjacent sides of metatarsals 1–5	1st and 2nd on either side, the base of the 1st phalanx of the 2nd toe; 3 and 4 on the lateral side of the proximal phalanx of toes 3 and 4	Abducts toes, flexes metatarso-phalangeal joints	Lateral plantar (S2, S3)

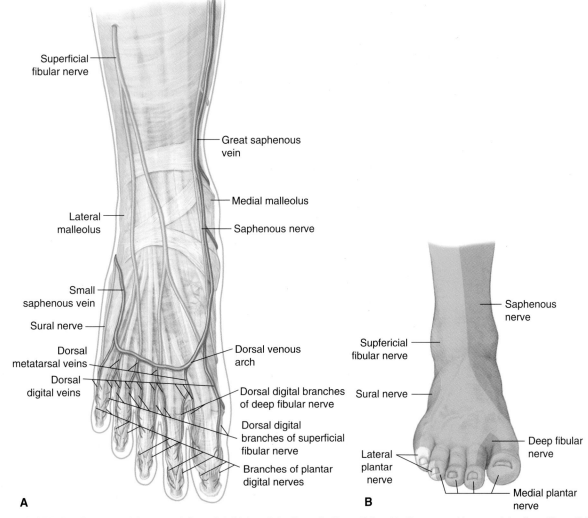

A

B

Figure 3.23A,B. Cutaneous Nerves and Superficial Veins of the Foot. **A.** Dorsal View. **B.** Cutaneous Nerves of the Foot, Dorsal View.

III. Arteries (Fig. 3.23E)

A. Dorsalis pedis (continuation of the anterior tibial artery at the ankle joint; midway between the malleoli): passes down the dorsum of the foot to the proximal end of the 1st intermetatarsal space and terminates as the 1st dorsal metatarsal and deep plantar arteries

B. Branches:

   1. Lateral tarsal

   2. Medial tarsal

   3. Arcuate

      a. Gives rise to 2nd, 3rd, and 4th metatarsal arteries

      b. These subsequently split to form the **dorsal digital arteries** to the adjoining sides of the toes

   4. Terminal branches

      a. 1st dorsal metatarsal to both sides of the big toe and adjoining sides of the big and 2nd toes

      b. Deep plantar form plantar arterial arch with deep branch of the lateral plantar artery

IV. Special Features: Insertions of Extensor Tendons

A. Extensor hallucis has medial and lateral expansions covering the metatarsophalangeal (MP) joint and a prolongation of tendon to the base of the 1st phalanx

B. Extensor digitorum longus

   1. Tendons to toes 2, 3, 4 are joined by extensor brevis

   2. Each receives fibers from lumbricales and interossei, spreads out on the dorsum of the 1st phalanx of each toe, and splits into 3 slips

      a. The intermediate to the base of the middle phalanx

      b. 2 collateral to the base of distal phalanx

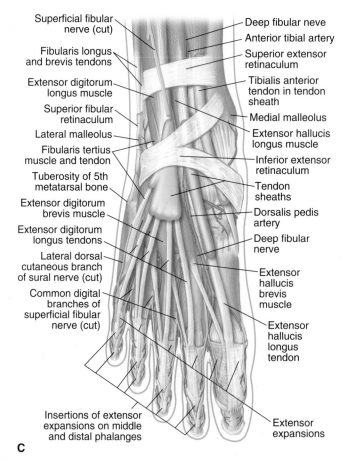

C

Figure 3.23C. Dorsum of the Foot. Superficial Dissection, Dorsal View.

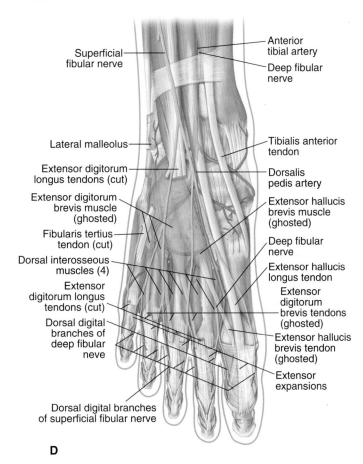

Superficial fibular nerve

Anterior tibial artery

Deep fibular nerve

Lateral malleolus

Tibialis anterior tendon

Extensor digitorum longus tendons (cut)

Dorsalis pedis artery

Extensor digitorum brevis muscle (ghosted)

Extensor hallucis brevis muscle (ghosted)

Fibularis tertius tendon (cut)

Deep fibular nerve

Dorsal interosseous muscles (4)

Extensor hallucis longus tendon

Extensor digitorum longus tendons (cut)

Extensor digitorum brevis tendons (ghosted)

Dorsal digital branches of deep fibular neve

Extensor hallucis brevis tendon (ghosted)

Extensor expansions

Dorsal digital branches of superficial fibular nerve

D

Figure 3.23D. Dorsum of the Foot. Deep Dissection, Dorsal View.

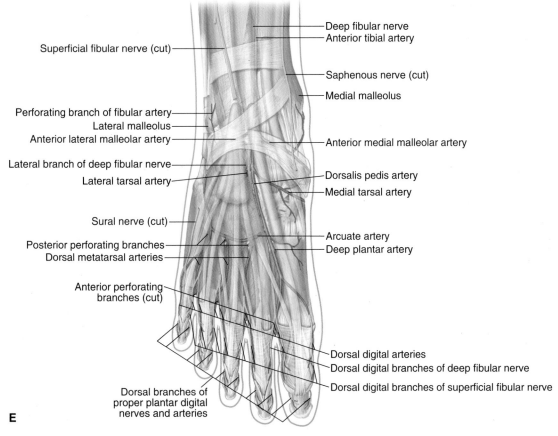

Deep fibular nerve

Anterior tibial artery

Superficial fibular nerve (cut)

Saphenous nerve (cut)

Medial malleolus

Perforating branch of fibular artery

Lateral malleolus

Anterior lateral malleolar artery

Anterior medial malleolar artery

Lateral branch of deep fibular nerve

Lateral tarsal artery

Dorsalis pedis artery

Medial tarsal artery

Sural nerve (cut)

Arcuate artery

Posterior perforating branches

Deep plantar artery

Dorsal metatarsal arteries

Anterior perforating branches (cut)

Dorsal digital arteries

Dorsal digital branches of deep fibular nerve

Dorsal digital branches of superficial fibular nerve

Dorsal branches of proper plantar digital nerves and arteries

E

Figure 3.23E. Arteries and Nerves of the Dorsum of the Foot.

Plantar Aponeurosis and Cutaneous Nerves of the Sole of the Foot

I. Plantar Aponeurosis (Fig. 3.24A)

A. Thickened deep fascia of the sole

B. Extends from tuberosity of calcaneus to end in 5 slips attached to the skin over heads of metatarsals and into flexor tendon sheaths (bands 2, 3, and 4 are stronger than 1 and 5)

II. Cutaneous Nerves (Fig. 3.24B)

A. Saphenous nerve (L3, L4) (from femoral) and sural nerve (S1, S2) (from both tibial and comon fibular nerves) supply small areas of skin on the medial and lateral parts, respectively, of the sole

B. Plantar surface of heel is supplied by the tibial (S1, S2) nerve

C. Most of the medial sole, including the toes to middle of 4th toe, are supplied by the medial plantar nerve, from tibial; the medial plantar nerve (L4, L5) accompanies the medial plantar artery and gives off branches:

    1. Plantar cutaneous branches to the medial side of the sole

    2. Proper digital nerve to the medial side of the big toe

    3. 3 common digital nerves, which split to give 2 proper digital nerves to adjacent sides of toes 1 to 4

D. Lateral half of the 4th toe and the lateral side of the foot are supplied by the lateral plantar nerve (S1, S2)

    1. Lateral plantar nerve is accompanied by the lateral plantar artery

    2. Nerve gives off a superficial branch, which sends proper digital nerves to the lateral side of the little toe, and common digital nerves, which divide to supply adjacent sides of toes 4 and 5

III. Clinical Considerations: Plantar Skin Reflex

A. When skin of the sole is slowly stroked along the outer border from heel forward, the toes flex

B. In patients with certain disorders of motor pathways, similar stimulation of the sole results in a slow dorsiflexion of hallux and a spreading of other toes—known as the **Babinski sign or reflex**

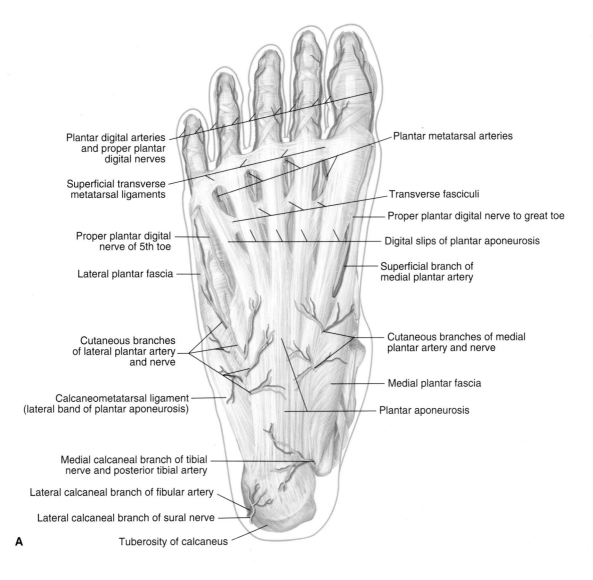

Plantar digital arteries and proper plantar digital nerves

Superficial transverse metatarsal ligaments

Proper plantar digital nerve of 5th toe

Lateral plantar fascia

Cutaneous branches of lateral plantar artery and nerve

Calcaneometatarsal ligament (lateral band of plantar aponeurosis)

Medial calcaneal branch of tibial nerve and posterior tibial artery

Lateral calcaneal branch of fibular artery

Lateral calcaneal branch of sural nerve

Tuberosity of calcaneus

Plantar metatarsal arteries

Transverse fasciculi

Proper plantar digital nerve to great toe

Digital slips of plantar aponeurosis

Superficial branch of medial plantar artery

Cutaneous branches of medial plantar artery and nerve

Medial plantar fascia

Plantar aponeurosis

A

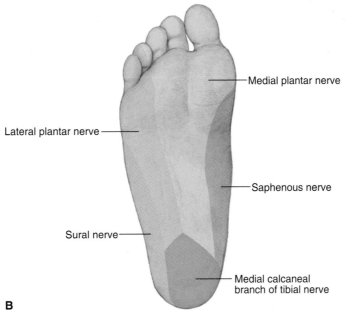

Medial plantar nerve

Lateral plantar nerve

Saphenous nerve

Sural nerve

Medial calcaneal branch of tibial nerve

B

Figure 3.24A,B. Cutaneous Nerves of the Sole of the Foot. **A.** Dissection. **B.** Distribution.

Muscles of the Sole of the Foot

I. Muscles (Fig. 3.25A–E)

Muscle	Origin	Insertion	Action	Nerve
Abductor hallucis	Medial process of tuberosity of calcaneus	Medial side of the base of the proximal phalanx of hallux	Flexes and abducts hallux	Medial plantar (S2, S3)
Flexor digitorum brevis	Medial process of tuberosity of calcaneus	Middle phalanx, lateral 4 toes	Flexes toes	Medial plantar (S2, S3)
Quadratus plantae	Lateral head: the lateral process of tuberosity calcaneus Medial head: the medial side of calcaneus	Lateral border of long flexor tendons	Flexes toes	Lateral plantar (S2, S3)
Flexor hallucis brevis	Cuboid, lateral cuneiform, the medial side of the 1st metatarsal	Medial belly: the medial side of the proximal phalanx of hallux Lateral belly: the lateral side of the proximal phalanx	Flexes the metatarsophalangeal joint of hallux	Medial plantar (S2, S3)
Adductor hallucis	Oblique head: bases of metatarsals 2–4; Transverse head: heads of metatarsals 3–5	Lateral side of the base of the proximal phalanx of hallux	Adducts hallux; helps maintain transverse arch of the foot	Lateral plantar (S2, S3)
Lumbricales				
1st	Medial side of the 1st long flexor tendon	Proximal phalanx and extensor tendons, toe 2	Flexes proximal, extends distal phalanges	Medial plantar (S2, S3)
2nd, 3rd, and 4th	Long flexor tendons 2–4	As above for toes 3–5	See above	Lateral plantar (S2, S3)
Abductor digiti minimi	Lateral and medial processes of tuberosity of calcaneus	Lateral surface of the proximal phalanx of the 5th toe	Abducts and flexes the proximal phalanx of the 5th toe	Lateral plantar (S2, S3)
Flexor digiti minimi brevis	Base of the 5th metatarsal bone	Lateral side of the base of the proximal phalanx of the 5th digit	Flexes the metatarsophalangeal joint of the 5th digit	Lateral plantar (S2, S3)
Plantar interossei (3)	Base and medial side of metatarsals 3–5	Medial side of bases of proximal phalanges and extensor expansions of digits 3–5	Adduct digits 3–5 (move these digits toward the midline of the foot as defined by a plane through 2nd digit); flex metacarpophalangeal and extend interphalangeal joints of digits 3–5	Lateral plantar (S2, S3)

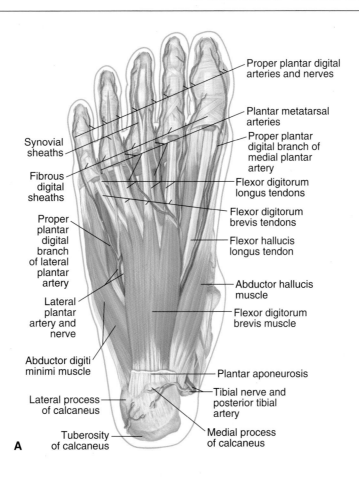

Proper plantar digital arteries and nerves

Plantar metatarsal arteries

Proper plantar digital branch of medial plantar artery

Flexor digitorum longus tendons

Flexor digitorum brevis tendons

Flexor hallucis longus tendon

Abductor hallucis muscle

Flexor digitorum brevis muscle

Plantar aponeurosis

Tibial nerve and posterior tibial artery

Medial process of calcaneus

Synovial sheaths

Fibrous digital sheaths

Proper plantar digital branch of lateral plantar artery

Lateral plantar artery and nerve

Abductor digiti minimi muscle

Lateral process of calcaneus

Tuberosity of calcaneus

A

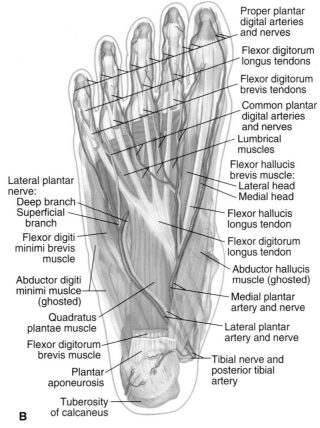

Proper plantar digital arteries and nerves

Flexor digitorum longus tendons

Flexor digitorum brevis tendons

Common plantar digital arteries and nerves

Lumbrical muscles

Flexor hallucis brevis muscle:
Lateral head
Medial head

Flexor hallucis longus tendon

Flexor digitorum longus tendon

Abductor hallucis muscle (ghosted)

Medial plantar artery and nerve

Lateral plantar artery and nerve

Tibial nerve and posterior tibial artery

Lateral plantar nerve:
Deep branch
Superficial branch

Flexor digiti minimi brevis muscle

Abductor digiti minimi muslce (ghosted)

Quadratus plantae muscle

Flexor digitorum brevis muscle

Plantar aponeurosis

Tuberosity of calcaneus

B

Figure 3.25A,B. Muscles of the Sole of the Foot. **A.** First Layer. **B.** Second Layer.

II. Special Features

A. Muscles and tendons of the plantar surface of the foot are arranged in 4 layers
  1. Layer 1: abductor hallucis, flexor digitorum brevis, abductor digiti minimi
  2. Layer 2: quadratus plantae, lumbricales, tendons of flexor digitorum longus and flexor hallucis longus
  3. Layer 3: flexor hallucis brevis, adductor hallucis, flexor digiti minimi brevis
  4. Layer 4: interossei, tendons of tibialis posterior and fibularis (peroneus) longus

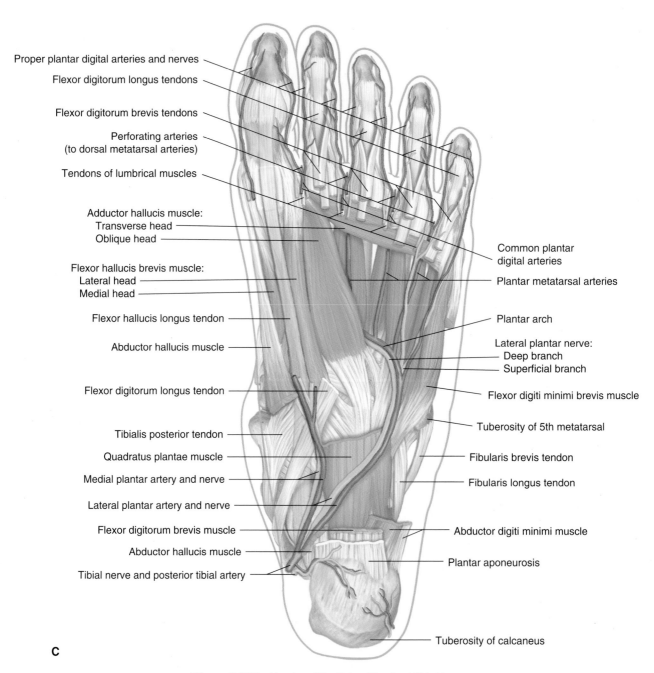

Proper plantar digital arteries and nerves

Flexor digitorum longus tendons

Flexor digitorum brevis tendons

Perforating arteries
(to dorsal metatarsal arteries)

Tendons of lumbrical muscles

Adductor hallucis muscle:
Transverse head
Oblique head

Flexor hallucis brevis muscle:
Lateral head
Medial head

Flexor hallucis longus tendon

Abductor hallucis muscle

Flexor digitorum longus tendon

Tibialis posterior tendon

Quadratus plantae muscle

Medial plantar artery and nerve

Lateral plantar artery and nerve

Flexor digitorum brevis muscle

Abductor hallucis muscle

Tibial nerve and posterior tibial artery

Common plantar
digital arteries

Plantar metatarsal arteries

Plantar arch

Lateral plantar nerve:
Deep branch
Superficial branch

Flexor digiti minimi brevis muscle

Tuberosity of 5th metatarsal

Fibularis brevis tendon

Fibularis longus tendon

Abductor digiti minimi muscle

Plantar aponeurosis

Tuberosity of calcaneus

C

Figure 3.25C. Muscles of the Sole of the Foot. Third Layer.

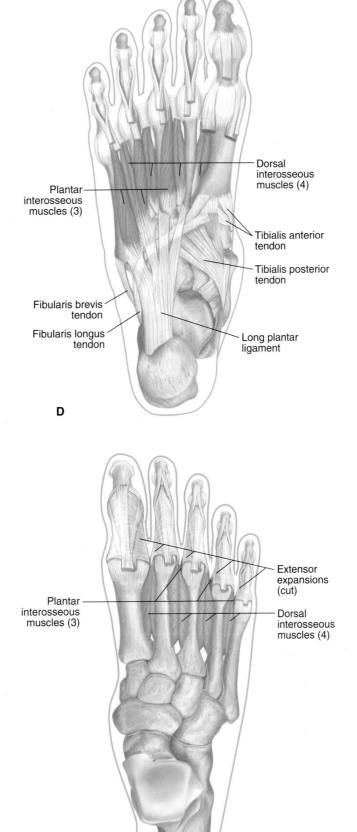

D

Dorsal interosseous muscles (4)

Plantar interosseous muscles (3)

Tibialis anterior tendon

Tibialis posterior tendon

Fibularis brevis tendon

Fibularis longus tendon

Long plantar ligament

Plantar interosseous muscles (3)

Extensor expansions (cut)

Dorsal interosseous muscles (4)

E

Figure 3.25D,E. Muscles of the Sole of the Foot. Fourth Layer. **D.** Plantar View. **E.** Dorsal View.

Vessels and Nerves of the Sole of the Foot

I. Arteries (Fig. 3.26A)

A. Posterior tibial divides beneath origin of abductor hallucis muscle into 2 branches

  1. Medial plantar: along the medial side of the foot and the medial border of the big toe

  2. Lateral plantar: courses obliquely lateralward to reach the base of 5th metatarsal and then arches medially to a point between the bases of the 1st and 2nd metatarsals; joins deep plantar branch of the dorsalis pedis artery to form **plantar arch**. Branches:

    a. Perforating to dorsal metatarsal arteries

    b. Plantar metatarsals (4) in interosseous spaces where they divide into **proper plantar digital arteries** to adjacent sides of toes; send **anterior perforating branches** to dorsal metatarsal arteries

    c. First plantar metatarsal supplies adjoining sides of the big and 2nd toes

    d. Proper plantar digital to the lateral side of the small toe

II. Nerves (Fig. 3.26B)

A. Tibial divides beneath origin of abductor hallucis muscle into 2 branches

  1. Medial plantar nerve: to abductor hallucis, flexor digitorum brevis, flexor hallucis brevis, and 1st lumbrical muscle

    a. Cutaneous branches: supply most of the medial sole, including the toes to the middle of 4th toe

    b. Medial plantar gives off branches: plantar cutaneous to the medial side of the sole; proper digital nerves to the medial side of the big toe; 3 common digital nerves, which split to give 2 proper digital nerves to adjacent sides of toes 1 to 4

  2. Lateral plantar nerve: to quadratus plantae and abductor digiti minimi muscles

    a. Superficial branch to flexor digiti minimi and the 2 interossei muscles of the 4th space

    b. Deep branch to adductor hallucis muscle, interosseous muscles of spaces 1, 2, and 3, and lumbrical muscles 2, 3, and 4

    c. Cutaneous branches:

      i. Supply the lateral half of the 4th toe and the lateral side of the foot

      ii. Give off a superficial branch, which sends proper digital nerves to the lateral side of the little toe and common digital nerves that divide to supply adjacent sides of toes 4 and 5

III. Clinical Considerations: Cuts of the Feet

  A. May bleed profusely

  B. Due to the numerous anastomoses between vessels, both ends of a severed artery must be ligated

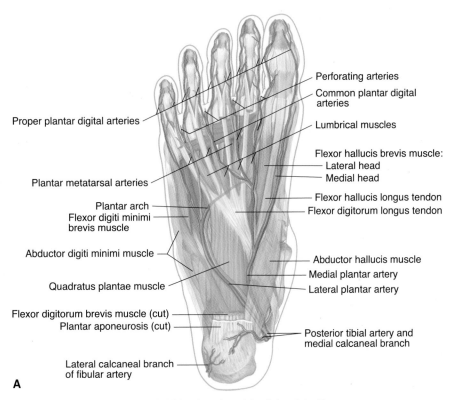

Perforating arteries

Common plantar digital arteries

Proper plantar digital arteries

Lumbrical muscles

Flexor hallucis brevis muscle:
Lateral head
Medial head

Plantar metatarsal arteries

Flexor hallucis longus tendon
Flexor digitorum longus tendon

Plantar arch
Flexor digiti minimi brevis muscle

Abductor digiti minimi muscle

Abductor hallucis muscle
Medial plantar artery
Lateral plantar artery

Quadratus plantae muscle

Flexor digitorum brevis muscle (cut)
Plantar aponeurosis (cut)

Posterior tibial artery and medial calcaneal branch

Lateral calcaneal branch of fibular artery

A

Figure 3.26A. Arteries of the Sole of the Foot.

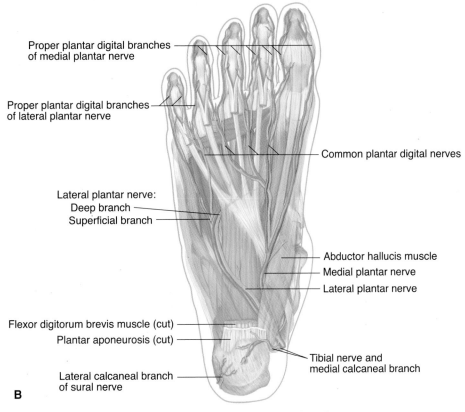

Proper plantar digital branches of medial plantar nerve

Proper plantar digital branches of lateral plantar nerve

Common plantar digital nerves

Lateral plantar nerve:
Deep branch
Superficial branch

Abductor hallucis muscle
Medial plantar nerve
Lateral plantar nerve

Flexor digitorum brevis muscle (cut)
Plantar aponeurosis (cut)

Tibial nerve and medial calcaneal branch

Lateral calcaneal branch of sural nerve

B

Figure 3.26B. Nerves of the Sole of the Foot.

The Hip Joint

I. Hip Joint

A. Type: enarthrosis (ball and socket)
B. Bones: head of the femur and acetabulum of the hip bone
C. Movements: circumduction of the lower limb, which is the combination of flexion, extension, abduction, and adduction that allows the limb to circumscribe a cone; lateral (external) rotation, and medial (internal) rotation

II. Ligaments (Fig. 3.27A–C)

A. Acetabular labrum: deepens acetabulum, helps to hold the head of the femur
B. Transverse acetabular: crosses acetabular notch to complete rim of acetabulum
C. Articular capsule
   1. Extends from rim of acetabulum to intertrochanteric crest and line
   2. Zona orbicularis: band of circularly arranged fibers on the inner aspect of the capsule, encircling the neck of the femur
D. Iliofemoral (Y-shaped ligament of Bigelow): from the anterior inferior iliac spine to intertrochanteric line, prevents overextension, abduction, and lateral rotation
E. Ischiofemoral: from ischium behind acetabulum to blend with the capsule, checks the medial rotation
F. Pubofemoral: from the superior pubic ramus, joins the iliofemoral ligament, checks abduction
G. Ligamentum capitis femoris (round ligament): intracapsular and 3.5 cm long; extends from the acetabular notch and transverse acetabular ligament to fovea of the femur; has little function as ligament but becomes taut in adduction of the femur

III. Synovial Membrane

A. Lines articular capsule
B. Covers the labrum, ligamentum capitis femoris, neck of the femur, from attachment of capsule, below, to articular cartilage of the head of the femur

IV. Muscles Acting on the Hip Joint

Flexion	Extension	Abduction	Adduction	Medial Rotation	Lateral Rotation
Iliopsoas	Gluteus maximus	Gluteus medius	Adductors (all)	Gluteus medius	Piriformis
Sartorius	Semitendinosus	Gluteus minimus	Gracilis	Gluteus minimus	Obturator internus
Pectineus	Semimembranosus	Tensor fasciae latae	Pectineus	Tensor fasciae latae	Gemelli
Rectus femoris	Biceps femoris	Piriformis	Obturator externus	Adductors (all)	Obturator externus
Adductors (all)	Adductor magnus (hamstring portion)	Sartorius	Quadratus femoris		Quadratus femoris
Tensor fasciae latae					Gluteus maximus

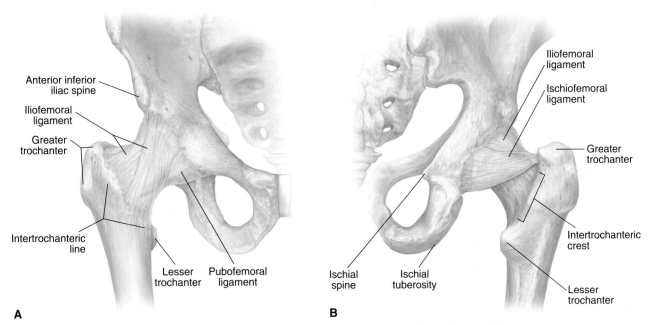

Anterior inferior iliac spine

Iliofemoral ligament

Greater trochanter

Intertrochanteric line

Lesser trochanter   Pubofemoral ligament

A

Iliofemoral ligament

Ischiofemoral ligament

Greater trochanter

Intertrochanteric crest

Ischial spine   Ischial tuberosity

Lesser trochanter

B

Figure 3.27A,B. Hip Joint, External Features. **A.** Anterior View. **B.** Posterior View.

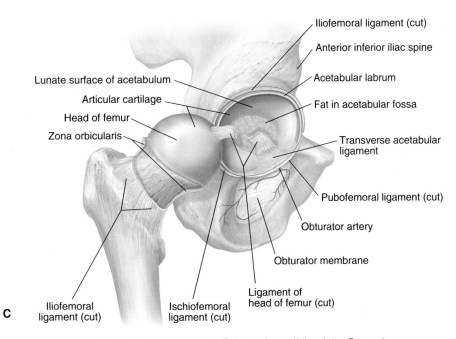

Lunate surface of acetabulum

Articular cartilage

Head of femur

Zona orbicularis

Iliofemoral ligament (cut)

Anterior inferior iliac spine

Acetabular labrum

Fat in acetabular fossa

Transverse acetabular ligament

Pubofemoral ligament (cut)

Obturator artery

Obturator membrane

Ligament of head of femur (cut)

Iliofemoral ligament (cut)

Ischiofemoral ligament (cut)

C

Figure 3.27C. Hip Joint, Internal Features. Lateral View, Joint Opened.

V. Hip Joint: Essentials of ROM

Flexion[a]	Extension	Abduction[b]	Adduction	Internal Rotation[c]	External Rotation[d]	Circumduction
135°	10°–30°	45°–50°	20°–30°	35°–45°	45°–60°	360°

Functional ranges:
[a]90° 117°–120° for squatting and lifting; 110° needed to arise from chair.
[b]20°.
[c]0°.
[d]20°.
Rotation in flexion: Internal and external, 45°.
Rotation in neutral: Internal rotation, 35°; external rotation, 50°.

A. **Degree of flexion and extension at the hip joint:** depends on the position of the knee; flexing the knee relaxes iliopsoas muscle, and the thigh can be actively flexed until it almost reaches the anterior abdominal wall (Note: some help in movement of the hip joint does result from flexion of the vertebral column)

B. **Extension of the hip joint:** iliofemoral ligament becomes taut and the hip can, thus, be extended only slightly beyond the vertical except by movement of bony pelvis with extension of lumbar vertebrae

C. **Abduction of the hip joint:** is somewhat freer than adduction of the joint

D. **Lateral rotation at the hip joint:** greater (more powerful) than medial rotation

E. **Stability of the hip joint:** relates to the fact that it is a deep-seated "ball-and-socket" joint
   1. Has greater stability than the shoulder joint but less mobility
   2. Labrum of the hip joint is of lesser importance to its stability than it is for the shoulder joint

F. **Instant center of movement:** point at which a joint rotates
   1. Movements generally take place about 3 axes, all running through the femoral head
   2. Simultaneous in all 3 planes for a ball-and-socket joint and therefore impossible to determine

G. **Innervation:** from L2 to S1 nerve roots but predominantly from L3, explaining why the medial thigh pain due to hip pathology is referred to L3 dermatome

H. **Hip difficulty symptoms on physical examination:** with turning, sitting with hip flexion, going up and down stairs, pulling on shoes, getting in and out of car, etc.

VI. Clinical Considerations (Fig. 3.27D,E)

A. **Dislocations:** because circulation to the head of the femur may be disrupted, reduction within 12 to 24 hours is mandatory
   1. **Congenital:** due to failure of acetabulum to deepen; more common in women (8:1)
   2. **Traumatic:** caused by a blow on the knee when the thigh is flexed, tearing capsule
      a. Head of the femur is usually dislocated posteriorly, with a tearing of the posterior part of capsule and frequently fracture of acetabulum
      b. In anterior dislocation, the head of the femur passes around the medial edge of the iliofemoral ligament and lodges against the body of pubic bone or obturator foramen

B. **Blood supply:** the medial circumflex femoral artery is the principal blood supply to the head of the femur
   1. **Retinacular (nutrient)** arteries pass along the femoral neck beneath capsule
   2. Other contributing arteries form the cruciate anastomosis: inferior gluteal, medial and lateral circumflex femoral, and the 1st perforating artery

C. **Fractures of the femoral neck** can disrupt blood supply to head, leading to avascular necrosis

D. **Referred pain to the knee in hip disease** is due to fact that both joints are supplied by femoral, sciatic, and obturator nerves

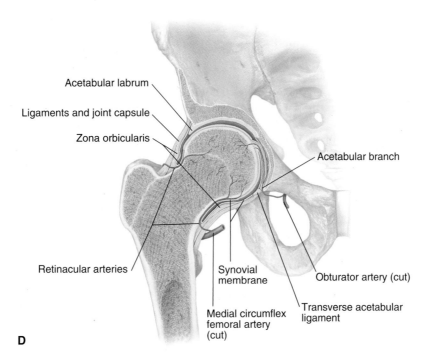

Acetabular labrum

Ligaments and joint capsule

Zona orbicularis

Acetabular branch

Retinacular arteries

Synovial membrane

Obturator artery (cut)

Medial circumflex femoral artery (cut)

Transverse acetabular ligament

D

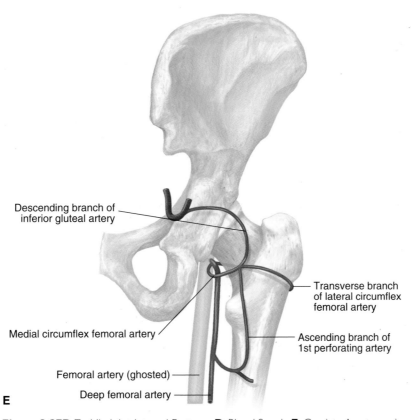

Descending branch of inferior gluteal artery

Transverse branch of lateral circumflex femoral artery

Medial circumflex femoral artery

Ascending branch of 1st perforating artery

Femoral artery (ghosted)

Deep femoral artery

E

Figure 3.27D,E. Hip Joint, Internal Features. **D.** Blood Supply. **E.** Cruciate Anastomosis.

The Knee Joint

I. Knee Joint

A. Type: ginglymus (hinge) between the femur and tibia, arthrodial between the femur and patella
B. Divisions: 3 joints in 1
   1. 2 between medial and lateral condyles of the femur and tibia
   2. 1 between the patella and the femur
C. Movements
   1. Femur-tibia permits flexion and extension with slight rotation when the leg is flexed
   2. Femur-patella permits sliding up and down

II. Ligaments (Fig. 3.28A–D)

A. Articular capsule: from the femur to tibia, strengthened by fibers from the fascia lata, iliotibial tract, and tendons of the vasti, hamstrings, and sartorius muscles
B. Patellar ligament: from the apex of patella to tuberosity of tibia; helps hold patella in place and serves as part of tendon of quadriceps muscle
C. Oblique popliteal: from the lateral femur, over condyles to the posterior head of tibia; checks extension
D. Arcuate popliteal: from the lateral condyle of the femur to the styloid process of fibula; may check medial rotation of leg
E. Tibial collateral (medial collateral): thickened portion of articular capsule from the medial side of medial femoral condyle to medial condyle and body of tibia; prevents lateral bending; checks extension, hyperflexion, and lateral rotation
F. Fibular collateral (lateral collateral): from the back of the lateral femoral condyle to the lateral side of the head and styloid process of fibula; checks hyperextension; relaxed in flexion
G. Coronary: from capsule to periphery of menisci and tibia; helps hold menisci in place
H. Anterior cruciate: from the front of intercondylar eminence to the medial surface of lateral femoral condyle posteriorly; checks extension, lateral rotation, and anterior slipping of tibia on the femur (or posterior displacement of the femur on tibia)
I. Posterior cruciate: from posterior intercondylar fossa and the posterior end of the lateral meniscus to the lateral surface of medial femoral condyle anteriorly; checks flexion, lateral rotation, and posterior slipping of tibia on the femur (or anterior displacement of the femur on tibia)
J. Medial meniscus: crescent-shaped (oval); attached to tibia anterior to the anterior cruciate ligament (ACL) and in posterior intercondylar fossa; deepens the medial tibial condyle
K. Lateral meniscus: nearly circular
   1. Attached to tibia anterior to the ACL, blending with the latter; posteriorly attached behind intercondylar eminence anterior to the medial meniscus
   2. Deepens the lateral tibial condyle
L. Transverse: interconnects anterior parts of 2 menisci

III. Synovial Membrane (Fig. 3.28E–K)

A. Largest and the most extensive in the body
B. Extends above patella and laterally and medially beneath vasti muscles
C. Extends downward under the patellar ligament; separated from latter by infrapatellar pad (fat)
D. Sends alar folds into joint cavity, which converge to form the **patellar fold**
E. Lines capsule, extends over menisci to free border and then under these to tibia
F. Forms blind sac behind the lateral meniscus between it and tendon of popliteus muscle
G. Reflected anteriorly over cruciate ligaments

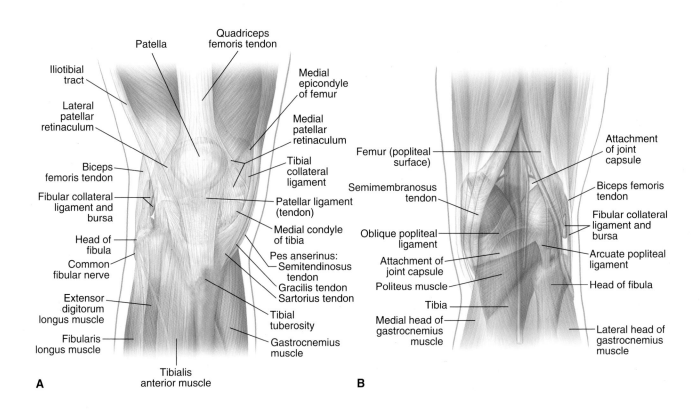

A

Iliotibial tract
Lateral patellar retinaculum
Biceps femoris tendon
Fibular collateral ligament and bursa
Head of fibula
Common fibular nerve
Extensor digitorum longus muscle
Fibularis longus muscle
Patella
Quadriceps femoris tendon
Medial epicondyle of femur
Medial patellar retinaculum
Tibial collateral ligament
Patellar ligament (tendon)
Medial condyle of tibia
Pes anserinus: Semitendinosus tendon
Gracilis tendon
Sartorius tendon
Tibial tuberosity
Gastrocnemius muscle
Tibialis anterior muscle

B

Femur (popliteal surface)
Semimembranosus tendon
Oblique popliteal ligament
Attachment of joint capsule
Politeus muscle
Tibia
Medial head of gastrocnemius muscle
Attachment of joint capsule
Biceps femoris tendon
Fibular collateral ligament and bursa
Arcuate popliteal ligament
Head of fibula
Lateral head of gastrocnemius muscle

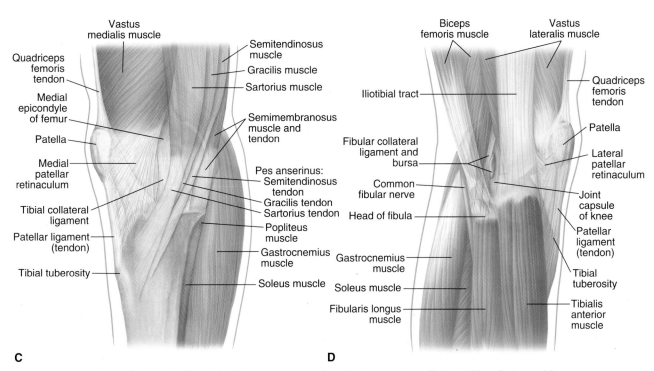

C

Quadriceps femoris tendon
Medial epicondyle of femur
Patella
Medial patellar retinaculum
Tibial collateral ligament
Patellar ligament (tendon)
Tibial tuberosity
Vastus medialis muscle
Semitendinosus muscle
Gracilis muscle
Sartorius muscle
Semimembranosus muscle and tendon
Pes anserinus: Semitendinosus tendon
Gracilis tendon
Sartorius tendon
Popliteus muscle
Gastrocnemius muscle
Soleus muscle

D

Iliotibial tract
Fibular collateral ligament and bursa
Common fibular nerve
Head of fibula
Gastrocnemius muscle
Soleus muscle
Fibularis longus muscle
Biceps femoris muscle
Vastus lateralis muscle
Quadriceps femoris tendon
Patella
Lateral patellar retinaculum
Joint capsule of knee
Patellar ligament (tendon)
Tibial tuberosity
Tibialis anterior muscle

Figure 3.28A–D. Knee Joint, Right. **A.** Anterior View. **B.** Posterior View. **C.** Medial View. **D.** Lateral View.

IV. Knee Joint (Between the Femur and Tibia): Range of Motion (ROM)

Flexion[a]	Extension[a]	Abduction[b]	Adduction[b]
130°–135°	0°–10°	0°[b]	0°[b]

[a]Flexion and extension of the knee are associated with rolling and gliding motions.
[b]Abduction and adduction are essentially 0°; however, a few degrees of passive motion is normally possible at 30° flexion.

A. Femur internally rotates (external tibial rotation) during the last 15° of extension (i.e., a "screw-home" mechanism, tightening the cruciate ligaments) related to size and convexity of the medial femoral condyle as well as the musculature around the joint

B. Posterior femur rollback on tibia during knee flexion increases maximum knee flexion

C. Functional flexion and extension ROM: from near full extension to about 90° of flexion

D. Rotation at the knee joint: does take place but varies with joint movement
   1. Rotation (polycentric rotation) varies with flexion: at 90° flexion, 30° internal and 45° external rotation is possible
   2. Minimal rotation takes place at full extension

E. Motion about the knee:
   1. Requires a very complex series of movements about a changing instant center of rotation
   2. 0.5 cm of excursion of medial meniscus and 1.10 cm excursion of lateral meniscus during 0°–120° of knee motion

F. Necessary functional degree of knee flexion required for:
   1. Squatting and lifting an object from floor: 117°
   2. Sitting and getting up from a chair: 93° to 110°
   3. Climbing stairs: 83°
   4. Descending stairs: 90°
   5. Bending over to tie one's shoes: 106°
   6. Normal walking: 67°

G. Full extension of the leg with the foot on ground passively "locks" the knee due to medial rotation of the femur on tibia
   1. In this position, thigh and leg muscles can briefly be relaxed without creating an unstable joint
   2. "Unlocking" the knee is accomplished by popliteus muscle contraction with rotation of the femur laterally (about 5° on the tibia so that flexion can take place)

H. Knee stabilizers:
   1. Medial: medial collateral ligament (MCL), joint capsule, medial meniscus, ACL, and posterior cruciate ligament (PCL)
   2. Lateral: joint capsule, iliotibial band, lateral collateral ligament, lateral meniscus, and ACL/PCL
   3. Anterior: ACL and joint capsule
   4. Posterior: PCL (tightens with internal rotation) and joint capsule
   5. Rotation: MCL checks external rotation; ACL checks internal rotation

I. Patello-femoral joint:
   1. Movement: sliding; patella and femur relations varies with knee position
      a. In full extension, patella moves superiorly with contraction of quadriceps muscle and is located just anterior to the most superior part of the femoral condyles
      b. In full knee flexion, quadriceps muscle relaxes and patella slides caudally, descending about 7 cm to be located anterior to the gap between tibia and femur
   2. Instant center of movement: located near posterior cortex above condyles of the femur
   3. Thickest cartilage in body because it bears the greatest load
   4. Patella helps in knee extension by increasing lever arm, as well as with stress distribution

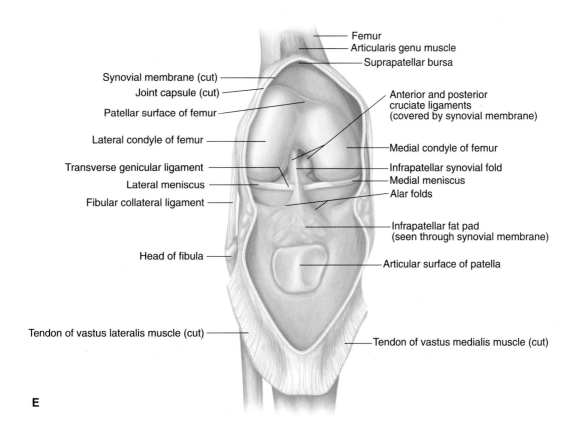

Femur
Articularis genu muscle
Suprapatellar bursa

Synovial membrane (cut)
Joint capsule (cut)
Patellar surface of femur

Anterior and posterior
cruciate ligaments
(covered by synovial membrane)

Lateral condyle of femur

Medial condyle of femur

Transverse genicular ligament
Lateral meniscus
Fibular collateral ligament

Infrapatellar synovial fold
Medial meniscus
Alar folds

Head of fibula

Infrapatellar fat pad
(seen through synovial membrane)

Articular surface of patella

Tendon of vastus lateralis muscle (cut)

Tendon of vastus medialis muscle (cut)

E

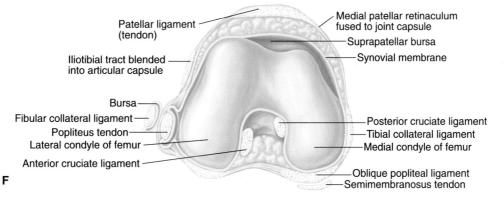

Patellar ligament
(tendon)

Medial patellar retinaculum
fused to joint capsule
Suprapatellar bursa
Synovial membrane

Iliotibial tract blended
into articular capsule

Bursa
Fibular collateral ligament
Popliteus tendon
Lateral condyle of femur
Anterior cruciate ligament

Posterior cruciate ligament
Tibial collateral ligament
Medial condyle of femur

Oblique popliteal ligament
Semimembranosus tendon

F

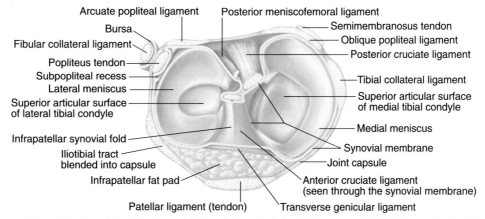

Arcuate popliteal ligament
Bursa
Fibular collateral ligament
Popliteus tendon
Subpopliteal recess
Lateral meniscus
Superior articular surface
of lateral tibial condyle
Infrapatellar synovial fold
Iliotibial tract
blended into capsule
Infrapatellar fat pad

Posterior meniscofemoral ligament
Semimembranosus tendon
Oblique popliteal ligament
Posterior cruciate ligament

Tibial collateral ligament

Superior articular surface
of medial tibial condyle

Medial meniscus
Synovial membrane
Joint capsule
Anterior cruciate ligament
(seen through the synovial membrane)
Transverse genicular ligament

Patellar ligament (tendon)

G

Figure 3.28E–G. Knee Joint, Right, Internal View. **E.** Anterior View, Joint Opened. **F.** Distal Femur, Inferior View.
G. Proximal Tibia, Superior View.

V. Muscles Acting on the Knee Joint

Flexion	Extension	Medial Rotation	Lateral Rotation
Semimembranosus	Quadriceps femoris	Popliteus	Biceps femoris
Semitendinosus	Tensor fasciae latae	Semimembranosus	
Biceps femoris		Semitendinosus	
Sartorius		Sartorius	
Gracilis		Gracilis	
Popliteus			
Gastrocnemius			
Plantaris			

VI. Clinical Considerations

A. Lesions of menisci
   1. Displacements and tears are most frequent type of damage; the medial involved 5 to 15 times as often as the lateral due to attachment of the MCL to the medial meniscus
   2. Meniscus, all or part, may become jammed between articular surfaces of condyles, "locking" the joint
B. Pain may be referred to the knee from hip disease
C. Knee joint injuries are common because it is a major weight-bearing joint and its stability depends on its associated muscles and ligaments
D. Traumatic dislocations of the knee are not common but can occur in accidents where there is disruption of ligaments
   1. Popliteal artery and the tibial nerve may be injured
   2. This trauma can lead to partial or complete paralysis of the muscles supplied by the nerve
E. Cavity of the knee joint can be examined for injury or disease with arthroscope (arthroscopy)
F. Tears of the ACL are fairly frequently associated with tears of other ligaments, particularly the tibial collateral and medial meniscus
   1. These 3 occurring together, a common sport injury caused by a blow to the lateral side of the knee, are called "terrible triad"
   2. Tibial collateral is particularly important to knee stabilization because the major part of the ligament is tense in all positions of the joint
G. Dislocation of patella: uncommon; more often seen in female due to angle of the femur
H. Fibular collateral ligament is not commonly torn, being very strong
I. Blood supply:
   1. Capsule of the knee joint is supplied by twigs from all vessels that enter into the genicular anastomosis around it
   2. In addition, the middle genicular artery penetrates the capsule posteriorly and is distributed, especially to the tissue of the intercondylar region
J. Nerve supply:
   1. Nerves to the knee joint are typically derived from femoral, obturator, and both parts of the sciatic nerve
   2. Many follow arteries, but some run directly to the capsule
K. Injections into the synovial cavity of the knee joint are made for diagnostic and therapeutic reasons; in addition, aspiration of synovial fluid may be necessary to relieve pressure (due to increased secretion), to sample fluid diagnostically, or to remove blood in the joint cavity as a result of soft tissue injury or fracture of a bone
   1. Injections are usually given laterally, with the knee flexed and the leg hanging

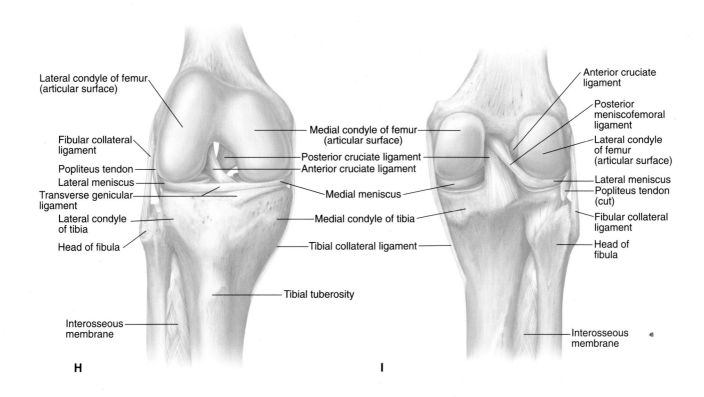

Lateral condyle of femur (articular surface)

Fibular collateral ligament

Popliteus tendon

Lateral meniscus

Transverse genicular ligament

Lateral condyle of tibia

Head of fibula

Interosseous membrane

Medial condyle of femur (articular surface)

Posterior cruciate ligament

Anterior cruciate ligament

Medial meniscus

Medial condyle of tibia

Tibial collateral ligament

Tibial tuberosity

H

Anterior cruciate ligament

Posterior meniscofemoral ligament

Lateral condyle of femur (articular surface)

Lateral meniscus

Popliteus tendon (cut)

Fibular collateral ligament

Head of fibula

Interosseous membrane

I

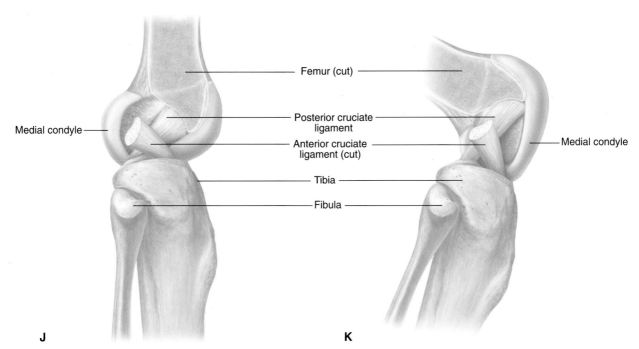

Femur (cut)

Medial condyle

Posterior cruciate ligament

Anterior cruciate ligament (cut)

Tibia

Fibula

Medial condyle

J

K

Figure 3.28H–K. Ligaments of the Knee, Right. **H.** Anterior View. **I.** Posterior View. **J.** Internal View, Knee Extended. **K.** Internal View, Knee Flexed.

VI. Clinical Considerations

    a. Location: into the center of the riangle marked by the apex of patella, lateral plateau of lateral tibial condyle, and anterior prominence of lateral femoral condyle

    b. Needle passes posteromedially

L. Popliteal (Baker) cyst: forms occasionally when synovial fluid escapes from the knee joint (synovial effusion) and accumulates in popliteal fossa

  1. Children: common; can be large but seldom produce symptoms

  2. Adults: can communicate with the synovial cavity via a narrow stalk, which passes through the fibrous capsule of the joint

M. 3 C's in knee examination: collateral ligaments, cruciate ligaments, and cartilages (menisci)

N. O'Donoghue "unhappy triad"

  1. Rupture of the medial tibial collateral ligament due to abduction and lateral rotation of the leg with the knee in a partially fixed position

    a. Ligament is crossed by tendons of sartorius, gracilis, and semitendinosus

    b. Abnormal mobility of the leg at the knee joint and the medial widening of the joint space on x-ray is seen

  2. Rupture of the ACL: results in increased mobility of the knee in flexion

  3. Damage to the medial meniscus: marked restriction of extension of the knee joint and displacement of fibrocartilage is seen

Bursae of the Knee Joint and the Tibiofibular Joints

I. Bursae of the Knee (usually named according to immediately adjacent structures, e.g., tendons) (Fig. 3.29A,B)

A. Anteriorly: 4
 1. Subcutaneous prepatellar bursa: between the front of patella and skin
 2. Suprapatellar or quadriceps bursa: between the front of the femur and quadriceps femoris muscle (generally communicates with the joint cavity)
 3. Deep infrapatellar bursa: between the patellar ligament and upper tibia
 4. Subcutaneous bursa: between tibial tuberosity and skin

B. Laterally: 3
 1. Between the fibular collateral ligament and biceps muscle
 2. Between the fibular collateral ligament and popliteus muscle
 3. Popliteus bursa: between popliteus muscle and lateral condyle of tibia (generally communicates with the joint cavity)

C. Medially: 3
 1. Anserine bursa: between the tibial collateral ligament and tendons of semitendinosus, sartorius, and gracilis muscles
 2. Between the tibial collateral ligament and the tendon of semimembranosus muscle
 3. Between tendon of semimembranosus muscle and tibia

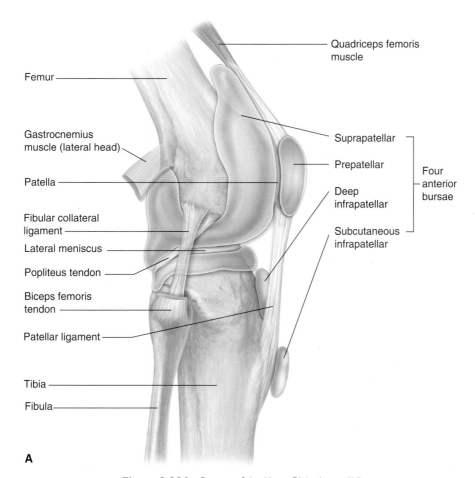

Figure 3.29A. Bursae of the Knee, Right. Lateral View.

> D. Posteriorly: 2
>   1. Gastrocnemius bursa: between the lateral head of the gastrocnemius muscle and the capsule (sometimes communicates with the joint)
>   2. Semimembranosus bursa: between the medial head of the gastrocnemius muscle and the capsule, extending under tendon of semimembranosus muscle (generally communicates with the joint cavity)

II. Tibiofibular Joint (Proximal) (Fig. 3.29C,D)

A. Type: diarthrodial
B. Bones: head of fibula and fibular facet, below the lateral condyle of the tibia
C. Movements: gliding up and down
D. Ligaments
  1. Articular capsule
  2. Anterior capitular
  3. Posterior capitular

III. Interosseous Membrane (Intermediate)

A. Type: synarthrosis
B. Function: holds shaft together, strengthens fibula, for muscle attachments
C. Ligament: interosseous membrane; fibers inclined downward and lateralward from the lateral border of the tibia to the anteromedial border of fibula
  1. Membrane separates anterior and posterior leg compartments and gives origin to muscles of both groups
  2. Upper margin of membrane does not reach tibiofibular articulation, allowing anterior tibial vessels to pass over the upper edge of membrane to the anterior leg compartment

IV. Tibiofibular Joint (Distal)

A. Type: syndesmosis
B. Movements: slight up and down
C. Ligaments
  1. Anterior tibiofibular (lateral malleolar)
  2. Posterior tibiofibular (lateral malleolar)
  3. Interosseous
  4. Transverse tibiofibular

V. Clinical Considerations

A. **Bursitis:** bursa most frequently involved
  1. Prepatellar: most common; becomes irritated by repeated or prolonged kneeling (thus, called "housemaid's knee" or "nun's knee"); between skin and patella
  2. Subcutaneous infrapatellar bursitis is due to excessive friction between skin and tibial tuberosity—**clergyman's knee**
  3. Deep infrapatellar bursitis: results in swelling between the patellar ligament and the tibia, above tibial tuberosity; enlargement obliterates "dimples" on each side of the patellar ligament when the leg is extended
B. **Genu valgum**
  1. "Knock knee" with the medial condyle and shaft of the femur protruding too far medially
  2. Excess stress is placed on lateral knee structures
C. **Genu varum**
  1. "Bowleg" with outward curving of the lower limb
  2. Causes unequal weight distribution, creating excess pressure on the medial side of the knee joint, which can lead to eventual destruction of the knee cartilage

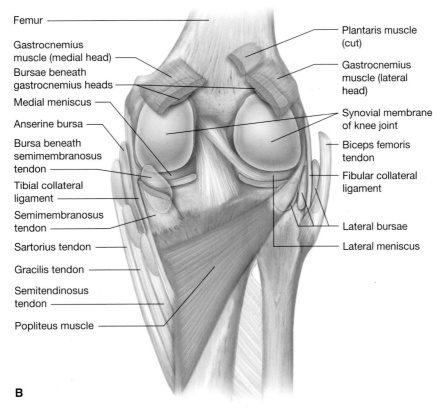

Femur

Gastrocnemius muscle (medial head)

Bursae beneath gastrocnemius heads

Medial meniscus

Anserine bursa

Bursa beneath semimembranosus tendon

Tibial collateral ligament

Semimembranosus tendon

Sartorius tendon

Gracilis tendon

Semitendinosus tendon

Popliteus muscle

Plantaris muscle (cut)

Gastrocnemius muscle (lateral head)

Synovial membrane of knee joint

Biceps femoris tendon

Fibular collateral ligament

Lateral bursae

Lateral meniscus

B

Figure 3.29B. Bursae of the Knee, Right. Posterior View.

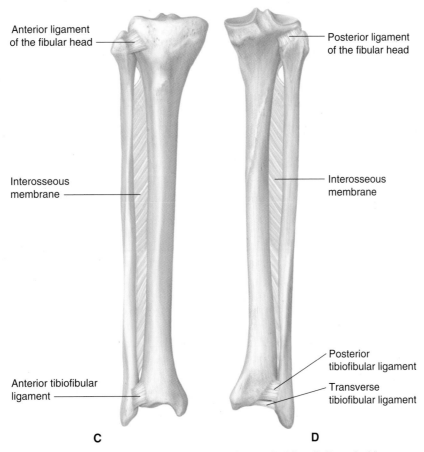

Anterior ligament of the fibular head

Interosseous membrane

Anterior tibiofibular ligament

Posterior ligament of the fibular head

Interosseous membrane

Posterior tibiofibular ligament

Transverse tibiofibular ligament

C

D

Figure 3.29C,D. Tibiofibular Joints, Right. **C.** Anterior View. **D.** Posterior View.

Joints of the Ankle and Foot

I. Ankle Joint (Talocrural) (Fig. 3.30A–C)

A. Type: ginglymus (hinge)
B. Bones: medial malleolus of tibia, lateral malleolus of fibula, and talus
C. Movements: dorsiflexion (extension) and plantar flexion (flexion)
D. Ligaments
  1. Articular capsule
  2. Medial collateral (deltoid) consists of 4 ligaments
    a. Anterior and posterior tibiotalar, tibionavicular, and tibiocalcaneal
    b. Anterior and posterior fibers check plantar and dorsiflexion, respectively; anterior fibers also limit abduction
  3. Lateral collateral ligaments: anterior and posterior talofibular and calcaneofibular

II. Subtalar (Talocalcaneal) Joint

A. Type: arthrodial
B. Bones: talus and calcaneus
C. Movements: gliding
D. Ligaments
  1. Anterior, posterior, medial, and lateral talocalcaneal
  2. Interosseous talocalcaneal

III. Talocalcaneonavicular Joint (Fig. 3.30D,E)

A. Type: arthrodial
B. Bones: talus, navicular, and calcaneus
C. Movements: gliding and some rotation; as part of the transverse tarsal joint, it allows most inversion/eversion
D. Ligaments
  1. Articular capsule
  2. Dorsal talonavicular
  3. Plantar calcaneonavicular (spring) ligament: supports the head of the talus

IV. Calcaneocuboid Joint

A. Type: arthroidial
B. Movements: gliding and slight rotation; as part of the transverse tarsal joint, it allows most inversion/eversion
C. Ligaments
  1. Dorsal and plantar calcaneocuboid
  2. Bifurcated: from calcaneus to cuboid and navicular
  3. Long plantar

V. Tarsometatarsal Joints

A. Between the bases of metatarsals, 3 cuneiforms, and cuboid
B. Type: arthrodial
C. Movements: slight gliding movements
D. Ligaments: each has dorsal, plantar, and interosseous

VI. Metatarsophalangeal Joints

A. Between the heads of metatarsals and bases of proximal phalanges
B. Type: condyloid
C. Movements: flexion, extension, abduction, and adduction
D. Ligaments: each has plantar and 2 collateral

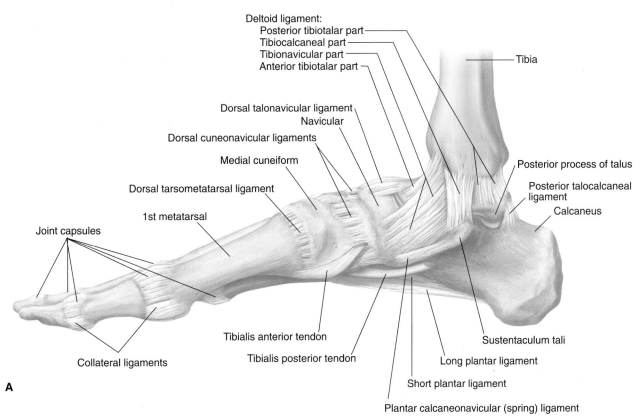

Deltoid ligament:
Posterior tibiotalar part
Tibiocalcaneal part
Tibionavicular part
Anterior tibiotalar part

Tibia

Dorsal talonavicular ligament
Navicular

Dorsal cuneonavicular ligaments

Medial cuneiform

Dorsal tarsometatarsal ligament

1st metatarsal

Posterior process of talus

Posterior talocalcaneal ligament

Calcaneus

Joint capsules

Collateral ligaments

Tibialis anterior tendon

Tibialis posterior tendon

Short plantar ligament

Plantar calcaneonavicular (spring) ligament

Sustentaculum tali

Long plantar ligament

Figure 3.30A. Ankle and Foot Joints, Right. Medial View.

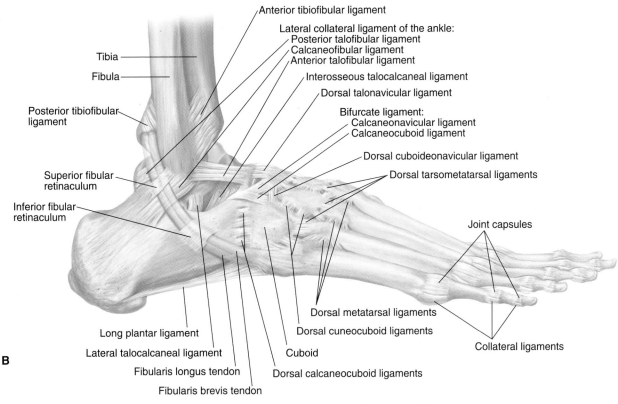

Anterior tibiofibular ligament

Lateral collateral ligament of the ankle:
Posterior talofibular ligament
Calcaneofibular ligament
Anterior talofibular ligament

Interosseous talocalcaneal ligament

Dorsal talonavicular ligament

Bifurcate ligament:
Calcaneonavicular ligament
Calcaneocuboid ligament

Dorsal cuboideonavicular ligament

Dorsal tarsometatarsal ligaments

Tibia

Fibula

Posterior tibiofibular ligament

Superior fibular retinaculum

Inferior fibular retinaculum

Joint capsules

Long plantar ligament

Lateral talocalcaneal ligament

Fibularis longus tendon

Fibularis brevis tendon

Dorsal metatarsal ligaments

Dorsal cuneocuboid ligaments

Cuboid

Dorsal calcaneocuboid ligaments

Collateral ligaments

Figure 3.30B. Ankle and Foot Joints, Right. Lateral View.

VII. Interphalangeal Joints

A. Between bases and heads of adjoining phalanges
B. Type: ginglymus
C. Movements: flexion and extension
D. Ligaments: each has plantar and collateral ligaments; extensor expansions act as dorsal ligaments

VIII. Ankle (Talocrural) Joint: ROM

Dorsiflexion (Extension)	Plantarflexion[a] (Flexion)	Rotation	Transverse Motion
20°–25°	35°–50°	5°	15°

[a]Hyperflexion: 90°.

A. Instant center of movement: is in the talus with, lateral and posterior points at the malleolar tips, which change slightly with movement
B. Ankle dorsiflexion and abduction: coupled movements in the ankle; the talus and fibula must externally rotate slightly with dorsiflexion
C. Tibial/talar articulation: major weight-bearing surface of the ankle capable of supporting compressing forces up to 5 times body weight on level surfaces and shear forces (backward-to-forward) up to body weight
D. Large weight-bearing surface area of the ankle joint allows for decreased stress (force per area) at this joint
E. Fibular/talar joint: transmits approximately 1/6 the force presented to the ankle joint
F. Stability of the joint is based on the shape of articulation (mortise maintained by the shape of talus) plus ligamentous support
   1. Dorsiflexion: best stability is in dorsiflexion, which is limited by plantar aponeurosis
      a. Further tension on aponeurosis causes the foot arch to rise (with the toe dorsiflexed)
      b. In addition, it is limited by passive resistance of triceps surae to stretching and tension in medial and lateral ligaments
   2. Plantar flexion is due to the muscles of the posterior and lateral leg compartments
   3. During weight bearing, the tibial and talar articulation are the key surfaces, which contribute most to joint stability
   4. When the the foot is plantarflexed (produced by the muscles in the anterior compartment of the leg), a "wobble" can occur in the joint due to instability of the joint, creating a small amount of abduction, adduction, inversion, and eversion
   5. Structures that limit movement
      a. Dorsiflexion
         i. Ligaments: Calcaneofibular ligament, medially; posterior talofibular; and the posterior joint capsule
         ii. Contact of bones (talus and tibia)
         iii. Tension of plantar flexors of ankle
      b. Plantar flexion
         i. Ligaments: anterior talofibular ligament, the anterior part of the medial anterior capsule
         ii. Contact of bones (talus and tibia)
         iii. Tension of dorsiflexors of ankle

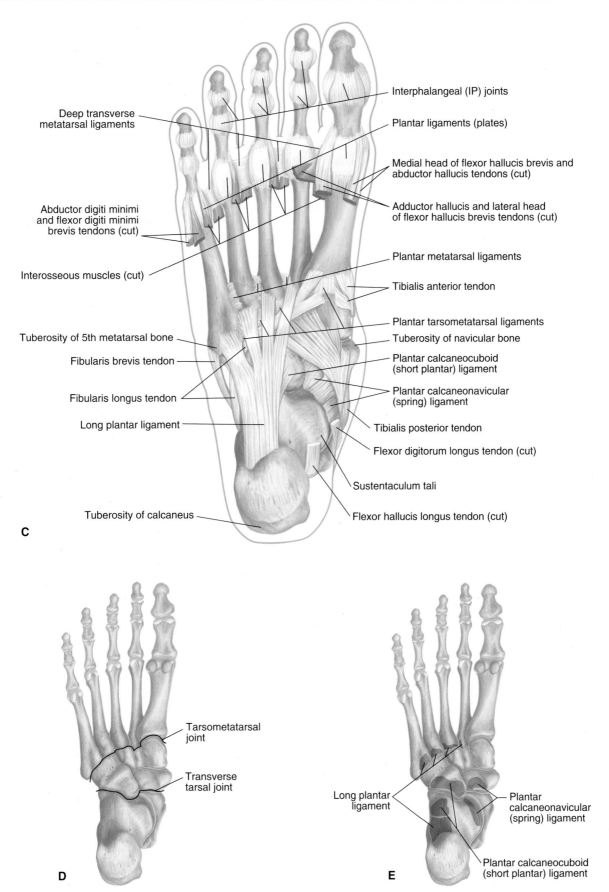

Interphalangeal (IP) joints

Plantar ligaments (plates)

Medial head of flexor hallucis brevis and abductor hallucis tendons (cut)

Adductor hallucis and lateral head of flexor hallucis brevis tendons (cut)

Plantar metatarsal ligaments

Tibialis anterior tendon

Plantar tarsometatarsal ligaments

Tuberosity of navicular bone

Plantar calcaneocuboid (short plantar) ligament

Plantar calcaneonavicular (spring) ligament

Tibialis posterior tendon

Flexor digitorum longus tendon (cut)

Sustentaculum tali

Flexor hallucis longus tendon (cut)

Deep transverse metatarsal ligaments

Abductor digiti minimi and flexor digiti minimi brevis tendons (cut)

Interosseous muscles (cut)

Tuberosity of 5th metatarsal bone

Fibularis brevis tendon

Fibularis longus tendon

Long plantar ligament

Tuberosity of calcaneus

C

Tarsometatarsal joint

Transverse tarsal joint

Long plantar ligament

Plantar calcaneonavicular (spring) ligament

Plantar calcaneocuboid (short plantar) ligament

D

E

Figure 3.30 C. Foot Joints. Right, Plantar View. **D.** Foot Joints. Foot Joints of Inversion and Eversion, Right, Plantar View. **E.** Foot Joints, Ligaments and Attachments. Right, Plantar View.

IX. Subtalar (Talo-calcaneo-navicular) Joint: ROM

Inversion (Supination)	Eversion (Pronation)	Functional ROM
20°–35°	5°–25°	6°

A. Primary action: Predominantly at posterior talocalcaneal and talonavicular joints; their action also involves transverse tarsal joints
B. Talocalcaneal part of the joint is a plane synovial joint, whereas the talonavicular part is a synovial ball-and-socket joint
C. Axis of rotation: 42° in sagittal plane, 16° in transverse plane
D. Joint motions are coupled: dorsiflexion and abduction during eversion (pronation); and plantar flexion and adduction during inversion (supination)

X. Transverse (Mid) Tarsal (Talo-naviculo-calcano-cuboid) Joint(s): ROM

A. Series of separate joints, anterior to the interosseous talocalcaneal ligament and sinus tarsi: middle and anterior talocalcaneal joints, the joints between the head of talus on one side and navicular and cuboid on the other, and the calcaneocuboid joint

Inversion[a]	Eversion[b]
33°	18°

[a]Inversion is combined with adduction (15°–20°), supination and plantar flexion.
[b]Eversion is combined with abduction (5°–20°), dorsiflexion and pronation.
Functional range of motion: 6°

B. Foot position governs motion
  1. 2 axes of rotation
     a. Talonavicular
     b. Calcaneocuboid
  2. With foot eversion, the 2 joints are parallel and the range of motion takes place
  3. With foot inversion: external rotation of the lower extremity results in joints not being parallel, and motion is limited
C. Calcaneocuboid joint: a plane synovial joint allowing inversion, eversion, and circumduction
D. Cuneonavicular joint: a plane synovial joint allowing very little movement
E. Tarsometatarsal joint: a plane synovial joint allowing gliding or sliding

XI. Metatarsophalangeal (MP) Joints: ROM

Dorsiflexion (Extension)	Plantarflexion (Flexion)
50°–70°	15°–25°

A. 2nd metatarsal (Lisfranc): At metatarsal-tarsal joint, the key stabilizing bone of the foot that carries most of the load with walking; the 1st metatarsal bears the most load while standing
B. Foot transmits approximately 1.2 times the body weight while walking and 3 times the body weight during running

XII. 1st Metatarsophalangeal Joint (at Big Toe): ROM

Flexion	Extension
45°	70°–90°

A. Joints between bases of proximal phalanges and heads of metatarsals allow much extension but rather limited flexion
B. Active abduction is usually accompanied by extension

XIII. Other Toes: ROM

A. Active flexion takes place in lesser toes at distal and proximal interphalangeal (PIP) joints

B. Active extension is seen only at MP joints

XIV. Structures Limiting Movement of the Joints of the Foot and Toes

A. Inversion: subtalar and transverse tarsal joints
1. Ligaments: the lateral collateral ligament of the ankle; the internal joint capsule
2. Other: tension of evertor muscles of the ankle

B. Eversion: the subtalar and transverse tarsal joint
1. Ligaments: the MCL of the ankle
2. Other: tension of tibialis posterior, flexor hallucis longus, and flexor digitorum longus muscles and tendons

C. Flexion:
1. MP: tension of the posterior part of the capsule, extensor muscles, and collateral ligaments
2. PIP: soft tissue apposition, tension of collateral ligaments, and the posterior joint capsule
3. Distal interphalangeal (DIP): tension in collateral ligaments, oblique retinacular ligaments, and the posterior joint capsule

D. Extension:
1. MP: tension of the plantar joint capsule, plantar ligaments, and flexor muscles
2. PIP: tension in the plantar joint capsule
3. DIP: ligaments and the joint capsule

E. Abduction:
1. MP: ligaments; collateral ligaments, medial joint capsule, tension of the adductor muscle, and skin between the web spaces of toes

F. Adduction:
1. MP: toe apposition

 **XV. Clinical Considerations: Sprains**

A. Usually is an inversion injury in which some part of a ligament is torn as a result of rocking the foot toward the midline

B. Ankle joint has least stability in plantar flexed position; an inversion strain in that position is most likely to injure the anterior talofibular ligament

C. Dislocation: usually occurs when the foot is forcibly everted, resulting in a severe pull on the medial ligament and frequently tearing off of the medial malleolus or breaking the fibula above the tibiofibular articulation (**Pott fracture**)

Arches of the Foot

I. Functional Considerations

A. Large number of bones allow for both great mobility and absorption of shock
B. Toes are important in balancing, running, and climbing

II. Structure of the Arches (Fig. 3.31A,B)

A. Longitudinal consists of 2 columns of bones, a medial and lateral
   1. Medial: calcaneus, talus, navicular, 3 cuneiforms, and 3 medial metatarsals
      a. Most important because it bears most of weight
      b. Talus and navicular are most subject to injury
   2. Lateral: calcaneus, cuboid, and 2 lateral metatarsals
      a. Balances weight
      b. Calcaneus most subject to injury
B. Transverse: 2nd and 3rd cuneiforms and 2nd to 4th metatarsals are wedge shaped, forming an arch

III. Weight Distribution and Support

A. Distribution (% of the total body weight): 25% to calcaneus and 25% to heads of metatarsals (10% to the head of the 1st and 3.75% to the more lateral metatarsals)
B. Support 80% stress on plantar ligaments, 20% on such muscles or tendons as tibialis posterior, fibularis (peroneus) longus, abductor and adductor hallucis for the medial longitudinal arch and adductor hallucis for the transverse arch

IV. Muscles Acting on the Ankle Joint

Dorsiflexion (Flexion)	Plantar Flexion (Extension)
Tibialis anterior	Gastrocnemius
Extensor digitorum longus	Soleus
Fibularis (peroneus) tertius	Plantaris
Extensor hallucis longus	Flexor hallucis longus
	Fibularis (peroneus) longus and brevis
	Tibialis posterior

V. Muscles Acting on Subtalar and Transverse Tarsal Joints

Inversion and Adduction	Eversion and Abduction
Tibialis anterior and posterior	Fibularis (peroneus) longus and brevis
Flexor hallucis longus	Fibularis (peroneus) tertius
Flexor digitorum longus and brevis	Extensor digitorum longus (lateral part)

VI. Clinical Considerations

A. **Flatfeet** (*pes planus*): condition in which the medial arch of the foot is nonexistent due to misalignment of bones and a stretching of ligaments
   1. In infants, flat appearance of the foot is normal due to subcutaneous fat pads in soles; may persist for 2 years
   2. In adolescents and adults, caused by fallen arches, usually the medial longitudinal arches
B. Flattening of the transverse arch of the foot may occur, and callus formation takes place under heads of the lateral 4 metatarsal bones as a protective measure for the abnormal pressure that is exerted
C. Sesamoids of the big toe take the weight of the body, especially during the latter part of walking phase; their mechanism may be altered in bunions and in hallux valgus

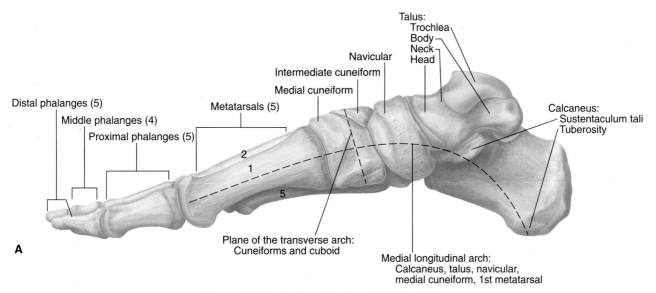

Figure 3.31A. Arches of the Foot, Right. Medial View.

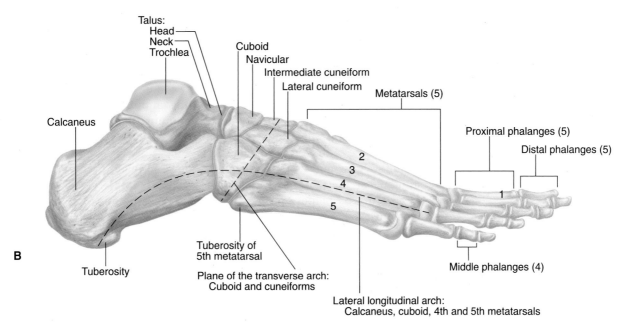

Figure 3.31B. Arches of the Foot, Right. Lateral View.

Disorders of the Feet

I. Posture of the Normal Foot

A. Long-axis direction of the normal postured foot is determined by rotation of the femur at the hip because talus is firmly held in mortise of the ankle

B. Long axis may be directed inward ("in-toeing") up to 15° or outward ("out-toeing") up to 25°; average posture when standing is a position of out-toeing of about 15°

II. Body Weight Distribution

A. Weight in the foot is distributed like a tripod: legs are the calcaneus, the 2 sesamoid bones under the head of the 1st metatarsal, and the heads of the 2 lateral metatarsals; thus, the axis of balance, *when standing*, passes through the center of the heel and forward between the 2nd and 3rd metatarsals

B. Ball of hallux sustains twice the pressure of that over each of the lateral metatarsal heads

III. Congenital Anomalies (Fig. 3.32A–F)

A. **Pes cavus:** very disabling deformity of the foot characterized by an exaggeration of the longitudinal arch (converse of the flatfoot)
  1. Inversion at the subtalar joint
  2. Possible calcaneal deformity
  3. Dropping of the forefoot (equinus) at the midtarsal joint
  4. Clawing of all toes

B. **Flatfeet:** weakening of supporting muscles and the plantar calcaneonavicular ligament removes support for the head of talus, which descends, stretching the ligament and flattening the longitudinal arch of the foot

C. **Talipes or clubfeet:** used in describing deformities of both the ankle and the foot (*pes* is term used when disorder is limited to the foot alone)
  1. Simple types
      a. Talipes equinus: the foot is in marked plantar flexion (like horse foot) with the heel abnormally elevated and weight placed on balls of toes
      b. Talipes calcaneus: dorsiflexion of the foot and prominence of the heel with weight of body resting on the heel alone
  2. Combined deformities
      a. Talipes equinovarus is the most common deformity and usually seen at birth: the heel is in varus (bent inward), the ankle is in equinus (plantar flexed), and the forefoot is in varus and supination; there is an equinus of the forefoot producing a cavus or an increase of the longitudinal arch
      b. Talipes equinovalgus: same as above except the heel is in valgus (bent outward) and the longitudinal arch is flattened (*pes valgus* or *planus*, flatfoot)
      c. Talipes calcaneovarus: talipes calcaneus and talipes varus combined; the clubfoot is dorsiflexed, inverted, and adducted
      d. Talipes calcaneovalgus: talipes calcaneus and talipes valgus combined; the clubfoot is dorsiflexed, everted, and abducted

IV. Disorders of the Toes (Fig. 3.32G,H)

A. **Hallux valgus (bunion):** long axis of the big toe is deviated laterally, toward other toes, and rotated internally in various degrees; condition may be either congenital or acquired

B. **Clawing of toes:** common; imbalance of short intrinsic muscles
  1. Consists of hyperextension or dorsiflexion of the proximal phalanx with plantar flexion of distal phalanges
  2. Result of overactivity of long and short extensors with reciprocal inhibition of corresponding flexors and weakness of interossei and lumbricals; high heels may be a cause

C. **Hammer and mallet toes:** clawing is confined to 1 toe
  1. Hammer type: marked dorsiflexion of the proximal phalanx with plantar flexion of the 2nd phalanx; the distal phalanx may be neutral, hyperflexed, or hyperextended
  2. Mallet type: deformity consists only of a marked plantar flexion of the distal phalanx

V. Nails (Fig. 3.32I)

A. **Ingrowing toenail:** common, congenital or traumatic, usually involves hallux; due to tight shoes, shrunken socks, or improper paring of nail corners

B. **Oxychogryphosis:** overgrowth of nail (like a ram's horn)

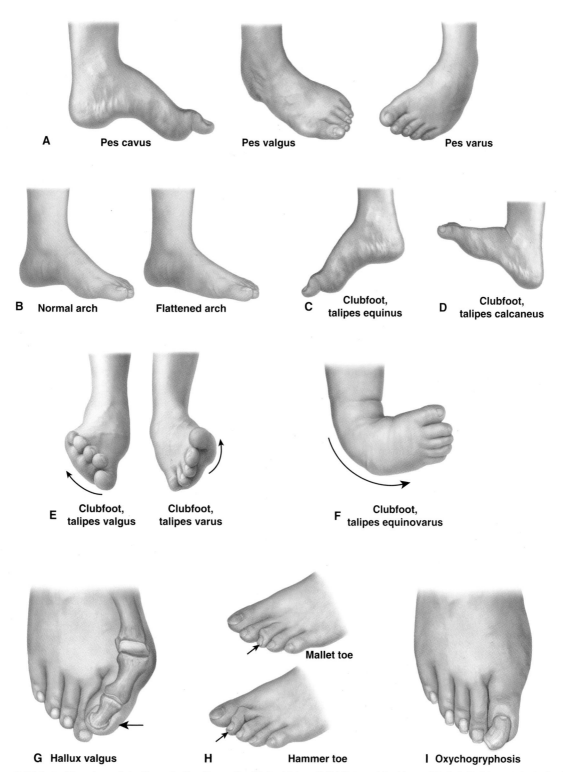

Figure 3.32A–I. Disorders of the Foot. **A.** Pes Cavus (**Left**), Pes Valgus (**Middle**), and Pes Varus (**Right**). **B.** Normal Arch (**Left**) and Flatfoot (**Right**). **C.** Clubfoot, Talipes Equinus. **D.** Clubfoot, Talipes Calcaneus. **E.** Clubfoot, Talipes Valgus (**Left**) and Varus (**Right**). **F.** Clubfoot, Talipes Equinovarus. **G.** Hallux Valgus. **H.** Mallet Toe (**Top**) and Hammer Toe (**Bottom**). **I.** Oxychogryphosis.

Walking (Bipedal Locomotion), Part 1

I. Introduction

A. Normal walking is a learned, complex behavior involving the balancing of body weight over a single support (one extremity) while controlling the forward motion

B. At least one foot is always in contact with ground and the forward fall of body weight is a major force that propels body forward during walking

C. Walking involves a complex series of muscle actions, postures, and bony adaptations to withstand forces transmitted across the hip joint and arrangement of ligaments and bones to maintain foot arches

II. Walking Cycle (Fig. 3.33)

A. Divided into **strides**—activities between successive heel strikes, on the same side

B. Stride is further divided into 2 distinct phases: stance and swing

1. **Stance phase:** begins with heel strike and ends when great toe leaves ground; uses 3/5 of the complete cycle
   a. Limb is supporting the body whose weight is transferred from the heel to head of metatarsals as the center of gravity passes forward over the foot
   b. Stance can be divided into 5 segments (phases):
      i. **Initial contact phase (IC)** or heel strike
      ii. **Loading response phase (LR)** or foot flat: the limb reacts to the weight of body by rolling forward on the heel (heel rocker action) to sustain body momentum and the foot is brought into full contact with ground; IC + LR make up the initial double stance interval (both feet are in contact with the ground)
      iii. **Midstance phase (MST):** begins interval of single stance (1 foot on ground); "ankle rocker" action occurs to bring the body weight over the planted foot and helps sustain forward body momentum
      iv. **Terminal stance phase (TST):** begins with raising of heel (heel-off); lower limb rolls forward on its forefoot ("forefoot rocker") and body advances ahead of the sole-supporting-foot; MST + TST make up single stance interval
      v. **Preswing phase (PSW):** last stance phase and last interval of double support (both feet in contact with ground); the lower limb is positioned to quickly swing forward beneath the body advancement as the body weight is unloaded from one limb and transferred to the opposite limb; ends with the forefoot rolling off ground, leading to beginning of the next phase (swing) or toe off; stance phase ends with no hip flexion, 40° knee flexion, and 15° ankle flexion

2. **Swing phase:** uses 2/5 of cycle and begins with toe off; consists of 3 segments (phases):
   a. **Initial swing phase (ISW):** begins with toe off; the foot is pushed off ground and the limb is accelerated forward, helping to provide the force to sustain the forward body momentum
   b. **Midswing phase (MSW):** the limb passes beneath body to where tibia of the leg is vertical
   c. **Terminal (final) swing phase (TSW):** the limb decelerates the forward movement to prepare for the IC of stance to initiate a new step

III. Normal Human Gait Determinants

A. Pelvic rotation: reflects thigh and leg lateral rotators
   1. Center of gravity to be displaced less far vertically
   2. Body pivots around the stance leg and the swing leg rotates laterally to start heel strike

B. Pelvic tilt: produced by abduction of the hip of the stance leg
   1. Without this abduction, the swing hip drops down abruptly as weight is transferred to the stance leg
   2. Abduction minimizes this drop by holding pelvis more horizontal

C. Knee flexion: produced by hamstrings and gastrocnemius muscles

 1. Important in the stance phase when the center of gravity reaches its highest point on the arc

 2. Bending knees flattens arc

D. Complex series of knee, ankle, and foot mechanisms that operate through the stance phase, involving slight flexions and extensions of these joints to modulate movements and smooth transitions at heel strike, foot flat, and toe off

E. Minimization of the lateral pelvic displacement: in normal walking, feet are kept near body's midline

 1. Carrying angle of the femur and abductors and adductors of the thigh at the hip minimize lateral displacement of the center of gravity in walking.

 2. Walking with feet planted directly below hip joints leads to a "lurching gait" because the body and center of gravity are thrown from side to side (in inebriation, in gait disorders, and in infants learning to walk)

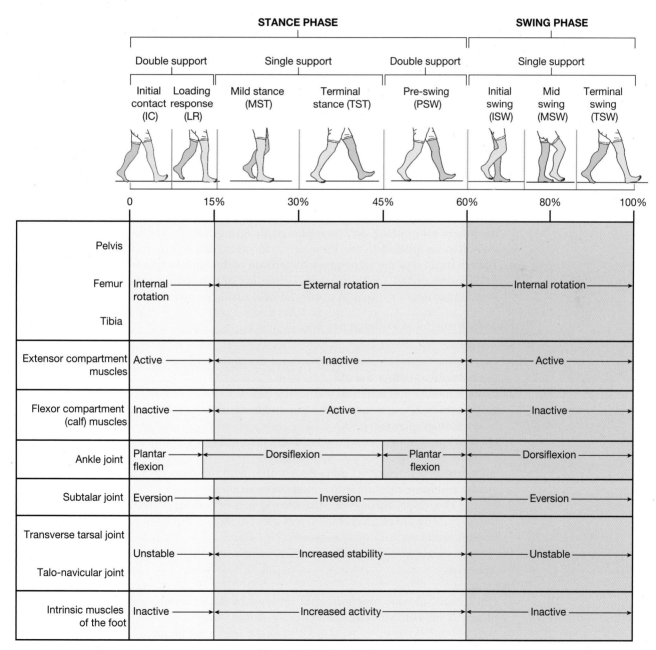

Figure 3.33. Phases of Walking.

Walking (Bipedal Locomotion), Part 2

I. Summary of Walking Movements

A. Stance phase: begins with heel strike (right extremity)

1. At right heel strike, the hip is semiflexed and laterally rotated, the knee is extended and locked by conjoint medial rotation of the femur on tibia, the ankle is dorsiflexed, and MP joints are extended

2. As heel begins to rise, the center of gravity of trunk moves forward, the hip extends, the knee remains extended, the foot first meets ground, and then plantar flexes toward toe off (swing phase)

3. During stance phase, the hip joint medially rotates: right acetabulum is significantly in front of the left at heel strike of the right foot, but behind it at toe off, accomplished by the medial rotation of the right hip

4. In middle of stance, as the center of gravity of trunk moves to the right over the fixed foot, the right hip also abducts, raising left acetabulum higher above ground than the right

B. Swing phase: begins at right toe off when the right hip is extended and medially rotated, the right knee starts to flex, and the ankle moves from plantar flexion to dorsiflexion

1. Hip then flexes with slight adduction in counteraction to abduction at the left hip: the hip starts to extend so that, at heel strike, it is semiflexed; in the swing phase, the hip is laterally rotated

2. Knee begins to extend and continues to extend until the swing phase starts: the knee unlocks and flexes, so toes can clear ground, and the limb is brought forward; the knee extends and locks again at heel strike (Note: there are 2 knee flex-extend cycles per step)

3. To prevent toes from dragging, the ankle dorsiflexes until the foot has gone through the lowest swing phase arc; then plantar flexion gradually begins and continues until the sole is on ground (Note: there are 2 dorsiflex plantar flex cycles per step)

4. Toward the end of the swing phase, extension of the knee by quadriceps femoris muscle (a bit less than 180°) causes passive tightening of hamstrings; this tension reverses the forward swing at the hip and plants the heel firmly on ground

II. Muscles Involved in Walking (Fig. 3.34)

A. Stance phase

1. Gluteus maximus and hamstrings extend the hip early in stance, and hip flexors check this movement before toe off

2. Gluteus medius and minimus abduct the hip, and the hip medial rotators act in the first half of stance; late in stance, adductors and lateral rotators check momentum generated by the former muscles

3. Quadriceps femoris muscle acts at the beginning of stance, extending the knee; hamstrings flex the knee just before toe off

4. Dorsiflexors of the foot act immediately after heel strike to check plantar flexion under gravity and bring the foot into contact with ground

5. Plantar flexors act throughout the second half of stance, powering forward thrust of the body using the thigh and the leg as a single unit; thus, the body is powered forward by plantar flexors and hip extensors

6. As body weight comes onto the foot, intrinsic foot muscles contract to support plantar ligaments

B. Swing phase

1. Hip flexors, already functioning at the end of stance, continue into the early swing phase, along with adductors and lateral rotators

   a. They are, however, essentially silent in the midswing phase

   b. Thigh momentum is checked at the end of the swing phase by extensors

2. Hamstrings function late in the stance phase and continue into the early swing phase to flex the knee
   a. Forward momentum of the limb in the swing phase results in the transition from flexion to extension at the knee (with little assistance from quadriceps femoris muscle)
   b. This momentum is checked by hamstrings before heel strike
3. Dorsiflexors of the ankle act throughout swing phase; intrinsic sole muscles are inactive

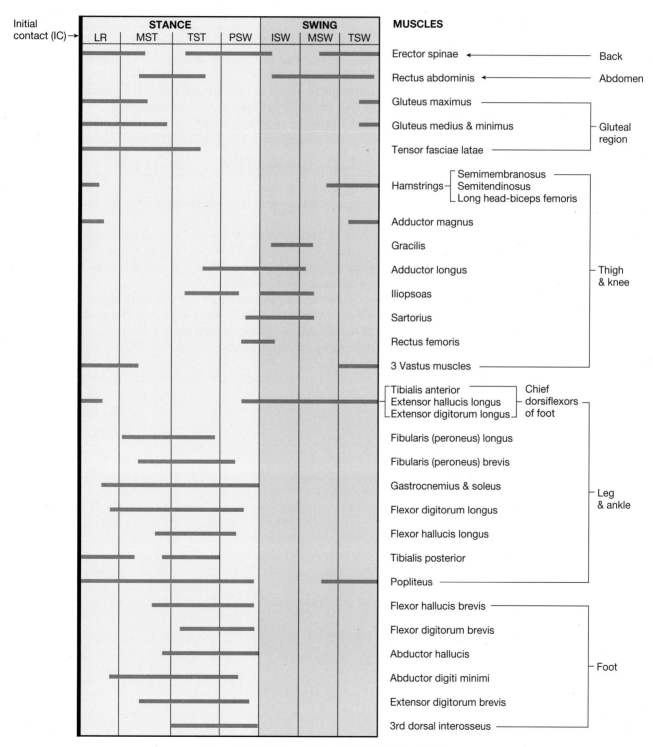

Figure 3.34. Timing of Muscle Activity During Walking.

Walking (Bipedal Locomotion), Part 3

I. Other Considerations in Walking (Fig. 3.35A)

A. Motion of pelvis: critical to normal locomotion

　1. As a balancing mechanism, the upper trunk rotates throughout the spinal column in an opposite direction from pelvis

　2. Motion of upper limbs is correlated with movement of the upper trunk

B. Center of gravity (in front of sacral promontory) rises in middle of each stance phase; as this happens twice per cycle, the head "bobs" twice per cycle

C. Lower limb is seldom fully extended when the body is over it in the stance phase; thus, an individual is usually slightly shorter while walking than in standing

D. Evertors and invertors of the foot stabilize and support arches with each step

E. The cycle is under CNS control

　1. Proprioceptive (stretch receptors) fibers of muscles and joints relay information as to the exact joint position; little occurs at the conscious level of control

　2. In tabes dorsalis (3rd-stage syphilis), proprioceptive fibers of cord are damaged; patient cannot judge position of muscles and joints, and gait is a "flail-like" slapping motion

II. Arches and Interosseous Ligaments in Walking (Fig. 3.35B)

A. Help create stability and flexibility to the foot

B. At heel strike: center of pressure (COP), where body weight acts, lies at the back end of the lateral longitudinal arch

C. From heel strike to foot flat: COP moves forward, with body weight under the lateral arch

D. Osseoligamentous arrangement: functions as a flexible unit from heel strike to foot flat to absorb some of the force of the upper body weight

E. From foot flat to heel rise: COP continues to move forward and medially from the lateral edge of the midfoot to a point midway between the bases of 1st and 2nd metatarsal bones

F. From heel rise to toe off: COP continues to move forward, from between metatarsals 1 and 2, to a point midway between the big toe and 2nd toe

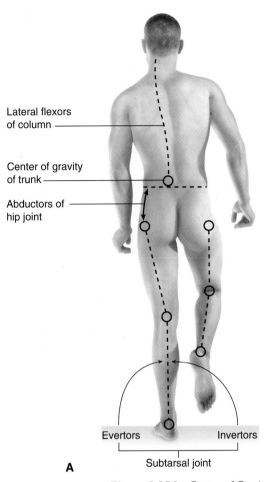

Lateral flexors
of column

Center of gravity
of trunk

Abductors of
hip joint

Evertors   Invertors

Subtarsal joint

A

Figure 3.35A. Center of Gravity During Walking.

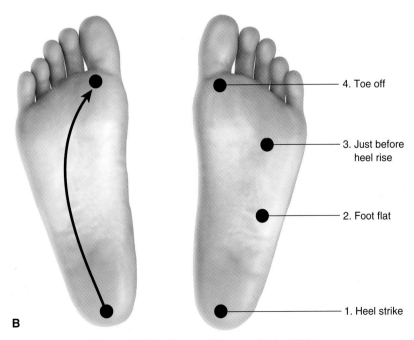

4. Toe off

3. Just before
heel rise

2. Foot flat

1. Heel strike

B

Figure 3.35B. Center of Pressure During Walking.

III. Clinical Considerations Relating to Muscle Activity (Fig. 3.35C,D)

A. Gluteus maximus paralysis: has a minimum effect on standing and walking; it is important in rising from a seated or crouched position

B. Gluteus medius and minimus: are of little importance in rising or standing, but paralysis hinders walking because pelvis can no longer be stabilized against body weight in a single stance phase

   1. Patient learns to swing trunk toward paralyzed side and there is a characteristic "waddling gait" (can also be associated with congenital hip dislocation)

   2. Trendelenberg sign: tests stability of the hip joint as patient stands on 1 leg

       a. Depends on normal gluteus medius and minimus muscles, a normally placed femoral head in acetabulum, and a normal angle of the femoral neck with its shaft

       b. If any 1 is defective, pelvis "sinks" down on the opposite, unsupported side, a (+) Trendelenberg sign

C. Quadriceps femoris paralysis: affects both standing and rising

   1. Most important effect is in a single stance phase of walking because it stabilizes supporting knee joint against body weight

   2. Without it, the knee can only be stabilized by being locked in full extension by bending the trunk forward or holding the knee back with one hand

D. Soleus and gastrocnemius paralysis: noticeable in walking

   1. Affected limb cannot impart a forward impetus to body by plantar flexion of the ankle at the end of the stance phase; thus, the normal limb is never advanced beyond the affected one because no force is available to propel body forward over it

   2. This is "staccato gait": the paralyzed limb always leads, while the sound limb trails

E. Extensor compartment muscle paralysis: results in foot drop (the foot tends to scrape on ground during the swing phase); if an individual tries to avoid this by exaggerated knee bending, the swing phase ends with the entire foot being "slapped" on ground instead of heel contact

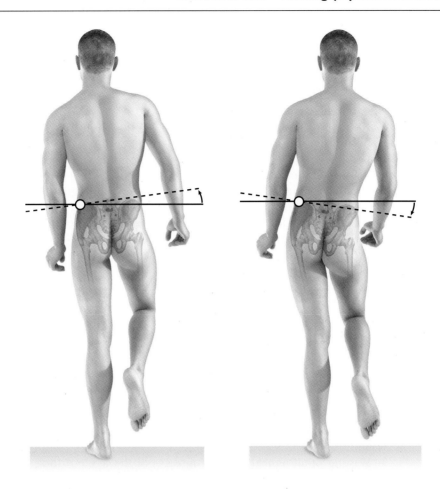

Trendelenberg sign is (–)
Patient can abduct pelvis on left femur

Trendelenberg sign is (+)
Patient unable to abduct pelvis on left femur - right buttock droops

C

Figure 3.35C. Trendelenburg Sign.

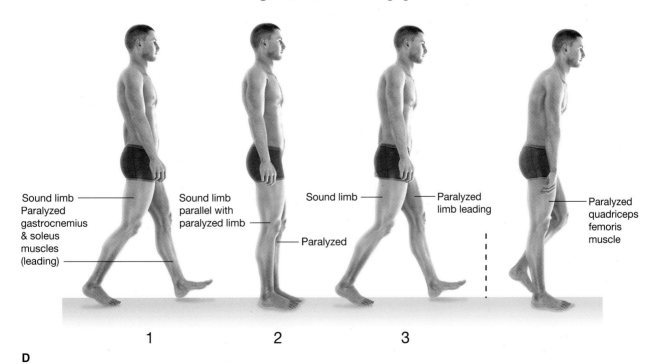

Sound limb
Paralyzed gastrocnemius & soleus muscles (leading)

Sound limb parallel with paralyzed limb

Paralyzed

Sound limb

Paralyzed limb leading

Paralyzed quadriceps femoris muscle

1   2   3

D

Figure 3.35D. Effects of Specific Muscle Paralysis on Walking.

Nerve Injuries in the Lower Limb

I. Specific Cases of Nerve Injury

A. Nerves to iliacus and psoas muscles
1. No superficial signs, but in walking, pelvis does not swing when extremity is fixed
2. No sensory loss

B. Femoral (Fig. 3.36A,B)
1. Wasting of the anterior thigh
2. Leg drop: an inability to extend the leg when the thigh is flexed
3. Weakness in flexion of the thigh due to loss of action of rectus femoris, sartorius, and pectineus muscles
4. Loss of sensation on the anterior thigh and the medial leg and foot

C. Obturator (Fig. 3.36C–E)
1. Wasting of the medial thigh
2. Loss of thigh adduction
3. Some loss of sensation on its upper medial thigh

D. Superior gluteal
1. Trendelenburg sign: significant weakness of abduction of the thigh so that pelvis tilts down on the opposite side of the injury
2. No sensory loss

E. Inferior gluteal
1. Wasting of the buttock
2. Weakness in extension of the thigh, as in climbing
3. No sensory loss

F. Sciatic
1. Wasting of all hamstrings and muscles of the leg and foot; except for flexion of the thigh and adduction of the thigh, no other activity in the lower extremity would be possible
2. Sensation loss on the leg and foot
   a. Common fibular (peroneal) (Fig. 3.36F–H)
      i. If damaged near point of division from sciatic, will result in foot-drop, loss of extension of all toes
      ii. Loss of sensation on the side of the leg
   b. Tibial division (Fig. 3.36I–M)
      i. If severed in upper popliteal fossa, there would be loss of flexion of toes and foot, no inversion of the foot
      ii. Wasting of calf
      iii. Loss of sensation on the sole of the foot and terminal parts of both surfaces of toes

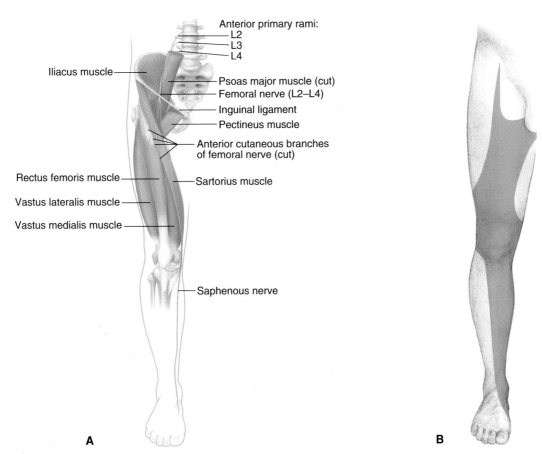

Anterior primary rami:
— L2
— L3
— L4

Iliacus muscle —

Psoas major muscle (cut)
Femoral nerve (L2–L4)

Inguinal ligament
Pectineus muscle

Anterior cutaneous branches
of femoral nerve (cut)

Rectus femoris muscle —
Vastus lateralis muscle —
Vastus medialis muscle —

Sartorius muscle

Saphenous nerve

A

B

Figure 3.36A,B. Femoral Nerve. **A.** Anterior View. **B.** Cutaneous Distribution, Anterior View.

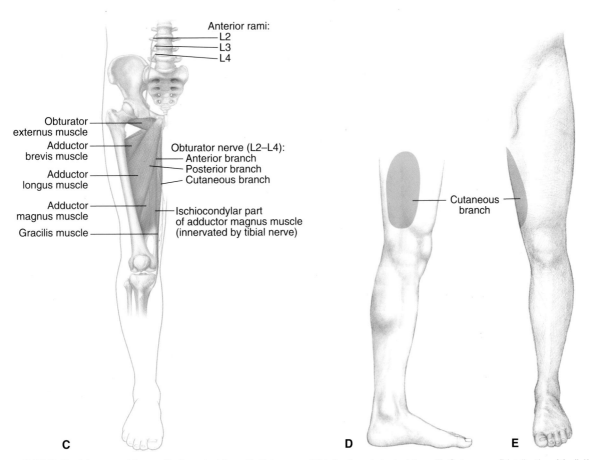

Anterior rami:
— L2
— L3
— L4

Obturator
externus muscle
Adductor
brevis muscle

Obturator nerve (L2–L4):
— Anterior branch
— Posterior branch
— Cutaneous branch

Adductor
longus muscle

Adductor
magnus muscle

Gracilis muscle

Ischiocondylar part
of adductor magnus muscle
(innervated by tibial nerve)

Cutaneous
branch

C

D

E

Figure 3.36C–E. Obturator Nerve. **C.** Anterior View. **D.** Cutaneous Distribution, Anterior View. **E.** Cutaneous Distribution, Medial View.

II. Anatomy of Straight-Leg-Raising Test

A. Investing sheath of the sciatic nerve (like all nerves) is continuous with coverings of CNS; thus, epineurium of the sciatic nerve is continuous with dura mater

B. If epineurium is pulled on, some degree of tension will be transmitted to nerve roots via dura mater

C. Clinically, one method of exerting tension on nerve roots is to exert a pull on the sciatic nerve by means of the straight-leg-raising test

    1. When the hip is flexed while the knee is extended, as in the straight-leg-raising test, tension is transmitted back to L4, L5, and S1-3 nerve roots and to dura

    2. Clinician may elicit pain not only from nerve roots but also from other structures; thus, clinical experience is necessary for interpretation of test results

III. Nerve Root Alignment in Relationship to Vertebrae

A. In lumbar region, the upward migration of cord during development causes lumbar nerve roots to slant downward at an acute angle; thus, although the 4th lumbar nerve root exits between 4th and 5th lumbar vertebrae, a disk herniation at this level will not affect 4th lumbar root because it exits above disk; instead, it would cause pressure on the 5th nerve root

B. A similar situation exists with subsequent disks and nerves

IV. Segmental Innervation of Joint Movements

A. In general, 2 adjoining spinal segments govern a specific joint movement: the 4 segments concerned in 2 opposing movements in a specific joint are in numerical sequence (e.g., hip flexion: L2, L3; hip extension: L4, L5)

B. In the lower limb, joint innervation is segmental, with each joint innervated by nerves arising one segment lower in the spinal cord than those that innervate the next proximal joint; 4 spinal segments control the hip, knee, and ankle

    1. Hip: L2, L3 govern hip flexion, internal rotation, and adduction; L4, L5 control hip extension, lateral rotation, and abduction

    2. Knee: L3, L4 control extension; L5, S1 govern flexion

    3. Ankle: L4, L5 control dorsiflexion; S1, S2 mediate plantar flexion

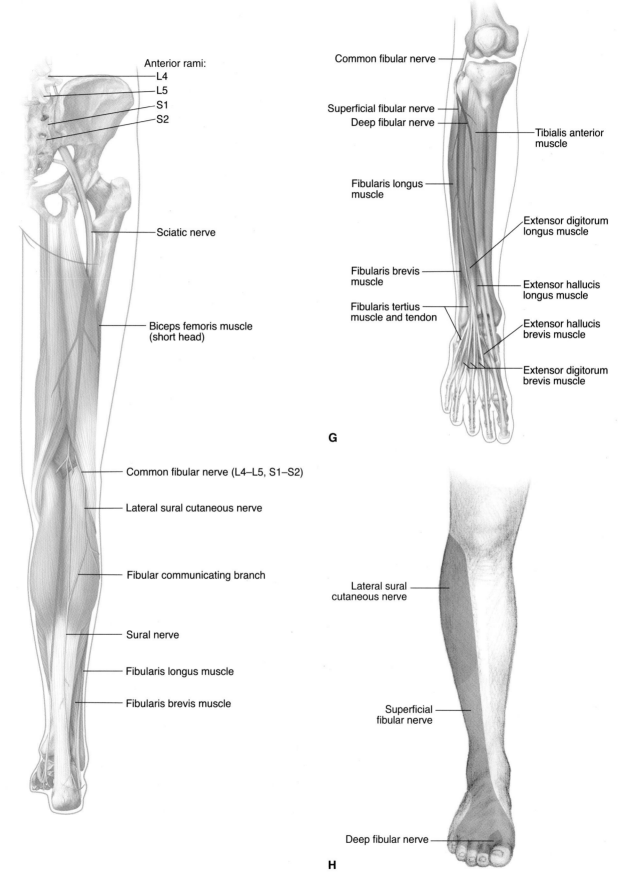

Figure 3.36F–H. Common Fibular Nerve. **F.** Posterior View. **G.** Anterior View. **H.** Cutaneous Distribution, Anterior View.

V. Summary of Muscle–Nerve Relationships in Lower Extremity

Segment	Muscle	Nerve
L2, L3	Adductor brevis	Obturator
L2, L3	Adductor longus	Obturator
L2, L3	Gracilis	Obturator
L2, L3	Sartorius	Femoral
L2-4	Iliacus	Femoral
L2-4	Psoas	Nerves to psoas
L3, L4	Obturator externus	Obturator
L3, L4	Pectineus	Femoral
L3, L4	Quadriceps femoris	Femoral
L3-S1	Adductor magnus	Obturator and tibial
L4, L5	Tibialis anterior	Deep fibular (peroneal)
L4-S1	Gluteus medius	Superior gluteal
L4-S1	Gluteus minimus	Superior gluteal
L4-S1	Inferior gemellus	Nerve to quadratus femoris
L4-S1	Plantaris	Tibial
L4-S1	Popliteus	Tibial
L4-S1	Quadratus femoris	Nerve to quadratus femoris
L4-S1	Tensor fasciae latae	Superior gluteal
L5-S1	Extensor digitorum longus	Deep fibular (peroneal)
L5-S1	Extensor hallucis longus	Deep fibular (peroneal)
L5-S1	Fibularis (peroneus) brevis	Superficial fibular (peroneal)
L5-S1	Fibularis (peroneus) longus	Superficial fibular (peroneal)
L5-S1	Tibialis posterior	Tibial
L5-S2	Gluteus maximus	Inferior gluteal
L5-S2	Obturator internus	Nerve to obturator internus
L5-S2	Biceps femoris	Tibial and common fibular (short head)
L5-S2	Semimembranosus	Tibial
L5-S2	Semitendinosus	Tibial
L5-S2	Soleus	Tibial
L5-S2	Superior gemellus	Nerve to obturator internus
S1, S2	Abductor digiti minimi	Lateral plantar
S1, S2	Abductor hallucis	Medial plantar
S1, S2	Adductor hallucis	Lateral plantar
S1, S2	Extensor digitorum brevis	Deep fibular (peroneal)
S1, S2	Extensor hallucis brevis	Deep fibular (peroneal)
S1, S2	Flexor digiti minimi	Lateral plantar
S1, S2	Flexor digitorum brevis	Medial plantar
S1, S2	Flexor digitorum longus	Tibial
S1, S2	Flexor hallucis brevis	Medial plantar
S1, S2	Flexor hallucis longus	Tibial
S1, S2	Gastrocnemius	Tibial
S1, S2	Lumbricales	Medial and lateral plantar
S1, S2	Interossei	Lateral plantar
S1, S2	Piriformis	Nerve to piriformis
S1, S2	Quadratus plantae	Lateral plantar

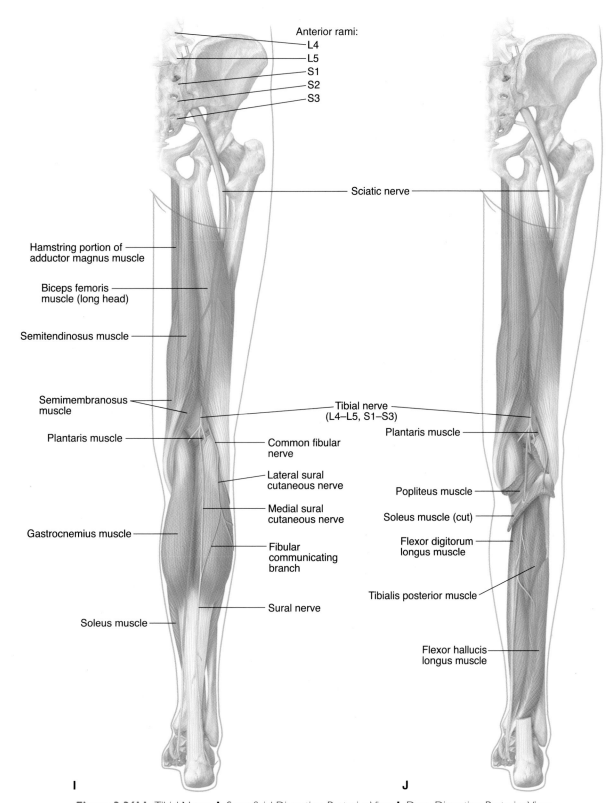

Anterior rami:
L4
L5
S1
S2
S3

Sciatic nerve

Hamstring portion of
adductor magnus muscle

Biceps femoris
muscle (long head)

Semitendinosus muscle

Semimembranosus
muscle

Tibial nerve
(L4–L5, S1–S3)

Plantaris muscle

Plantaris muscle

Common fibular
nerve

Popliteus muscle

Lateral sural
cutaneous nerve

Soleus muscle (cut)

Medial sural
cutaneous nerve

Flexor digitorum
longus muscle

Gastrocnemius muscle

Fibular
communicating
branch

Tibialis posterior muscle

Sural nerve

Flexor hallucis
longus muscle

Soleus muscle

I

J

Figure 3.36I,J. Tibial Nerve. **I.** Superficial Dissection, Posterior View. **J.** Deep Dissection, Posterior View.

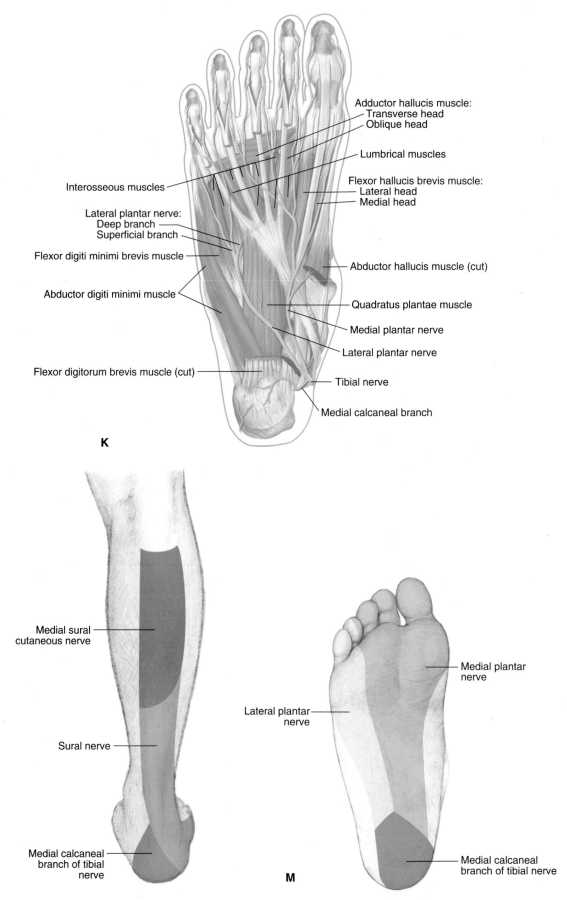

K

Adductor hallucis muscle:
  Transverse head
  Oblique head

Lumbrical muscles

Flexor hallucis brevis muscle:
  Lateral head
  Medial head

Abductor hallucis muscle (cut)

Quadratus plantae muscle

Medial plantar nerve

Lateral plantar nerve

Tibial nerve

Medial calcaneal branch

Interosseous muscles

Lateral plantar nerve:
  Deep branch
  Superficial branch

Flexor digiti minimi brevis muscle

Abductor digiti minimi muscle

Flexor digitorum brevis muscle (cut)

L

Medial sural
cutaneous nerve

Sural nerve

Medial calcaneal
branch of tibial
nerve

M

Medial plantar
nerve

Lateral plantar
nerve

Medial calcaneal
branch of tibial nerve

Figure 3.36K–M. Tibial Nerve. **K.** Plantar View. **L.** Cutaneous Distribution, Posterior View. **M.** Cutaneous Distribution, Plantar View.

Essential Terms of Direction and Movement

Abduction: movement away from midline
Adduction: movement toward midline
Anatomical position: standing erect with upper limbs at the side and palms facing forward
Anterior (ventral): front or forward facing
Coronal (frontal): plane dividing the body into front and back portions
Deep: farther from the surface
Depression: movement inferiorly
Distal: farther from body core; relative term used in limbs
Dorsal (posterior): back or rear facing
Eversion: movement of the foot to face the sole outward (away from midline)
External: outside
Flexion: movement to decrease the angle between two parts of the body
Frontal (coronal): plane dividing the body into front and back portions
Horizontal (transverse): plane dividing the body into upper and lower parts
Inferior: lower, farther from top of the head
Internal: inside
Inversion: movement of the foot to face the sole inward (toward the midline)
Lateral: farther from midline
Longitudinal: along the long axis of a body part
Medial: nearer the midline
Median (midline or midsagittal): plane dividing the body into right and left halves
Midline (median or midsagittal): plane dividing the body into right and left halves
Midsagittal (median or midline): plane dividing the body into right and left halves
Oblique: plane passing at noncardinal angle through a body part
Palmar (volar): anterior or palm side of the hand
Plantar: sole of the foot
Posterior (dorsal): back or rear facing
Pronation: movement of the hand to face the palm backward (when in anatomical position)
Proximal: nearer to the body core; relative term used in limbs
Sagittal: vertical plane dividing the body into right and left portions
Superficial: nearer to the surface
Superior: higher, or closer to the top of the head
Supination: movement of the hand to face the palm forward (when in anatomical position)
Transverse (horizontal): plane dividing the body into upper and lower parts
Ventral (anterior): front or forward facing
Volar (palmar): anterior or palm side of the hand

Fundamentals of Joints

I. Introduction

A. Joint or articulation: the junction between two or more bones of the skeleton

B. Joints can be classified in one of two ways

   1. By the movement they permit

   2. By the tissue joining the bones of the joint

Note: Each of these systems of classification provides useful information about the joint, but the systems do not necessarily correspond

II. Classification by movement

A. Synarthroses: Immovable joints. Examples: suture joints (the joints in the skull) and synchondroses (the type of joint found in growth plates)

B. Amphiarthroses: Slightly moveable joints. Example: symphysis (such as the joint between two vertebrae)

C. Diarthroses: Freely moveable joints. Examples: typical synovial joints such as the shoulder and wrist

Note: An important concept to remember is that joint strength and flexibility are opposed. Greater joint strength comes at the cost of less flexibility and vice versa. Movement allowed at a particular joint depends on the shape of the bones and articular surfaces, the ligaments crossing the joint, and the muscles crossing the joint

III. Classification by type of tissue

A. Fibrous joints: bones of these joints are connected by fibrous ligaments—dense connective tissues that connect bone to bone (as opposed to tendons, which connect muscles to bones). Ligaments are named based on their position or based on the bones they attach. Three distinct types:

   1. Suture joints connect the flat bones of the skull, which meet in a tooth-like pattern

      a. The fibrous tissue of these joints is continuous with the periosteum, and the joints are **synarthroses** (immovable)

      b. Suture joints undergo changes throughout childhood and into early adulthood. At birth, the sutures have broad spaces of fibrous tissue called fontanelles. These joints close down and undergo ossification (becoming fused with bone) beginning in childhood and continuing into a person's 20s. A joint that has ossified over time is called a **synostosis**

   2. Gomphoses: joints that anchor the teeth in the alveolar processes (sockets) of the mandible and the maxilla

      a. Amphiarthroses (slightly moveable), although the normal movement of this joint is not what we consider a "loose tooth"

      b. Allow microscopic movements that enable us to gauge how hard we are biting or if food is stuck in our teeth

   3. Syndesmoses: apposed bones are joined by a fibrous membrane (interosseous membrane) or ligament

      a. Amphiarthroses (slightly moveable) and maintained as fibrous unions throughout life (i.e., syndesmoses do not become synostoses)

      b. Examples include the attachment of the borders of the radius and ulna, which are connected with an interosseous membrane; the attachment of the borders of the tibia and fibula, which are connected with an interosseous membrane; and the inferior tibiofibular joint, which is connected by a ligament

B. **Cartilaginous joints:** bones are joined by either hyaline cartilage or fibrocartilage that is avascular and anervous except at the margins

1. Hyaline cartilage is slippery and strong when compressed but has little tensile strength (strength against being stretched)

2. Fibrocartilage, on the other hand, is tough and strong both when compressed and when stretched (high tensile strength)

3. Two distinct types of cartilaginous joints:

   a. **Synchondroses:** a temporary type of cartilaginous joint seen at **epiphyseal plates** (growth plates) during development

      i. Allow for growth of long bones by flexibly joining the epiphysis, or end, of a growing long bone to the diaphysis, or shaft, of a long bone

      ii. Made of hyaline cartilage that is eventually replaced by bone after growth is complete (synchondroses become synostoses)

      iii. Children are particularly susceptible to breaking bones at their growth plates because that region of the bone is actually hyaline cartilage, which has little tensile strength

      iv. Synchondroses are also found at the union between the first rib and the sternum

   b. **Symphyses:** permanent cartilage unions characterized by fibrocartilage disks separating bones covered by hyaline cartilage

      i. Amphiarthroses (slightly moveable)

      ii. Examples include pubic symphysis and the intervertebral disks between vertebral bodies

C. **Synovial joints:** the most common, most moveable, and most complex type of joint

1. Most are diarthroses (freely moveable)

2. Characterized by a joint cavity between the bones that has a synovial membrane and is lubricated with synovial fluid

3. All synovial joints have

   a. A **joint cavity** between the bones: The space between articulating bones that is lined with the synovial membrane. The joint capsule surrounding the joint cavity provides support for the delicate synovial membrane where it is not in contact with the bone

   b. A **synovial membrane lining** that secretes synovial fluid to lubricate and nourish the joint (syn = like, ovial = egg-white)

   c. **Articular cartilage** that covers the ends of bones that articulate with each other. It consists of hyaline cartilage lubricated with synovial fluid to reduce friction in the joint

   d. Some also have accessory structures, which play key roles when they are present

      i. **Accessory ligaments** may connect bone to bone and stabilize the joint by limiting motion in unwanted directions. Accessory ligaments may be

         a) **Capsular:** a thickening of the joint capsule itself

         b) **Extracapsular:** outside the joint capsule

         c) **Intracapsular:** inside the joint capsule

      ii. **Articular disks or menisci** may intervene between joint spaces. Examples are the lateral and medial menisci in the knee and the articular disks in the sternoclavicular joints

      iii. **Muscles and tendons** can be very important for the integrity of many joints. Examples are the rotator cuff muscles in the shoulder, which support the humerus and keep it in the glenoid cavity, and the popliteus muscle in the knee

4. **Six subclassifications of synovial joints** based on their structure and how much movement each allows; listed below from least to most amount of movement allowed

   a. **Plane joints** allow only gliding or sliding motions in any direction of a single plane. Thus, it is a uniaxial joint

      i. Articular surfaces in plane joints are flat or slightly curved, and movement is restricted by a tight fibrous capsule

    ii. Examples: facet joints (those between articulating surfaces on the vertebrae), intercarpal joints, carpometacarpal joints, intermetacarpal joints, intermetatarsal joints, acromioclavicular joints

  b. **Hinge joints (a.k.a. ginglymus)** allow flexion and extension only. Movement is around one axis that is perpendicular to the bones of the joint, making hinge joints another example of uniaxial joints

    i. The capsule is thin and flexible on the surfaces where bending occurs but is reinforced with strong laterally placed collateral ligaments

    ii. Examples: elbow, knee, interphalangeal joints (the joints between finger and toe segments)

  c. **Pivot joints (a.k.a. trochoidal)** allow rotary movement around one axis that is longitudinal through the bone; they are also uniaxial joints

    i. A process of one bone rotates in a ring formed by another bone and a ligament

    ii. Examples: proximal radioulnar joint, atlantoaxial joint (the joint between the first and second cervical vertebrae)

  d. **Condyloid joints** allow flexion, extension, abduction, adduction, and circumduction. (Circumduction* is a combination of flexion, extension, abduction, and adduction)

    i. Consist of oval surfaces that allow for movement in two planes perpendicular to each other. Thus, this is a **biaxial joint**

    ii. Rotation at this joint is not allowed due to the shape of the articulating surfaces

    iii. Examples: wrist, metacarpophalangeal joints of the fingers and toes

  e. **Saddle joints (a.k.a. sellar)** allow flexion, extension, abduction, adduction, and circumduction

    i. Biaxial, but here articulating surfaces are concavoconvex (one bone shaped like a saddle and the other shaped like a horse's back)

    ii. Example: carpometacarpal joint of the thumb

  f. **Ball and socket joints** allow flexion, extension, abduction, adduction, circumduction, and rotation

    i. Multiaxial, allowing movement in an almost infinite number of axes through the ball of the joint. Ball and socket joints allow for more flexibility than any other type of joint

    ii. Examples: hip, shoulder (glenohumeral)

D. Bursae: sacs of synovial membrane that lie between moveable structures in order to reduce friction

  1. Examples: subacromial bursa that lies between the acromion and supraspinatus tendon and the prepatellar bursa that overlies the patellar ligament

  2. Synovial sheaths: bursae that surround long tendons as they cross joints Examples: the radial and ulnar bursae of the flexor muscles at the wrist

E. Blood supply of joints: Joints are relatively poorly supplied with blood vessels

  1. In general, blood supply comes from collateral branches of larger vessels

  2. Freely moveable joints are surrounded by **collateral vessels**, systems of anastomoses that allow blood flow around the joint regardless of the position of the limb

F. Nerve supply of joints: In contrast to blood supply, joints are very well supplied with sensory nerves

  1. The major sensation from joints is proprioception, which allows us to know what position our limbs are in

  2. Pain sensation in joints is carried by branches of larger nerves in the area. Thus, joint pain is often referred to the skin overlying the joint or the muscles around the joint

  3. The main point to remember about joint innervation is **Hilton's law**: A nerve innervating muscles that act across a joint must also supply sensory fibers to that joint. So, for example, the femoral nerve that supplies the quadriceps muscles also sends sensory branches to the knee joint

---

*To demonstrate the difference between circumduction and rotation: With your arm pointed straight ahead, trace a large circle in the air with your finger (using your whole arm). This is circumduction of the shoulder. Then with the same arm, pretend to turn a screwdriver with your elbow straight. This is rotation of the shoulder. Also, remember that the metacarpophalangeal joints are capable of circumduction (tracing out circles), but cannot do rotation.

Note: Page numbers in *italics* refer to figures

A

Abduction, 261
    and flexion, 132
Accessory ligaments, 264
Acromioclavicular joint, 129, 130
Adduction, 261
Adductor (Hunter's) canal, 180
Adductor hiatus, 182
Adductor-interosseous compartment, 120
Alar ligaments, 20
Allen test, 124
Amphiarthroses, 263
Anatomical position, 261
Anatomical snuffbox, 112
Angle of inclination, 168
Ankle, 150, *151*
    bones, 172, *173*
    joint (talocrural), 236, *237*, 238, *239*
Ankylosing spondylitis, 28
Antebrachial fascia, 68
Anterior (ventral), 261
Anterior arch, 12
Anterior atlantoaxial ligament, 20
Anterior atlanto-occipital membrane, 20
Anterior forearm
    muscles, 100, *101*, 102, *102*
    neurovasculature, 103, 104, *105*
Anterior funiculus, 52
Anterior horns, 50
Anterior intermuscular septum, 198
Anterior lateral spinal vein, 60
Anterior longitudinal ligament, 22
Anterior median fissure, 50
Anterior median spinal vein, 60
Anterior ramus, 54
Anterior (ventral) root, 54
Anterior (pelvic) sacral foramina, 18
Anterior shoulder. *see also* Shoulder
    muscles, 82, *83*
    special features, 82
Anterior thigh muscles, 178, *179*. *see also*
        Thigh
Anterior tibial artery, 207–208
Anterolateral sulcus, 50
Anulus fibrosus (fibrous ring), 22
Apical ligament, 20
Arachnoid mater, 46
Arm
    bone of, 74, *75*
    brachium, 64
    cutaneous nerves, 66
    humerus, 74, *75*
    lymphatics, 70
    muscles, 95, *95*, 96, *97*
    neurovasculature, 98, *99*
Articular cartilage, 264
Articular disks or menisci, 264
Articular processes, 10
Articulated vertebral column, 8, *9*
Articulations. *see* Joints

Auricular surface, 18
Auscultation, triangle of, 32
Axilla, 87, *89*
    armpit, 64
Axillary
    artery, 92, *93*
    lymph nodes, 70
    nerve (C5-6), 91

B

Babinski sign/reflex, 214
Ball and socket joints, 265
Basilic vein, 68
Basivertebral veins, 60
Biaxial joint, 265
Bipedal locomotion. *see* Walking (bipedal
        locomotion)
Blood supply
    hip joint, 224, *225*
    knee joint, 230
    shoulder, 92, 94, *94*
    spinal cord, 58, *59*
    upper limb, 92, 94, *94*
Bones
    arm, 74, *75*
    forearm, 76, *77*, 78, *78*
    hand, 79, *79*, 80, *81*
    lower limb
        ankle, 172, *173*
        foot, 172, *173–175*
        leg, 169, 170, *171*
        thigh, 166, *167*, 168
    pectoral (shoulder) girdle, 72, *73*
    vertebrae, *9*, *17*
    wrist, 79, *79*, 80, *81*
Brachial fascia, 68
Brachial plexus, 56, 87, *89*
    injuries, 88
Bursae, 265
Bursitis, 234

C

Calcaneocuboid joint, 236
Calcaneus, heel bone, 172
Calf bone, fibula, 169
Capitate, 79
Carpal bones (wrist bones), 79
Carpal tunnel, 80
Carpal tunnel syndrome, 142
Carpometacarpal joint, 136
Carrying angle, 134
Cartilaginous joints, 264
Caudal anesthesia, 48
Center of pressure (COP)
    walking, arches and interosseous liga-
        ments, 250, *251*
Central canal, 50
Cephalic vein, 68
Cervical
    cord neuropraxia, 90

curvatures, 7
cutaneous nerves, 4
enlargement, 50, *51*
plexus, 56
rib syndrome, 90
spine, ROM, 42
vertebrae, 10, *11*, 12, *13*
Charley horse, 178, 194
Clavicle (collar bone), 72
Clavicle fractures, 72
Clavipectoral fascia, 68
Clergyman's knee, 234
Clubfeet, 244
Coccydynia, 18
Coccygeal injury, 18
Coccyx vertebrae, 18
Collateral vessels, 265
Condyloid joints, 265
Congenital anomalies, feet,
        244, *245*
Congenital dislocations, 224
Conus medullaris, 50, *51*
Cordotomy, 52
Coronal (frontal), 261
Coronoid process, 76
Costotransverse
    joint, 26, *27*
    ligament, 26
Costovertebral joint, 25, *25*, *27*
Coxa
    valga, 168
    vara, 168
Cruciate
    hip joint, anastomosis, 224, *225*
    ligament, 20
Crural fascia, 156
Crutch palsy, 90
Cuboid, 172, *173*
Cuneiforms (wedge-shaped), 172
Cutaneous innervation
    arm, 66
    back, 4, *5*
    dermatomes, 66, *67*, 153, *154*
    forearm, 66
    hand, 66
    lower limb, 152, *153*, 154
    origin and distribution, 152, *153*
    shoulder and pectoral region, 66
    source, 152
    spinal-vertebral segments, 154
Cutaneous nerves, 4, *5*, 110,
        116, *117*
    foot dorsum, 211, *211*
    foot sole, 214–215
Cuts of feet, 220

D

Deep brachial artery, 98
Deep fascia, 6
Deep femoral artery, 184

Deep fibular (peroneal) nerve (L4, L5, Sl-2), 210
Deep palmar arch, 124
Deep vessels accompany deep blood vessels, 158
Denticulate ligaments (bilateral), 48
Denticulations, 48
Depression, 261
Diarthroses, 263
Digital flexion creases, 114
Dinner fork, deformity, 78
Distal, 261
Distal row, wrist bones, 79
Dorsal (posterior), 261
Dorsal carpal arch, 123
Dorsal metatarsal veins, 155
Dorsal scapular nerve (C5), 90
Dorsal subaponeurotic space, 112
Dorsal venous arch, 155
Dorsal venous network, 110
Down syndrome, 118
Dura mater, 46
Dural sac, visualization of, 48

E
Elbow
    joint, 135
        humeroulnar joint, 133
        pulled elbow, 134
        radioulnar joint, 133–134
        ROM, 134
    median nerve (C5-T1), injury, 141
    ulnar nerve (C8, T1), injury, 144, 145
Epidural anesthesia, 48
Epidural space, 46
Epiphyseal plates, 264
Erb-Duchenne palsy, 88
Erector spinae
    intermediate group, 36
    muscle, 2, 2
Eversion, 261
Extension
    thoracolumbar spine, 42
    vertebral column movements, 42
Extensor retinacula, 156, 206
External, 261
External vertebral venous plexus, 60

F
Fascia
    lata, 156, 176, 177
    lower limb, 156
Fasciae, 6, 6
Femoral
    artery, 184, 185
    canal, 180
    head, avascular necrosis of, 168
    neck fracture, 168
    nerve, 186, 187
    sheath, 180, 181
    triangle, 180, 181
    vein, 184
Fibrous digital sheaths, 116
Fibrous joints
    gomphoses, 263
    suture joints, 263
    syndesmoses, 263–264
Fibula (calf bone), 169

Fibular
    (peroneal) artery, 207
    neck fractures, 170
    (peroneal) nerve (L4, L5, Sl-2), 196, 208, 210
    retinacula, 156
Filum terminale internum, 48
Fissures and sulci, external appearance, 50, 51
Flatfeet, 242, 244
Flexion, 261
    cervical spine, 42
    thoracolumbar spine, 42
    vertebral column movements, 42
Flexor retinacula, ankle, 156
Flexor retinaculum, wrist (transverse carpal ligament), 116
Foot, 150, 151
    arches of
        ankle joint, muscles acting on, 242
        flatfeet, 242
        functional considerations, 242
        structure of, 242, 243
        subtalar and transverse tarsal joints, muscles acting on, 242
        weight distribution and support, 242
    bones, 172, 173–175
    disorders, 244, 245
    dorsum, 211, 211, 212, 212, 213
    drop, 206
    muscles, 211, 212, 213
    overinversion, 170
    sole
        cutaneous nerves, 214, 215
        muscles, 216, 217–219
        plantar aponeurosis, 214, 215
        vessels and nerves, 220, 221
    and toes, 241
Forearm
    antebrachium, 64
    anterior forearm muscles, 100, 101, 102, 102
    bones of, 76, 77, 78, 78
    lymphatics, 70
    neurovasculature, 103, 104, 105, 108, 109
    posterior forearm, 106, 107
    radial nerve (C5-T1), injury, 148
Frontal (coronal), 261

G
Genicular anastomosis, 197
Genu
    valgum, 234
    varum, 234
Ginglymus, 265
Glenohumeral joint, 129–130
Gluteal region
    arteries, 190, 191
    cutaneous nerves, 152, 153, 154
    muscles, 188, 189
    sacral plexus and derivatives, 190, 191, 192
    sciatica, 192
    trendelenburg sign/gluteal gait, 192
Gluteus
    maximus, 188, 189, 191, 193, 195, 222, 248

    maximus paralysis, 252
    medius and minimus, 252
Gomphoses, 263
Gray
    commissure, 50
    matter, 50
    ramus communicans, 54
Great saphenous vein, 155, 157, 158
Greater occipital nerve, 56
Groin strain, 182

H
Hallux valgus (bunion), 244
Hamate, 79
Hammer and mallet toes, 244
Hand, 64
    dorsum, 112, 113
        anatomical snuffbox, 112
        cutaneous nerves, 110, 111
        dorsal subaponeurotic space, 112
        extensor retinaculum and extensor expansions, 112
        knuckles, 112
        lymphatics, 110
        skin, 110
        vessels, 110
    joints, 136, 138, 139, 140
    nerves, 126, 127, 128, 128
    palm of, 115, 117
        cutaneous nerves, 116
        deep palmar fascia, 116
        digital flexion creases, 114
        palmar flexion creases, 114
        skin, 114
    palmar hand, 119, 119, 120, 121, 122, 122
    vessels, 123, 123–125, 125
Head, muscles producing movements of, 44
Heel bone, calcaneus, 172
Herniated (slipped) disc, 22
Hilton's law, 265
Hinge joints/ginglymus, 265
Hip, 150, 151
    joint
        blood supply, 224, 225
        cruciate anastomosis, 224, 225
        ligaments, 222, 223
        muscles acting, 222
        ROM, 224
        synovial membrane, 222
    pointer, 178
Horizontal (transverse), 261
Horizontal axis, 130
Humeral shaft fracture, 74
Humeroulnar joint, 133
Humerus, 74, 75
Hypothenar compartment, 120

I
IC. see Initial contact phase (IC)
Iliac crest, 2
Iliolumbar joints, 164, 165
Iliopsoas, 178
Iliotibial tract, 156
Inferior, 261
Inferior fibular retinacula, 204
Inferior gluteal, 190, 191

Inferior longitudinal band, 20
Inferior radioulnar joint, 138
Inferolateral angle, 18
Ingrowing toenail, 245, *245*
Inguinal nodes, lymph nodes, 158, *159*
Initial contact phase (IC), 246
Initial swing phase (ISW), 246
Intercarpal articulation, 136
Intercostal nerves, 56
Intermediate sacral crests, 18
Intermetacarpal joints, 136
Intermuscular septa, 198, *199*
   medial and lateral, 176, *177*
Internal, 261
Internal pudendal, 190, *191*
Internal vertebral venous plexus, 60
Interossei muscles, 122, *122*
Interosseous artery, 103
Interphalangeal joints, 136, 238
Interpubic joints, 164, *165*
Interspinous ligament, 22
Intertransverse ligament, 22
Interval behind inguinal ligament, 180, *181*
Intervertebral
   discs, 22
   joints, 22, *23*
   veins, 60
Intra-articular ligament, 25
Inversion, 261
ISW. *see* Initial swing phase (ISW)

J

Joints
   acromioclavicular joint, 129, 130
   ankle joint (talocrural), 236, *237*, 238, *239*
   atlantoaxial joints, 20, *21*
   atlanto-occipital joint, 20, *21*
   blood supply
      hip joint, 224, *225*
      knee joint, 230
   calcaneocuboid joint, 236
   carpometacarpal joint, 136
   cavity, 264
   classification by movement, 263
   classification by tissue type
      blood supply, 265
      bursae, 265
      cartilaginous joints, 264
      fibrous joints, 263–264
      nerve supply, 265
      synovial joints, 264–265
   costotransverse joint, 26, *27*
   costovertebral joints
      rib movement, 26
      ribs *vs.* vertebrae, 25, *25*, 27
   elbow, *135*
      humeroulnar joint, 133
      pulled elbow, 134
      radioulnar joint, 133–134
      ROM, 134
   foot joints, 241
   glenohumeral joint, 129–130
   hand joints, 136, 138, *139*, 140
   hip
      blood supply, 224, *225*
      cruciate anastomosis, 224, *225*
      ligaments, 222, *223*
      muscles acting, 222

ROM, 224
   synovial membrane, 222
iliolumbar joints, 164, *165*
inferior radioulnar joint, 138
intermetacarpal joints, 136
interphalangeal joints, 136, 238
interpubic joints, 164, *165*
intervertebral joints, 22, *23*
knee
   blood supply, 230
   bursae of, *233*, 233–234, *235*
   divisions and movements, 226
   ligaments, 226, *227*
   nerve supply, 230
   synovial membrane, 226, *229*, *231*
metacarpophalangeal joints, 136
1st metatarsophalangeal joint (big toe), 240
metatarsophalangeal (MP) joints, 236, 240
pelvic girdle, articulations, 164, *165*
sacrococcygeal joints, 164, *165*
sacroiliac joints, 164, *165*
shoulder joint, 130
sternoclavicular joint, 129, 130
subtalar (talocalcaneal or
   talo-calcaneo-navicular) joint,
   ROM, 236, 240
talocalcaneonavicular joint, 236, 239
tarsometatarsal joints, 236
tibiofibular joints, *233*, 234, *235*
transverse (mid) tarsal
   (talo-naviculo-calcano-cuboid)
   joint(s), 240
wrist joints, 136, *137*, 138, 140
zygapophyseal joints, 22

K

Klumpke palsy, 90
Knee, 150, *151*
   cap, patella, 169
   flexion, 246
   joint
      blood supply, 230
      bursae of, *233*, 233–234, *235*
      divisions and movements, 226
      ligaments, 226, *227*
      synovial membrane, 226, *229*, *231*
   popliteal region and anastomosis, 196,
      197, *197*
Knuckles, 112
Kyphosis, 8
   dowager hump, 28

L

Laminae, 10
Laminectomy, 52
Lateral, 261
Lateral atlanto-occipital ligament, 20
Lateral bending
   cervical spine, 42
   thoracolumbar spine, 43
Lateral costotransverse ligament, 26
Lateral flexion
   vertebral column movements, 42
Lateral funiculus, 52
Lateral horns, 50
Lateral sacral crests, 18
Latissimus dorsi muscle, 2

Leg, 150, *151*
   compartments, 198, *199*
   fibula (calf bone), 169
   fibular neck, fractures, 170
   foot, overinversion of, 170
   lateral and anterior leg muscles, 204,
      205, 206
   ossification, 169
   patella (knee cap), 169
   patella fracture, 170
   posterior muscles, 200, *201*, *202*, *203*
   Pott fracture, 170
   spiral fracture, 170
   tibia (shin bone), 169, *171*
   vessels and nerves
      anastomoses, 208
      anterior tibial artery, 207–208
      calcaneal tendon, 210
      deep fibular (peroneal) nerve (L4,
         L5, Sl-2), 210
      fibular (peroneal) artery, 207
      fibular (peroneal) nerve (L4, L5,
         Sl-2), 208, 210
      posterior tibial artery, 207, *209*
      superficial fibular (peroneal) nerve
         (L4, L5, Sl-2), 210
      tibial nerve (L4, L5, Sl-3), 208, *209*
Leptomeningitis, 48
Ligamenta flava, 22
Ligamentum nuchae, 22
Loading response phase (LR), 246
Long thoracic nerve (C5-7), 90
Longitudinal, 261
Longitudinal ligament, 22
Lordosis, 8
LR. *see* Loading response phase (LR)
Lumbar
   cistern, 46
   curvatures, 7
   cutaneous nerves, 4
   plexus (L1-4), 56, 152, *153*
   puncture, 48, *49*
   triangle, 32
   vertebrae, 16, *16–17*
Lumbosacral
   articular surface, 18
   enlargement, 50, *51*
Lumbricals, 122
Lunate, 79
Lymph nodes, 158, *159*
Lymphatic divide, 158
Lymphatic drainage
   deep vessels accompany deep blood
      vessels, 158
   lymph nodes, 158, 159
   lymphatic divide, 159
   superficial fascia, superficial vessels lie,
      158, *159*
Lymphatics, 6, *71*
   axillary lymph nodes, 70
   deep lymphatics, 70
   forearm and arm, 70
   hand, dorsum of, 110
   superficial lymphatic vessels, 70

M

Mammillary process, 16
Marie-Strümpell disease, 28

Medial, 261
Medial epicondyle fracture/trauma, 74
Medial thigh
    adductor hiatus, 182
    muscles, 182, *183*
Median (midline/midsagittal), 261
Median antebrachial vein (variable), 68
Median cubital vein, 68
Median furrow, 2, *2*
Median nerve (C5-T1), 104, 126, 127, 141,
    142, *143*
Median nerve injury, 128
Median nerves, 98
Median sacral crest, 2, 18
Meningitis, 48
Meningocele, 52
Meningomyelocele, 52
Metacarpals, 79
Metacarpophalangeal joints, 136
Metatarsals, 172
Metatarsals fractures, 174
1st Metatarsophalangeal joint (big toe),
    240
Metatarsophalangeal (MP) joints, 236, 240
Middle cluneal nerves, 56
Midline (median/midsagittal), 261
Midpalmar space, 116
Midsagittal (median/midline), 261
Midstance phase (MST), 246
Midswing phase (MSW), 246
Minor deep back muscles, 40, *40*
MP joints. *see* Metatarsophalangeal (MP)
    joints
MST. *see* Midstance phase (MST)
MSW. *see* Midswing phase (MSW)
Muscles
    anterior forearm, 100, *101*, 102, *102*
    anterior shoulder, 82, *83*
    anterior thigh muscles, 178, *179*
    arm, 95, *95*, 96, *97*
    erector spinae, 2, *2*
    foot, 211, *212*, *213*
    gluteal region, 188, *189*
    interossei muscles, 122, *122*
    latissimus dorsi muscle, 2
    leg
        lateral and anterior leg muscles, 204,
            205, 206
        posterior muscles, 200, *201*, 202, *203*
    medial thigh, 182, *183*
    nerve relationships, lower extremity, 258
    palmar hand, 119, *119*, 120, *121*,
        122, *122*
    posterior forearm, 106, *107*
    posterior shoulder, 84, *84*, *85*, 86, *86*
    posterior thigh muscles, 194, *195*
    shoulder girdle, 130
    shoulder joint, 130
    sole of foot, 216, *217–219*
    and tendons, 264
Musculocutaneous nerves (C5-7), 91, 98
Myelography, 48

N

Nails, 245, *245*
Nerve injuries
    lower limb
        common fibular (peroneal), 254, *257*
        femoral, 254, *255*
        iliacus and psoas muscles, 254
        inferior gluteal, 254
        joint movements, segmental innerva-
            tion of, 256
        muscle–nerve relationships, 258
        nerve root alignment, 256
        obturator, 254, *255*
        sciatic, 254
        straight-leg-raising test, anatomy, 256
        superior gluteal, 254
        tibial division, 254, *260*
    upper limb
        median nerve (C5-T1), 141, 142, *143*
        radial nerve (C5-T1), 146, *147*, 148
        ulnar nerve (C8, T1), 144, *145*
Nerve supply, knee joint, 230
Nerves, foot sole, 220–221. *see also specific
    nerves*
Neurovasculature
    anterior forearm, 103, 104, *105*
    arm, 98, *99*
    posterior forearm, 108, 109, *109*
Nodose lumbago (rheumatism), 30
Nuchal, 30
Nucleus pulposus, 22
Nutrient arteries, 168

O

Oblique, 261
Obturator membrane, pelvic girdle articu-
    lations, 164
Obturator vessels and nerve, 186
Occipital nerve, 56
Olecranon, 76
Ossification
    ankle and foot, 172, 174
    carpals, 80
    forearm, 76
    humerus, 74
    leg bones, 169
    metacarpals, 80
    pectoral (shoulder) girdle, 72
    pelvic girdle, 160
    phalanges, 80
    thigh bones, 166
    ulna and radius, 76
Oxychogryphosis, 245, *245*

P

Pachymeningitis, 48
Painful arc syndrome, 132
Palmar
    aponeurosis, 116, 118
    carpal arch, 123
    digital arteries, 123
    fascia, 116
    flexion creases, 114
    hand, 119, *119*, 120, *121*, 122, *122*
    volar, 261
Patella (knee cap), 169
Patella fracture, 170
Patellar (knee) reflex, 170
Patellar retinacula, 156
Pectineus, 178
Pectoral
    girdle, 129, 130, *131*, 132
        shoulder girdle, 64
    (shoulder) girdle bones, *73*
        clavicle (collar bone), 72
        clavicle fractures, 72
        ossification, 72
        scapula (shoulder blade), 72
    nerves, 90
Pectoralis fascia, 68
Pedicles, 10
Pelvic
    rotation, 246
    tilt, 246
Pelvic cancers, 60
Pelvic girdle
    articulations
        greater sciatic foramen, 164
        joints, 164, *165*
        lesser sciatic foramen, 164
        obturator membrane, 164
        sacroiliac strain, 164
    bursitis, 162
    definition, 160
    false pelvis, 162
    fractures, 162
    hip girdle, 150, *151*
    os coxae or hip bone, 160, *161*, *163*
    ossification, 160
    pelvic inlet/outlet, 162
    true pelvis, 162
Pes cavus, 244
Phalanges, 79–80
Phalanges fractures, 174
Phlebothrombosis, 156
Pia mater, 48, *49*
Pisiform, 79
Pivot joints/trochoidal, 265
Plane joints, 264–265
Plantar, 261
Plantar aponeurosis
    foot sole, 214–215
Plantar ligament, 204
Popeye deformity, 96
Popliteal
    artery, 196–197, *197*
    (Baker) cyst, 232
    fascia, 156
    fossa, 196, *197*
    nodes, lymph nodes, 158, *159*
    vein, 196
Posterior (dorsal), 261
Posterior arch, 12
Posterior atlantoaxial ligament, 20
Posterior atlanto-occipital membrane, 20
Posterior forearm
    muscles, 106, *107*
    neurovasculature, 108, 109, *109*
Posterior funiculus, 50
Posterior horns, 50
Posterior intermuscular septum, 198
Posterior interosseous artery, 108
Posterior lateral spinal vein, 60
Posterior leg muscles, 200, *201*, 202, *203*
Posterior longitudinal ligament, 22
Posterior median spinal vein, 60
Posterior median sulcus, 50
Posterior ramus, 54
Posterior (dorsal) root, 54
Posterior sacral foramina, 18
Posterior superior iliac spine, 2

Posterior thigh muscles, 194, *195*
Posterior tibial artery, 207, *209*
Posterolateral sulcus, 50
Pott fracture, 170, 241
Preswing phase (PSW), 246
Primary curvatures, 7
Pronation, 261
Proper digital branches, 126
Proximal, 261
Proximal row, wrist bones, 79
PSW. *see* Preswing phase (PSW)

Q
Quadriceps femoris muscle paralysis, 178, 252

R
Radial
    artery, 103, 110, 124
    groove, radial nerve (C5-T1), injury, 146, 148
    nerves (C5-T1), 98, 104, 108, 146, *147*, 148
    notch, 76
    styloid process, 78
Radiate ligament, 25
Radicular veins, 60
Radiocarpal articulation, 136
Radioulnar joint, 133–134, 136
Radius, 76
Range of motion (ROM)
    ankle (talocrural) joint, 238
    elbow joint, 134
    hand, 136, 138, *139*, 140
    hip joint, 224
    knee joint, 228
    pectoral girdle and shoulder, 130, 132
    toes, 240, 241
    vertebral segments, 42–43
    wrist joints, 136, *137*, 138, 140
Ribs, 2
    movement of, 26
ROM. *see* Range of motion (ROM)
Rotation
    cervical spine, 42
    thoracolumbar spine, 43
    vertebral column movements, 42
Rotator cuff muscles, 84, *84*, *85*, 86, *86*
Rotatory dislocation, 28

S
Sacral
    canal, 18
    curvatures, 7
    cutaneous nerves, 4
    plexus (L4-S3), 56, 152, *153*
    tuberosity, 18
Sacrococcygeal joints, 164, *165*
Sacroiliac
    joints, 164, *165*
    strain, 164
Sacrum vertebrae, 18, *19*
Saddle joints/sellar, 265
Sagittal, 261
Saphenous
    hiatus (fossa ovalis), 156
    vein, 155, *157*
Scaphoid, 79
Scapula (shoulder blade), 72

Sciatica, 192
Scoliosis, 8
Secondary curvatures, 7
Sellar, 265
Sensory fibers, 4
Shin bone, tibia, 169, *171*
Shin splints, 206
Shoulder
    anterior shoulder, 82, *83*
    articulations, 129, 130, *131*, 132
    axillary artery, 92, *93*
    blood supply, 92, 94, *94*
    dislocation, 132
    pectoral (shoulder) girdle, 72, *73*
    posterior shoulder, 84, *84*, *85*, 86, *86*
Small saphenous vein, 155, *157*
Smith fracture, 78
Sole of foot, muscles, 216, *217–219*.
    see also Foot
Soleus and gastrocnemius paralysis, 252
Spina bifida
    cystica and occulta, 52
Spinal anesthesia, 48
Spinal cord
    blood supply
        anterior spinal artery, 58, *59*
        posterior spinal arteries, 58, *59*
        radicular arteries, 58, *59*
    clinical considerations, 52
    description, 50, *51*
    fissures and sulci, 50, *51*
    internal structure, 50, 52
    segment, 54
    visualization of, 48
Spinal (dorsal root) ganglion, 54
Spinal meninges
    arachnoid mater, 46
    comments, 46, *47*
    dura mater, 46
    lumbar puncture, 48, *49*
    pia mater, 48, *49*
Spinal nerves, 53, *53*, 54
    anterior and posterior rami, 56, *57*
    to vertebral column, 54, *55*
Spinous processes, 2, 10
Spiral fracture, 170
Splenius (superficial group), 36
Spondylolisthesis, 28
Spondylolysis, 28
Spondylomalacia, 28
Sprains, 241
Stance phase, 246, 248
Sternoclavicular joint, 129, 130
Straight-leg-raising test, anatomy, 256
Subarachnoid space, 46
Subclavius muscle (C5), 91
Subcostal nerve, 56
Subdural space, 46
Subluxation, 28
Suboccipital muscles, 41, *41*
Subtalar (talocalcaneal or
    talo-calcaneo-navicular) joint,
    ROM, 236, 240
Subtrochanteric fracture, 166
Superficial, 261
Superficial back muscles, *33*
    characteristics, 32
    features, 32, *33*

2nd layer, 34, *34*
3rd layer, 35, *35*
1st layer, 32
Superficial fascia, 6, 156
Superficial fibular (peroneal) nerve (L4,
    L5, Sl-2), 210
Superficial lymphatic vessels, 70
Superficial palmar space, 119
Superficial transverse metacarpal ligament,
    116
Superior, 261
Superior cluneal nerves, 56
Superior costotransverse ligament, 26
Superior fibular retinacula, 204
Superior gluteal, 190, *191*
Superior longitudinal band, 20
Supination, 261
Suprascapular nerve (C5-6), 90
Supraspinous ligament, 22
Surgical neck fracture, 74
Suture joints, 263
Swing phase, 246, 248–249
Sympathetic fibers, 4
Symphyses, 264
Synarthroses, 263
Synchondroses, 264
Syndesmoses, 263–264
Synostosis, 263
Synovial joints
    accessory ligaments, 264
    articular cartilage, 264
    classifications
        ball and socket joints, 265
        condyloid joints, 265
        hinge joints/ginglymus, 265
        pivot joints/trochoidal, 265
        plane joints, 264–265
        saddle joints/sellar, 265
    joint cavity, 264
    synovial membrane lining, 264
Synovial membrane, 130, 222, 226, *229*,
    231
Synovial membrane lining, 264
Synovial tendon sheaths, 204, 206
Syringomyelia, 52

T
Talipes/clubfeet, 244
Talocalcaneonavicular joint, 236, 239
Talus, ankle bone, 172, *173*
Tarsometatarsal joints, 236
Tectorial membrane, 20
Tendon sheaths, 202
Tennis elbow, 109
Terminal stance phase (TST), 246
Terminal (final) swing phase (TSW), 246
Thenar compartment, 119
Thenar space, 116
Thigh, 150, *151*
    anterior thigh, muscles, 178, *179*
    compartments
        anterior compartment, 176, *177*
        definition, 176
        hip/gluteal region, 176, *177*
        medial compartment, 176, *177*
        posterior compartment, 176, *177*
    femur bones, 166, *167*
    medial thigh muscles, 182, *183*

Thigh (*Continued*)
  posterior thigh muscles, 194, *195*
  subtrochanteric fracture, 166
Thoracic curvatures, 7
Thoracic vertebrae, 14, *14–15*
Thoracodorsal (C6-8), 91
Thoracolumbar aponeurosis (fascia), 30
Thoracolumbar spine, ROM, 42
Thrombophlebitis, 156
Tibia (shin bone), 169, *171*
Tibial nerve, 196, 208–209
Tibiofibular joints, *233*, 234, *235*
Toes
  clawing of, 244
  disorders, 244, *245*
Transverse (horizontal), 261
Transverse intermuscular septum, 198
Transverse ligament, 20
Transverse processes, 10
Transverse (mid) tarsal
    (talo-naviculo-calcano-cuboid)
    joint(s), 240
Transversospinal muscles, 38, *39*
Trapezium, 79
Trapezius muscle, 2
Trapezoid, 79
Traumatic dislocations, 224, 230
Triceps muscle
  radial nerve (C5-T1), injury, 146
Triquetrum, 79
Trochlear notch, 76
Trochoidal, 265
TST. *see* Terminal stance phase (TST)
TSW. *see* Terminal (final) swing phase (TSW)
T2-weighted MRI, 48

U
Ulna, 76
Ulnar
  artery, 103, 123
  nerves (C8, T1), 98, 104, 126, 127,
    144, *145*
  tuberosity, 76
Unique cervical vertebrae,
    12, *13*
Upper brachial plexus injuries, 88
Upper subscapular nerve (C5-6), 91

V
Varicose veins, 156
Veins
  grafts, 156
  hand, 124
  spinal cord, 60, *61*
  vertebral column, 60
Venipuncture, 68
  great saphenous vein, 156
Ventral (anterior), 261
Vertebra prominens, 12
Vertebral
  arch, 10
  body, 10
  column
    abnormal curvatures, 8
    ankylosing spondylitis, 28, *29*
    articulated vertebral column, 8, *9*
    clinical considerations, 28, *29*
    composition and length, 7, *7*
    curvatures, 7
    dislocations of, 28, *29*
    fractures of, 28, *29*

  spinal nerves, 54, *55*
  whiplash, 28, *29*
  foramen, 10
  notches, 10
  segments, ROM, 42–43
Vertical axis, 130
Volar (palmar), 261

W
Walking (bipedal locomotion)
  arches and interosseous ligaments, 250,
    251
  human gait determinants, 246–247
  motion of pelvis, 250
  muscle activity, 252, *253*
  muscles involved in, 248, 249, *249*
  stance phase, 248
  swing phase, 248
  walking cycle, 246, 247, *247*
Walking cycle, 246–247, *247*
Whiplash, 28
White matter, 50, 52
White ramus communicans, 54
Winged scapula, 90
Wrist
  arthrodesis, 140
  bones, 79, *79*, 80, *81*
  drop, 90
  joints, 136, *137*, 138, 140
  median nerve (C5-T1), injury, 141
  ulnar nerve (C8, T1), injury,
    144, *145*

Z
Zygapophyseal joints, 22